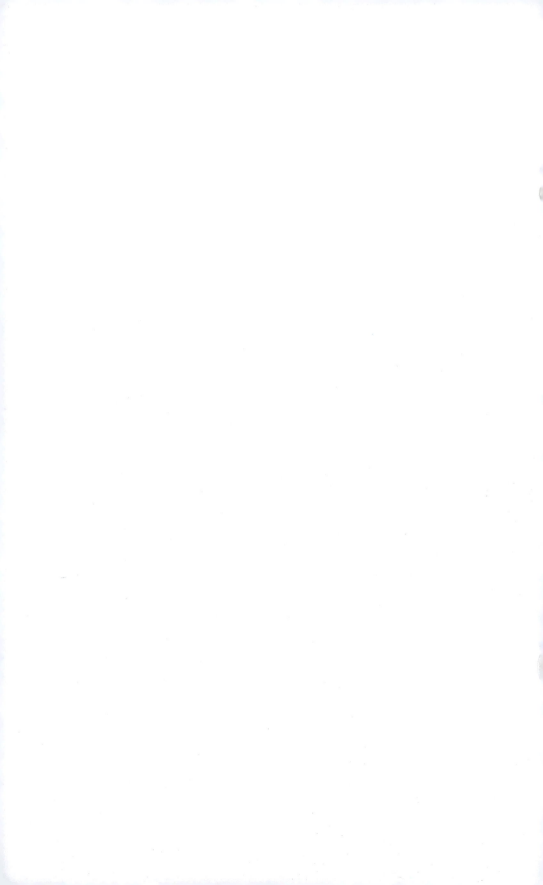

Informal Caregivers: From Hidden Heroes to Integral Part of Care

Andreas Charalambous
Editor

Informal Caregivers: From Hidden Heroes to Integral Part of Care

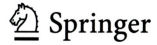 Springer

Editor
Andreas Charalambous
Nursing
Cyprus University of Technology
Limassol, Cyprus

ISBN 978-3-031-16744-7   ISBN 978-3-031-16745-4   (eBook)
https://doi.org/10.1007/978-3-031-16745-4

This Springer imprint is published by the registered company Springer Nature Switzerland AG
The registered company address is: Gewerbestrasse 11, 6330 Cham, Switzerland

Forward

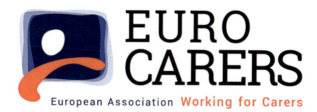

In many ways, this book seeks to explore fundamental and pressing questions for our post-pandemic societies and care systems. The first concern is the nature of informal, unpaid, long-term care. Across ages, the provision of care to a loved one with care needs—be it a family member, a friend or a neighbour—has been seen as the right and normal thing to do; something that is just part of the natural order of things. Caregiving has always been a central life activity, almost as if the desire to care for others is an essential component of the human experience. It binds people together, creates a sense of belonging and helps us overcome social injustices. To put it simply, without care, society as we know would likely cease to exist.

But historically, caregiving has also been an undervalued task, entrusted on groups of people who are not in a very high-status position in our society (e.g. women, migrants, working class) Moreover, when not adequately supported (as is regularly the case), carers face a long list of negative consequences: caring can indeed impact on their health and well-being; it can lead to difficulties in balancing paid work with care responsibilities (which in turn can impact on their labour market participation), and it can generate financial difficulties and poverty, due to limited social provision and direct costs of care. Importantly, the COVID-19 crisis has done nothing but exacerbate these issues. As a result, informal carers often find themselves having to show inventiveness, bravery and strength in the face of adversity—a combination of traits that some may define as heroic. As one of the carers in our network put it once: "the constant search for support is much more of a burden than the actual caregiving". This book therefore also explores the question of whether informal carers are the unsung heroes—and heroines—of our societies.

It is now commonly agreed by policy makers and researchers that the bulk of all care in Europe is provided by informal carers, and by women in particular. If these people are expected to keep providing care—and they are—their needs and require-ments should be an inherent part of health and social policy development, and their contribution should be properly considered as part of the economic equation. Caregiving is a personal and collective journey that deserves urgent political atten-tion and resolute support from the cradle to the grave.

This book provides a comprehensive overview of the aspects that should be taken into consideration when developing measures that are likely to make an actual dif-ference in the daily life of millions of carers across Europe.

Brussels, Belgium   Stecy Yghemonos

Contents

Caregiving and Caregivers: Concepts, Caregiving Models, and Systems

Andreas Charalambous 🄳

1   Introduction

The world is facing many and constant sociodemographic changes, such as an increased average life expectancy and the presence of chronic and noncommunicable diseases, which in turn, lead to an enhanced dependency on others. On a global scale, it is estimated that the number of people aged 60 years or older is expected to grow expediently by 2030. This demographic shift is accompanied by a health transition, whereby 23% of the total global burden of disease is now attributable to disorders in older adults including cancer. As cancer is largely a disease of the older population, a significant increase in the incidence and chronicity of cancer in this population is predicted. Under the scenario where global prevalence of disabilities and diseases remain stable, the growth in the number of older adults alone is expected to increase demands for healthcare beyond the capacity of healthcare systems. Even in today's conditions, healthcare systems are already facing significant challenges in corresponding to the current needs, a fact that has resulted in changes in the delivery models in place. Therefore, these changes aimed to achieve less reliance on specialized care settings and more focus on delivering care in the community. Within this context, informal caregivers (or family caregivers) provide a high proportion of the care needed and are an essential extension of the healthcare system. Despite the fact that informal caregivers are a critical resource to their care recipients and an essential component of the healthcare systems around the world,

A. Charalambous (✉)
Department of Nursing, School of Health Sciences, Cyprus University of Technology, Limassol, Cyprus

Department of Nursing Science, Faculty of Medicine, University of Turku, Turku, Finland
e-mail: andreas.charalambous@cut.ac.cy

yet their role and importance to society as a whole have only recently been appreciated. An informal caregiver, often a family member, provides care, typically unpaid, to someone with whom they have a personal relationship.

2   The Concept of Caregiving

The etymology of the word "care" comes from the Old English term "wicim" meaning "mental suffering, mourning, sorrow, or trouble." "Give" is also Old English, from "eo-, iofan, iaban," meaning "to bestow gratuitously." When the two root meanings are assimilated, caregiving is the action/process of helping those who are suffering [1]. Drentea [2] refers to caregiving as "the act of providing unpaid assistance and support to family members or acquaintances who have physical, psychological or developmental needs" (p. 1).

In a conceptual analysis, caregiving within the context of family caregiving [3] was found to have four characteristics: tasks, transition, roles, and process. Tasks identified include activities of daily living, instrumental activities of daily living, the amount of care provided, and direct and indirect care. Transitions focused on care management, delegation, and transfer from family to institutional care. Caregiving roles recognized the extension of normal, family care and involved "mutual nurturing behaviors" (p. 68).

Nursing is not the only discipline where the concept of caregiving has been utilized and studied. Within the context of sociology, for example, caregiving has been defined as the care provided by unpaid workers such as family members, friends, and neighbors as well as individuals affiliated with religious institutions [2]. Psychology is another discipline where the concept of caregiving has been a focal point, however from a different perspective, that of the psychological ramifications of the act of caregiving. Within this context, preceding studies have demonstrated that being an informal caregiver puts a person at risk of poorer mental health [4–6]. A review described depression as the most common studied cancer caregiver outcome, with prevalence rates ranging from 20 to 73% [7]. Furthermore, depressive symptoms in cancer caregivers have been associated with greater difficulties related to sleep, anxiety, and fatigue and lower levels of quality of life and life satisfaction. These studies have been extended to identify caregiver-related characteristics building this way the profile of those who are more likely to assume the role. Furthermore, these studies have placed emphasis on the effects of caregiving on the caregiver, caregiver burden, coping strategies, challenges, and the rewards of caregiving [8, 9].

3   What Is an Informal Caregiver or a Family Caregiver?

Family members (as family caregivers) consist of the backbone of a society's care supply, and despite this being a prevalent perspective, an official definition of informal care is lacking [1]. Therefore, in order to comprehensively capture the core meaning of the caregiving concept, it is necessary not only to briefly review the official definitions adopted by relevant institutions and civil society stakeholders but also to review those more frequently reported by the scientific community.

According to the United Nations definition, "informal caregiving" primarily stands for all nonprofessional care provided—by choice or by default—by family members, friends, neighbors, or other persons caring for people with long-term care needs at all ages, usually in private households [10]. The Organisation for Economic Co-operation and Development (OECD) has a twofold definition of an informal caregiver. Primarily, an informal caregiver includes those who provide care to friends or family members or may do so as part of noncontractual voluntary work [11], but also it includes undeclared or illegal caregivers who receive a salary or compensation from the care recipient, but do not have an official contract with them and are not registered with relevant social security offices [12].

In the EU, 60% of all care is provided by informal caregivers, and a report funded by the European Commission [13] identified a certain set of characteristics that can be considered as typical of an informal caregiver: a close relationship with the care receiver, no professional training, no working contract, no equivalent pay, a wide range of care giving duties, no official hours, and no entitlement to social rights.

Similarly, Lilleheie et al. [14] defined informal caregivers as individuals who have a significant personal relationship with and provide a broad range of unpaid assistance to an older person or an adult with a chronic or disabling condition outside of a professional or formal framework. In the same light, informal caregivers have been identified as individuals voluntarily caring for a relative or a friend facing illness, disability, or any condition requiring particular attention [15]. The caring occasion/caring moment becomes transpersonal when "two persons (caregiver and other) together with their unique life histories and phenomenal field (of perception) become a focal point in space and time, from which the moment has a field of its own that is greater than the occasion itself. As such, the process can (and does) go beyond itself, yet arise from aspects of itself that become part of the life history of each person, as well as part of some larger, deeper, complex pattern of life" [16, p. 59].

According to Revenson et al. [17], informal caregiving can be defined as the provision of usually unpaid care to a relative or friend with a chronic illness, disability, or other long-lasting health and care needs. A preceding notable definition includes the one proposed by Swanson et al. [3] who conceptualized family caregiving as: "Provision by a family care provider of appropriate personal and health care for a family member or significant other" (p. 68) and the one proposed by Bowers [9] who included five distinctive categories of roles that provide meaning or purpose for the caregiver: anticipatory, preventive, supervisory, instrumental, and protective.

Although these definitions have common elements, they tend to vary across studies and within official recording systems of different countries that makes attempts to operationalize and measure the concept difficult. Nevertheless, taking into consideration these definitions, it can be concluded that, taking into account both a societal and a scientific perspective, the following essential characteristics can be used to define an informal caregiver, as someone who provides care (1) systematically (at least weekly) (2) to someone with a chronic illness, disability, or other long-lasting health, social or long-term care needs, (3) as part of an unpaid noncontractual voluntary work outside a professional or formal framework [18].

4   The Scale of Caregiving

According to the "Caregiving in the US 2020" report, by the National Alliance for Caregiving (NAC) and AARP, more than one in five Americans (21.3%) are caregivers, having provided care to an adult or child with special needs at some time in the past 12 months. This totals an estimated 53.0 million adults in the United States, up from the estimated 43.5 million caregivers in 2015 [19]. In terms of caregivers for adults only, the prevalence of caregiving has risen from 16.6% in 2015 to 19.2% in 2020—an increase of over eight million adults providing care to a family member or friend age 18 or older, primarily driven by a significant increase in the prevalence of caring for a family member or friend who is age 50 or older [19]. Compared to 2015, a greater proportion of caregivers of adults are providing care to multiple people now, with 24% caring for two or more recipients (up from 18% in 2015). This finding, in combination with the increased prevalence of caregiving, suggests a nation of Americans who continue to step up to provide unpaid care to family, friends, and neighbors who might need assistance due to health or functional needs [19].

In the European Union, estimates suggest that as much as 60% of all long-term care is provided by informal carers [13]. The available estimates of the number of informal caregivers range from 10% to 25% of the total population in Europe. The average varies significantly between countries, groups of countries, and depending on how informal care is defined and measured.

In the United Kingdom, a national report on the value of caring, commissioned by Carers UK in 2015, found that carers are providing informal (unpaid) care with an estimated value of £132 billion annually, compared to £134 billion total annual government spending on the National Health Service (NHS) [20]. The high level of informal care may be partly due to the fact that the number of people aged 85 years and over in the United Kingdom has increased by 38% to over 431,000 from 2001 to 2015 and the number of people with a life-limiting long-term illness has increased by 16% to 1.6 million over the same period [20]. The report notes that the situation may be being exacerbated by cuts in the levels of formal (paid) homecare support available from central and local government [20]. Although the UK Care Act (2014) was designed to provide greater support for those in need of care and their informal carers and to give informal carers similar legal rights to those they care for, there has been little new government money to support the introduction of the legislation [21]. As a consequence, many carers are still struggling to get the support from health and care services that they need [22].

5 The Financial Impact of Caregiving

The economic impact of caregiving can be complex and poses challenges in its defining, although it can be defined through two main channels, direct and indirect. The direct economic impact accounts for the influence caregiving has on decisions around work, absenteeism, and productivity. The second channel by which the economic impact of caregiving can be defined is the indirect consequence of poorer health on those providing care [23]. Workers who are less healthy also tend to be much less productive, generating lower per capita incomes and being employed less often [24]. When caregivers become less healthy as a result of increased caregiver burden and poor support, they are more likely to miss work or stop working altogether. The increased concerns over their own health as well as the health of the person who take care of might contribute to them becoming progressively less productive. This estimated indirect economic effect totals nearly $221 billion, bringing the overall economic impact of caregiving to $264 billion [23].

Although family caregivers are not generally paid for their services, spending time helping family and friends with long-term services and supports (LTSS) needs is often costly. Therefore, with regard to employment, absenteeism, and productivity, it is frequent that some caregivers may have to reduce their work hours when they provide care, switch to part-time work, or temporarily dropout of the labor force. Reduced work hours lead to lower earnings and may force caregivers to forfeit employer-sponsored health insurance. Temporary labor supply reductions can have long-lasting repercussions, because people who leave their jobs often struggle to find alternative employment and must accept lower-paying positions. Lost earnings can also reduce future retirement income, as people are forced to save less for retirement and accumulate fewer Social Security credits. Reduced employment from caregiving can also have macroeconomic consequences, reducing government tax revenue and potentially slowing economic growth [25]. The direct economic effect resulting from caregiving is estimated at nearly $44 billion through the loss of 656,000 jobs and an additional 791,000 caregivers suffering from absenteeism issues at work [23].

6 Informal Caregiving During the COVID-19 Pandemic

The COVID-19 pandemic has complicated the practice of informal caregiving in several unique ways [26]. Despite the limited data available, there is evidence that throughout those measures, that is, contact restrictions, informal caregiving still took place [27]. Health policies and mandates designed to slow the spread of COVID-19, such as social distancing, quarantining, and physical isolation, complicated informal caregiving and imparted additional challenges. Informal caregivers may have relied on the support of additional volunteer services and social care to fulfil their caregiving responsibilities that were halted when these policies were implemented [28].

In addition to these indirect effects of the pandemic, there are direct effects of the virus itself on physical health that might influence the provision of personal care [29]. Caregivers who provide personal care to family members outside their own household are at higher risk of retracting COVID-19 themselves, as they regularly travel to and meet with care recipients and accompany them to hospital visitations. The natural fear of an infection as well as fearing infecting someone close might therefore also have an impact on the frequency and amount of informal care provision and the use of it [30].

According to Bergman [29], the accumulating outcome of these direct and indirect effects of the pandemic can impact the intensity and burden for caregivers resulting in the worsening of the situation for those who rely on personal care, as less care will be provided. A multicenter online survey regarding psychosocial consequences due to the COVID-19 restrictions (ECLB-COVID19) showed that informal caregivers have a higher burden regarding mental and physical health [31]. Within the context of informal caregivers, persons with dementia who are more concerned about the pandemic were more likely to experience an overload or distress regarding to their role as caregiver [32]. Cohen et al. [33] conducted a cross-sectional study of 835 informal caregivers in the United States and assessed changes in caregiving intensity and the resultant caregiver burden due to the pandemic. The majority reported experiencing increases in caregiving intensity (55.7%) and caregiver burden (53.1%).

7 Family Caregiving Models

The need to provide adequate care to vulnerable groups (e.g., elderly, cancer patients) is a major challenge facing our society on many levels. The assumption of our current health care system is that close family members will provide the majority of day-to-day assistance and manage the wide array of problems confronted by these groups of people. However, most healthcare delivery models focus primarily on individual patients and do not properly engage, educate, or support family caregivers or other informal care providers resulting in an increased caregiver burden.

The impact of caregiving is a complex process that is somewhat challenging to understood how it occurs and affects the individual. The efforts to comprehensively understand the topic at hand gave birth to conceptual models such as the stress process model [34] and the appraisal model [35]. Within the context of neurodegenerative disease, an integrative model of the caregiver stress has been developed by Sorensen [36] through the combination of the stress process model and the appraisal model.

According to Sorensen et al [36] the caregiving process is influenced by six different interacting elements, including primary and secondary stressors, background and contextual factors, exacerbating or ameliorating factors, and the appraisal and the outcomes. Within the primary stressors, the objective elements in the caregiving setting are included, which in turn lead to secondary stressors (i.e., the consequences of the objective elements). The appraisal included in the model encapsulates a subjective evaluation by the caregiver of what is perceived as demands at hand and their available resources for dealing with the caregiving role [37]. The evaluation process concludes in varying outcomes, which can be psychosocial, behavioral, or physiological. The outcomes can vary according to the presence of exacerbating and mitigating factors facilitating or inhibiting the onset of the above outcomes. Additionally, background and contextual factors such as sociodemographic and cultural or ethnic determinants frame the caregiver's experience [37].

With the latter being acknowledged as a significant contributor to the caregiver experience, the Revised Sociocultural Stress Model poses as an example that demonstrates how cultural values, caregiver burden, coping, social support, and mental and physical health outcomes interact [38]. Based on the model, the cultural values indirectly influence caregivers' mental and physical health through two possible pathways: coping and social support [39, 40]. Therefore, according to the Revised Sociocultural Stress Model, cultural values, such as familism and filial piety, are expected to indirectly affect caregivers' mental health outcomes through the coping style utilized by the caregiver. Familism is largely understood as the individual's multifaceted identity with the family and may include the strength of dedication, loyalty, and obligation the individual has toward their family [41].

Subsequent efforts to increase the understanding of the caregiving process and the generation of caregiver burnout have resulted in the development of the Job Demands-Resources Model (JD-R) model, which introduces a two-dimensional process of burnout. On the one dimension, there is exhaustion and the depletion of the caregiver's emotional resources, and on the other one, there is engagement in the job and the willingness to find new positive and constructive challenges within the work [42]. The consideration of the JD-R model and the caregiver stress model [36] has provided new insights to the conceptualization of caregiver burnout. Gerain and Zech [37] argue that the conceptualization of caregiving should extend the already identified principles of the caregiver stress model within a more contextual depth. This new conceptual perspective has been introduced as the Informal Caregiving Integrative Model (ICIM), which poses as a theoretical framework to guide future research. As part of this theoretical framework, the stressors and resources are considered in the caregiver's psychosocial characteristics, and the relationship with the care recipient is also considered in the construction of the caregiver's experience. Furthermore, burnout is taken into consideration as a key mediator between stressors and outcomes, whereas the caregiver's appraisal is integrated as an integral part of the model. Finally, feedback loops are integrated in the model to allow a more comprehensive construction of the caregiving experience [37].

8 Tasks Performed by Informal Caregivers

As patients with cancer benefit from advances in therapy and extended survival, treatment is shifting from inpatient to outpatient settings, and more daily caregiving now occurs in the home, and the pattern is likely to continue across different diagnoses (e.g., cancer and dementia) and patients' groups (e.g., elderly). Family caregivers are increasingly asked to perform clinical care tasks that until recently would have been performed by trained healthcare professionals [43]. For example, they are expected to deliver a wide range of tasks such as medication management, physical care, and financial management as well as emotional support [44]. However, without the appropriate support, these daily burdens leave family caregivers with their own needs for support and assistance that, when left unmet, can lead to poorer quality of life and higher levels of distress [45], which can result in an undesired care breakdown for the person they care for [46]. A review by Ullgren et al. [47] in the context of informal caregivers of cancer patients identified various areas where they performed tasks of varying complexity and intensity. The most prevalent areas of caregiving included "psychosocial support" (e.g., supporting during anxiety), motivating and maintaining social engagement, and physical support (e.g., including medicine administration). The researchers found that assessing and monitoring symptoms were reported frequently, relating both to the symptoms and the medication side effects.

A role often assumed by family caregivers includes the role of the decision maker, a rather demanding role that requires caregivers to being alert, watching and waiting and deciding when to act and when not to act. Finally, a rather prevalent role assumed by informal caregivers included that of the liaison between formal care providers (and different healthcare professionals) on a variety of issues, for example, communicating the type of medication that had been given and what should be given in a specific situation [47].

Within the context of progressing Parkinson's disease, a study in the United Kingdom by Hand et al. [48] demonstrated that over 80% of carers provided help in housework/domestic tasks (e.g., cleaning, washing up, and cooking) and companionship activities (e.g., listening, friendship). However, assistance with personal care (bathing, 41.2%; dressing, 63.2%; and toileting, 37.7%), feeding (49.1%), and during sleep (45.6%) was less common. The majority of informal caregivers perceived the need to observe the participant constantly [Hand et al].

Within the context of elderly care, a cross-sectional study in 25 geriatric day hospitals (GDH) in Belgium explored the type of assistance provided by informal caregivers [49]. The study showed that informal caregivers were involved in care for basic activities of daily living (ADL) but more for instrumental ADLs (IADL). Adult children were more involved in transportation for obligatory tasks and help organization, and spouses were more in charge of meal preparation, managing medication, and doing household chores. Incontinence management, bathing, medication management and household chores were the main activities that the informal caregivers no longer wished to do. Adult children wished more often to stop feeding their relative and manage medication than spouses.

9   Conclusion

The world is experiencing rapidly significant demographic, technological, and social challenges with profound changes in the current systems of care. This transformation has resulted in long-term care systems evolving into mixed models in which care is considered to be a shared responsibility. In this transformation, informal care is and will be a key element of such systems resulting in an increase in the demand for and the complexity of such care. The provision and context of informal caregiving is not without challenges and the sustainable support of the caregivers calls for more attention by policy-makers, role recognition, and integration of the role in the healthcare delivery systems.

References

1. Hermanns M, Mastel-Smith B (2012) Caregiving: a qualitative concept analysis. Qual Rep 17(Art. 75):1–18. Retrieved from http://www.nova.edu/ssss/QR/QR17/hermanns.pdf
2. Drentea P (2007) Caregiving. In Ritzer R (ed) Blackwell encyclopedia of sociology [Caregiving]. Blackwell reference online. Retrieved http://www.blackwellreference.com/subscriber/book?id=g9781405124331_9781405124331
3. Swanson EA, Jensen DP, Specht J, Johnson ML, Maas M, Saylor D (1997) Caregiving: concept analysis and outcomes. Scholarly Inquiry Nurs Pract 11(1):65–76
4. Pottie CG, Burch KA, Montross Thomas LP, Irwin SA (2014) Informal caregiving of hospice patients. J Palliat Med 17:845–856. https://doi.org/10.1089/jpm.2013.0196
5. Sallim AB, Sayampanathan AA, Cuttilan A, Chun-Man Ho R (2015) Prevalence of mental health disorders among caregivers of patients with alzheimer disease. J Am Med Dir Assoc 16:1034–1041. https://doi.org/10.1016/j.jamda.2015.09.007
6. Papastavrou E, Charalambous A, Tsangari H (2009) Exploring the other side of cancer care: the informal caregiver. Eur J Oncol Nurs 13(2):128–136. https://doi.org/10.1016/j.ejon.2009.02.003
7. Fletcher BAS, Dodd MJ, Schumacher KL, Miaskowski C (2008) Symptom experience of family caregivers of patients with cancer. Oncol Nurs Forum 35:23–44
8. Papastavrou E, Charalambous A, Tsangari H (2012) How do informal caregivers of patients with cancer cope: a descriptive study of the coping strategies employed. Eur J Oncol Nurs 16(3):258–263. https://doi.org/10.1016/j.ejon.2011.06.001
9. Bowers BJ (1987) Intergenerational caregiving – adult caregivers and their aging parents. Adv Nurs Sci 2(2):20–31
10. United Nations (2017) Expert group meeting on care and older persons: links to decent work, migration and gender. United Nations UN Department of Economic and Social Affairs, New York. [(accessed on 27 December 2021)]. Available online: https://www.un.org/development/desa/ageing/wp-content/uploads/sites/24/2018/03/17-EGM-Care-Report-7-March-2018.pdf
11. OECD (2019) Health at a glance 2019: OECD indicators. OECD Publishing, Paris
12. OECD (2018) Care needed: improving the lives of people with dementia, OECD health policy studies. OECD Publishing, Paris
13. Triantafillou J, Naiditch M, Repkova K, Stiehr K, Carretero S, Emilsson T, Di Santo P, Bednarik R, Brichtova L, Ceruzzi F, Cordero L, Mastroyiannakis T, Ferrando M, Mingot K, Ritter J, Vlantoni D (2010) Informal care in the long-term care system. Interlinks European Overview Paper, Athens
14. Lilleheie I, Debesay J, Bye A, Bergland A (2020) Informal caregivers' views on the quality of healthcare services provided to older patients aged 80 or more in the hospital and 30 days after discharge. BMC Geriatr 20(1):97. https://doi.org/10.1186/s12877-020-1488-1
15. Schulz R, Tompkins CA (2010) Informal caregivers in the United States: prevalence, caregiver characteristics, and ability to provide care. In: Olson S (ed) The role of human factors in home health care: workshop summary. National Academies Press, Washington, DC, p 322
16. Watson J (1985) Nursing: human science and human care, a theory of nursing. Appelton-CenturyCrofts, Norwalk

17. Revenson T, Griva K, Luszczynska A, Morrison V, Panagopoulou E, Vilchinsky N, Hagedoorn M et al (2016) Caregiving in the illness context. Springer, London
18. Tur-Sinai A, Teti A, Rommel A, Hlebec V, Lamura G (2020) How many older informal caregivers are there in Europe? Comparison of estimates of their prevalence from three European surveys. Int J Environ Res Public Health 17(24):9531. https://doi.org/10.3390/ijerph17249531
19. National Alliance for Caregiving (NAC) and AARP (2020) Caregiving in the U.S. Available online https://www.caregiving.org/wp-content/uploads/2021/01/full-report-caregiving-in-the-united-states-01-21.pdf
20. Yeandle S, Buckner L (2015) Valuing carers: the rising value of carers' support. Carers UK, London
21. UK Department of Health (2014) The care act, chapter 23. The Stationery Office Ltd, London
22. Carers UK (2019) Facts about carers 2019 (Policy briefing, August, pp. 1–11). Retrieved from https://www.carersuk.org/images/Facts_about_Carers_2019.pdf
23. White D, DeAntonio D, Ryan B, Colyar M (2021) The economic impact of caregiving. Blue Cross Blue Shield Association Report. Available at https://www.bcbs.com/sites/default/files/file-attachments/health-of-america-report/HOA_Economics_of_Caregiving_0.pdf
24. Healthy people, healthy economies (2016) The Blue Cross Blue Shield Association and Moody's Analytics
25. Mudrazija S, Johnson RW (2020) Economic impacts of programs to support caregivers: final report. U.S. Department of Health and Human Services. Available at https://aspe.hhs.gov/reports/economic-impacts-programs-support-caregivers-final-report-0
26. Cohen SA, Nash CC, Greaney ML (2021) Informal caregiving during the COVID-19 pandemic in the US: background, challenges, and opportunities. Am J Health Promot 35(7):1032–1036. https://doi.org/10.1177/08901171211030142c
27. Lorenz-Dant K (2020) Germany and the COVID-19 long-term care situation: Country report in LTCcovid.org, International Long Term Care Policy Network, CPEC-LSE. https://ltccovid.org/wp-content/uploads/2020/04/Germany_LTC_COVID-19-15-April-new-format.pdf. Accessed 28 Dec 2021
28. Armitage R, Nellums LB (2020) COVID-19 and the consequences of isolating the elderly. Lancet Public Health 5(5):e256
29. Bergmann M, Wagner M (2021) The impact of COVID-19 on informal caregiving and care receiving across Europe during the first phase of the pandemic. Front Public Health 9:673874. https://doi.org/10.3389/fpubh.2021.673874
30. Giebel C, Hanna K, Cannon J, Eley R, Tetlow H, Gaughan A, Komuravelli A, Shenton J, Rogers C, Butchard S, Callaghan S, Limbert S, Rajagopal M, Ward K, Shaw L, Whittington R, Hughes M, Gabbay M (2020) Decision-making for receiving paid home care for dementia in the time of COVID-19: a qualitative study. BMC Geriatr 20(1):333
31. Ammar A, Chtourou H, Boukhris O, Trabelsi K, Masmoudi L, Brach M et al (2020) COVID-19 home confinement negatively impacts social participation and life satisfaction: a worldwide multicenter study. Int J Environ Res Public Health 17(17):6237. https://doi.org/10.3390/ijerph17176237
32. Savla J, Roberto KA, Blieszner R, McCann BR, Hoyt E, Knight AL (2020) Dementia caregiving during the "stay-at-home" phase of COVID-19 pandemic. J Gerontol B Psychol Sci Soc Sci 76(4):e241–e245. https://doi.org/10.1093/geronb/gbaa129
33. Cohen SA, Kunicki ZJ, Drohan MM, Greaney ML (2021) Exploring changes in caregiver burden and caregiving intensity due to COVID-19. Gerontol Geriatr Med 7:2333721421999279
34. Pearlin LI, Mullan JT, Semple SJ, Skaff MM (1990) Caregiving and the stress process: an overview of concepts and their measures. Gerontologist 30:583–594. https://doi.org/10.1093/geront/30.5.583
35. Lawton MP, Moss M, Kleban MH, Glicksman A, Rovine M (1991) A two-factor model of caregiving appraisal and psychological well-being. J Gerontol 46:P181–P189. https://doi.org/10.1093/geronj/46.4.p181

36. Sörensen S, Duberstein P, Gill D, Pinquart M (2006) Dementia care: mental health effects, intervention strategies, and clinical implications. Lancet Neurol 5:961–973. https://doi.org/10.1016/S1474-4422(06)70599-3
37. Gérain P, Zech E (2019) Informal caregiver burnout? Development of a theoretical framework to understand the impact of caregiving. Front Psychol 31(10):1748. https://doi.org/10.3389/fpsyg.2019.01748
38. Knight BG, Sayegh P (2010) Cultural values and caregiving: the updated sociocultural stress and coping model. J Gerontol 65:5–13
39. Mitchell AM (2015) Cancer caregiving: an exploration of values, burden, repetitive thinking, and depression. Electronic Theses and Dissertations. Paper 2234. https://doi.org/10.18297/etd/2234
40. Bauer J, Sousa-Poza A (2015) Impacts of informal caregiving on caregiver employment, health, and family. Popul Ageing 8:113–145. https://doi.org/10.1007/s12062-015-9116-0
41. Sayegh P, Knight BG (2010) The effects of familism and cultural justification on the mental and physical health of family caregivers. J Gerontol Psychol Sci 66:3–14
42. Demerouti E, Bakker AB, Nachreiner F, Schaufeli WB (2001) The job demands-resources model of burnout. J Appl Psychol 86:499–512
43. van Ryn M, Sanders S, Kahn K, van Houtven C, Griffin JM, Martin M, Atienza AA, Phelan S, Finstad D, Rowland J (2011) Objective burden, resources, and other stressors among informal cancer caregivers: a hidden quality issue? Psychooncology 20(1):44–52
44. Lamura G, Mnich E, Wojszel B, Nolan M, Krevers B, Mestheneos L, Döhner H (2006) The experience of family carers of older people in the use of support services in Europe: selected findings from the EUROFAMCARE project. Zeitschrift Fur Gerontologie Und Geriatrie 39(6):429–442
45. Printz C (2011) Cancer caregivers still have many unmet needs. Cancer 117(7):1331
46. Potier F, Degryse J, Bihin B et al (2018) Health and frailty among older spousal caregivers: an observational cohort study in Belgium. BMC Geriatr. 18(1):291. https://doi.org/10.1186/s12877-018-0980-3
47. Ullgren H, Tsitsi T, Papastavrou E, Charalambous A (2018) How family caregivers of cancer patients manage symptoms at home: a systematic review. Int J Nurs Stud. 85:68–79. https://doi.org/10.1016/j.ijnurstu.2018.05.004
48. Hand A, Oates LL, Gray WK, Walker RW (2019) The role and profile of the informal carer in meeting the needs of people with advancing Parkinson's disease. Aging Mental Health 23(3):337–344. https://doi.org/10.1080/13607863.2017.1421612
49. Eyaloba C, De Brauwer I, Cès S et al (2021) Profile and needs of primary informal caregivers of older patients in Belgian geriatric day hospitals: a multicentric cross-sectional study. BMC Geriatr 21:315. https://doi.org/10.1186/s12877-021-02255-1

Caregiving Burden and Other Psychosocial Considerations

Dégi László Csaba

1   Introduction

Cancer is a significant cause of informal caregiving [1]. In 1930, about 20% of people diagnosed with cancer lived another 5 years [2]. In the United States, the 5-year survival rate for all malignancies has increased from 49% in 1975 to 69% in 2013 [3]. By 2020, it is projected that more than 53 million Americans will serve as informal caregivers, including approximately 3 million caring for a person with cancer [4, 5]. By 2030, 22.1 million Americans are expected to be cancer survivors, most of whom will be 65 years of age or older [6]. As a result, a significant number of families are forced to deal with caregiving and grief due to cancer. The study found that 84% of the elderly received support from family members and other unpaid caregivers before diagnosing cancer. Spouses were the primary informal caregivers, followed by children, friends, siblings, and parents [7]. In addition, cancer survivors who rated their health as poor or fair were more likely to report having an informal caregiver than those who rated their health as good to excellent [7]. In addition, nearly 56% of care recipients had more than one caregiver [8]. In addition, informal caregivers are the backbone of the palliative care workforce and the primary providers of end-of-life care [9]; they are thought to provide 75–90% of home care for people at the end of life [10]. Despite growing evidence that caring for cancer patients severely impacts caregivers' well-being and quality of life, informal caregivers are among the "invisible" or "hidden" workforce providing support and direct care to cancer patients [11].

By 2040, the burden of disease from cancer in Europe is expected to increase by 21%, while the annual number of cancer deaths will increase by 31% [12]. The impact and burden on informal caregivers will increase as the prevalence of cancer

D. L. Csaba (✉)
Faculty of Sociology and Social Work, Babes Bolyai University, Cluj Napoca, Romania
e-mail: laszlo.degi@ubbcluj.ro

A. Charalambous (ed.), *Informal Caregivers: From Hidden Heroes to Integral Part of Care*, https://doi.org/10.1007/978-3-031-16745-4_2

increases, patient prognoses, and life expectancies improve, and patient reliance on ambulatory care services increases [12]. At this point, it is worth noting that previous research on pre-cancer health-oriented caregiving tasks and the relationship between caregiver activity patterns and caregiver burden has shown that a significant proportion of caregivers are already overloaded with tasks and burdens, which may be exacerbated by the additional responsibilities associated with the patient's new cancer diagnosis and subsequent treatment [6].

2   Cancer Caregivership Burden

Cancer patient caregiving, the process by which family members and friends help a cancer patient, is a unique and special type of stress due to the fear of death associated with a cancer diagnosis and treatment [13]. Informal caregivers of cancer patients are family members, partners, or friends who provide unpaid help in several categories, including social support, help with activities of daily living, and clinical care tasks [14]. Cancer patients' and caregivers' more extensive social networks are indeed becoming more important [15]. More than 40% of American adults are now single [16], and it is essential to consider other forms of supportive partnerships. Informal caregivers, who may or may not be family members, have been characterized as laypersons who play a critical supporting role in the patient's cancer experience, providing essential labor and emotion management [17]. In addition, informal caregivers are critical in the care of older patients and often meet the complicated demands associated with functional dependence, cognitive impairment, and various chronic illnesses [18].

Although the prevalence of psychosocial problems among informal caregivers of older cancer survivors is still unknown, there appear to be a higher prevalence of stress, decreased quality of life, and increased anxiety among informal caregivers of older cancer survivors compared with the general population [19].

The stress experienced by caregivers of cancer patients is greater than that of caregivers of older adults and comparable to that of caregivers of dementia patients [20]. For example, in the 2016 National Alliance for Caregiving study [1], cancer caregivers were significantly more likely than noncancer caregivers to assist with activities such as bed and chair transfers (57% vs. 42%), toileting (46% vs. 26%), dressing (42% vs. 31%), and feeding (39% vs. 22%). Caregiver burden is complex and includes social, physical, economic, and psychological aspects, even when there is no comprehensive description [21, 22].

Analyzing the impact of informal caregivers' perceived difficulties in cancer care is critical to discover benefits throughout the caregiving experience [23]. Caregivers who engage in religious coping and feel the availability of social support are more likely to report discovering benefits [13]. In addition, a representative prospective study examining the relationship between the presence of an informal caregiver and all-cause mortality among older adults, as well as the relationship between caregivers' perceptions of burden and benefits and care recipient mortality, found that caregivers of older adults who report only benefits or with caregivers who report only burden have an increased risk of mortality. In contrast, this risk is increased but lower for care recipients with informal caregivers who perceive both burden and benefits [24]. Even after adjusting for health, socioeconomic, and demographic factors associated with mortality, this pattern of informal caregivers remained associated with higher mortality risk among older persons, suggesting that interventions aimed at both reducing caregiver burden and increasing perceived benefits when burden reduction is not possible may support recipient longevity [24]. Therefore, caregiver burden may contribute to death through psychological and physiological systems that need further investigation [24].

2.1   Physical and Sleep Burden

Although informal caregiving has been the primary source of protection for those struggling with health difficulties since prehistoric times, informal caregiving of relatives with cancer has been associated with poor physical health. Subjective caregiver stress was related to physical impairments during the 2 years of cancer caregiving and the later onset of these impairments. For example, caregivers who returned to care over time and widowed were more likely to develop arthritis and heart disease [25]. Cancer caregivers have increased electrodermal and cardiovascular reactivity compared with controls [26, 27]. The extent to which the survivor and their caretaker spouse were comparable in their physical and mental health and relationship satisfaction was examined. The research shows that the survivor's physical and psychological health significantly impacts the spouse's satisfaction with the marriage. Survivor physical and mental health has also been associated with poorer quality of life and increased caregiver distress [28].

While caregivers' health has been shown to deteriorate due to cancer caregiving, the demographic and psychosocial predictors of long-term deterioration in their health are less well understood in terms of the unique contribution of caregivers' depressive symptoms to their physical decline. For example, in observing the physical and mental health of cancer patients and their informal caregivers over a year after diagnosis, it was found that patients' and caregivers' reports of physical health at each time point were unrelated. In contrast, their reports of mental health at each time point were positively associated to a small to moderate degree [29]. Psychosocial variables are known to impact the deterioration of caregivers' physical health significantly, and caregivers are at increased risk for premature illness compared with non-caregivers [30].

Numerous informal caregivers, even those who do not perceive caregiving as a burden, struggle with various issues, including anxiety, depression, practical and financial challenges, and insomnia [31]. Sleep is a critical component of health and health-related quality of life, and sleep disturbances can adversely affect physical and psychological well-being. Between 36% and 95% of caregivers reported that their nightly sleep was interrupted due to poor sleep quality. Depending on disease stage, prevalence rates ranged from 36% to 80% in the early stages of cancer and from 42% to 95% when patients with advanced disease were treated. During active treatment of patients, 37–59% of caregivers reported sleep problems before the start of treatment, while more than 70% of respondents reported sleep problems during patient treatment [32].

Sleep disturbances commonly experienced by caregivers include difficulty falling asleep and staying asleep due to frequent interruptions from patient care and nocturnal hypervigilance due to constant monitoring of the patient or the caregiver's concerns, resulting in a significant reduction in total sleep time [33]. In addition, numerous urgent or ongoing patient demands can disrupt caregiver sleep patterns, while increasing caregiver stress can decrease caregiver ability to provide care and perpetuate patient sleep disturbances due to unresolved symptoms or unmet concerns [34]. Disrupted sleep can be so debilitating that it jeopardizes both the patient's well-being and the caregiver's ability to provide effective care [35]. In addition, less than 20% of caregivers take a prescription or over-the-counter sleep medication [32].

2.2   Psychosocial and Spiritual Burden

Cancer is a traumatic experience for both patients and family caregivers, who assist with self-care and medical activities and offer knowledge, emotional support, and financial assistance. Caregivers of cancer or palliative care patients have been shown to have increased levels of anxiety, depression, and strain, as well as unmet needs for knowledge and psychological and physical support [17]. While information needs are high in the initial phase of cancer, they gradually decrease in the posttreatment phase as caregivers obtain knowledge from medical professionals and the internet [31]. To what extent the demands of caregivers providing ongoing, resuming, or emerging care differ from those providing end-of-life care remains unclear [3]. In conversations with social workers, the most commonly expressed concerns (49%) were psychological, followed by physical (28%), social (22%), and spiritual (2%) [36]. A few studies found a high incidence of cancer-related communication problems and the distress associated with these challenges. These studies focused on cancer patients' difficulties talking about their disease with family members and friends who do not have cancer. The majority of patients and partners who reported communication problems did so an average of 9 months after completing treatment, suggesting that even after completing treatment, either painful memories of cancer-related communication problems persist or communication problems have persisted during past treatment [37].

A negative attribution style does appear to exacerbate the association between informal cancer caregiver stress and cortisol levels but does not affect informal caregivers' depressive symptoms [38]. In addition, the literature on cancer survivors has shown that cancer-related stress may even cause patients' fruit and vegetable consumption to decrease and family caregivers' fruit and vegetable consumption to increase after treatment [39].

A loved one's cancer diagnosis causes significant emotional distress for family caregivers. This experience is compounded by the obligation to provide clinical and health care, impacting caregiver's well-being, the safety of care, and care outcomes

[40]. In addition, there is a disproportionately strong association between mothers' psychological distress and their adult caregiver daughters' quality of life, as mothers are likely to share their psychological concerns about cancer diagnosis, treatment, and survival with their adult daughters, as sharing emotional experiences is common in female relationships [41, 42]. Male caregivers view their involvement in cancer care positively, whereas adult daughters view it negatively [43]. In addition, wives, husbands, daughters, and sons tend to approach caregiving differently, affecting caregivers' emotional well-being [44]. For example, male caregivers were more likely to report higher levels of caregiver appreciation than female caregivers, which was associated with lower levels of caregiving stress [45].

Caregivers' cultural views and values affect their assessment of the caregiving situation [46–48]. In a study highlighting the depression and social support of caregivers of elderly cancer patients from Israel, depression was prevalent among both caregivers (76%) and patients (85%); moreover, the majority of caregivers lived with the patient in a shared apartment [18]. All of these findings suggest that when a family is struggling with a life-threatening illness such as cancer, patients' depressive symptoms are critical to their well-being and that of their family caregivers [49].

In addition, a cancer diagnosis can lead to an increase in existential concerns. Because cancer is often a life-threatening illness, family caregivers have existential concerns impacting their spiritual well-being. Spirituality has been highlighted as a psychological resource that can help family caregivers cope with stressful situations [50]. In addition, the spiritual well-being of cancer caregivers has received less attention in studies. A few studies concluded that the harmful effects of caregiving stress on mental health were less pronounced in caregivers with higher levels of spirituality [13]. Spiritual well-being among caregivers is similar to that of cancer patients and is mainly constant over time [51]. Moreover, spiritual well-being, mental health, and physical health are modestly associated between survivors and caregivers, indicating that survivors and caregivers have comparable levels of spiritual well-being and quality of life [52].

Evidence suggests that a strong sense of meaning and purpose in life is associated with improved mental health and physical symptoms [53]. Family support is critical to the spiritual well-being of family caregivers in the months following a cancer diagnosis in a family member. A study examining the extent to which caregiver experiences were associated with changes in spiritual well-being in the months following a family member's cancer diagnosis found that a perceived lack of family support for caregiving was associated with a decrease in caregivers' sense of meaning in life and peace over the 4-month study period. At the 4-month follow-up, a lack of family support in caregiving was significantly associated with lower levels of meaning and peace but not with faith. This conclusion is consistent with the hypothesis that low levels of social support impair meaning-making by limiting people's ability to process stressful experiences [51]. Specific data support the notion that lower social support and higher caregiver burden are products of profoundly rooted personality traits that contribute to the development or exacerbation of depressive symptoms, as both lower social support and higher caregiver burden mediate the relationship between neuroticism, interpersonal self-efficacy, and depression [54]. In addition, caregivers with high levels of neuroticism or low inter-personal self-efficacy see less accessible social support and experience more per-sonal and role pressures, leading to or exacerbating depressive symptoms in the caregiving setting [54]. Kim and Carver (2007) have shown that the attachment theory provides a robust framework for understanding caregiving behaviors and dif-ficulties. They have also shown that individuals who are more likely to be ineffec-tive caregivers of cancer patients can be identified by their attachment orientation, particularly insecure attachment qualities [23]. Therefore, it is essential to empha-size that attachment orientation toward the cancer patient is a critical predictor in the level of distress, in addition to the caregiver-reported level of physical function-ing [55].

Cancer caregivers and cancer patients often view the realities of treatment efforts as a release from the cognitive burden imposed by the existential threat of cancer. Patients and informal caregivers often use the metaphor of "treatment as hope" and may be reluctant to discontinue treatment despite potentially fatal side effects [56]. Similarly, related research on caregiver motivation has found that autonomous rea-sons do not predict spirituality or mental health [57].

2.3   Financial Burden and Caregiver Guilt

Financial toxicity is a term that refers to the psychological distress, negative coping behaviors, and material circumstances experienced by cancer patients due to high treatment costs, increased cost-sharing, and reduced household income as a result of cancer and its treatment. Family caregivers may suffer the adverse consequences of the high co-payments and reduced work hours associated with cancer treatment [58]. For example, caregivers reported spending a significant amount of time pro-viding medical, emotional, instrumental, and other material support to cancer patients in the 2 years following diagnosis, with average time costs ranging from $38,334 for breast cancer caregivers to $72,702 for lung cancer caregivers. These figures were comparable to direct medical expenditures associated with cancer care in the United States [59]. In Europe, informal caregivers contribute an estimated one-third of total cancer treatment expenditures [60]. These long treatment times are reflected in the high costs reported for informal cancer care [61]. For cancer caregivers, time is structured differently, and they cannot anticipate future life goals or decisions. This temporal anomie requires caregivers to live in the present moment, which offers several benefits and comes with a fair amount of discomfort and obli-gation [62]. According to one study, caregivers miss approximately 50% of their potential workdays each month to assist with patient care [63]. Caregiving that dis-rupted daily caregiver routines was associated with lower self-reported mental health and dysregulated cortisol patterns in older caregivers but better-regulated cortisol patterns in younger caregivers [64]. Working younger adult caregivers who had to balance the demands of work and family were shown to be more prone to feelings of guilt [65, 66]. A more significant impact on the caregiver's schedule was strongly associated with greater feelings of caregiver guilt [66]. Guilt as a significant emotional phenomenon in cancer caregiving has not been adequately explored. However, data suggest that higher levels of psychological distress and impaired mental, social, and physical functioning are significantly associated with caregiver guilt, above and beyond the variance explained by covariates [66].

Nonetheless, family caregiving's financial costs and consequences are increasingly well understood. For example, the Comprehensive Score for Financial Toxicity study found a modest association between patient and caregiver financial burden and identified characteristics associated with caregiver financial burden. For example, older adult caregivers may have particular financial difficulties [67]. In addition, financial toxicity was associated with higher patient nonadherence to treatment, increased lifestyle-altering behaviors, and poorer quality of life in both patients and caregivers [21].

There is a dearth of research using standardized approaches to determine the economic value of psychological support [10, 68, 69]. The financial cost of care should be considered alongside other well-documented inequities in palliative care and a significant social determinant of the end-of-life experience [10]. Informal caregivers appear to make a substantial financial contribution to the broader health care system. Some research suggests that informal care accounts for up to 70% of total health care expenditures [10, 70]. However, those from lower socioeconomic backgrounds continually face the most significant financial burden. This relates to education per se. Across Europe, there is a significant correlation between education and wealth; those with high levels of education earn up to 70% more than those with low levels of education [71].

Cost figures are one approach to quantifying the value of caregivers; however, patients' and caregivers' narratives about the impact of cancer on their lives are much more meaningful [5]. The lived experience of being an informal caregiver can be understood when compared to the idea of co-dependency [12]. A consensus study found that the financial burden of caregiving deserves a more substantial research focus, with regular examinations of critical outcomes reported by caregivers and clinician education. Priorities will vary depending on the caregiver at risk [72].

2.4 Long-Term and Quality-of-Life-Related Burden

Five years after diagnosis, 40% of current caregivers and 50% of survivor caregivers had a significant prevalence of depressive symptoms severe enough to be considered clinically significant. However, the incidence was much lower among patients in remission (20%) [73]. In addition, physical morbidity among cancer caregivers was related to their long-term caregiving role and, more specifically, to chronic or developing depressive symptoms 5 years after the initial cancer diagnosis [30]. In addition, the stress of caregiving 3–6 years earlier was significantly related to the unmet needs of bereaved caregivers [3].

While previous research suggests that the quality of life of cancer patient caregivers varies over time due to coping with the stressor [74], caregiver burden over time is significantly associated with anxiety and depression [75]. In addition, the early physical health of cancer caregivers deteriorates compared to demographically comparable non-caregivers due to long-term caregiving responsibilities and depressive symptoms [76]. A study examining changes in caregivers' physical health 2–8 years after cancer diagnosis in their family members and prospective predictors of these changes found that caregivers play a critical role in cancer patients' treatment outcomes. However, caregiving experience increases the risk of long-term deterioration in caregivers' health [30].

The long-term impact of cancer caregiving on family caregivers' quality of life is now well established [25, 77]. One study showed that caregiver age and prior caregiving stress were significant predictors of quality of life in all groups of caregivers, underscoring the substantial impact of caregiving status on quality of life at the 5-year time point [78]. At the 5-year evaluation, caregivers who would become active caregivers or bereaved were more likely to be older and female and less likely to be educated and employed than at baseline. As a result, the bereaved were less likely than other caregivers to be wealthy or the deceased's husband but more likely to be the dead's mother or child [73]. At the eight-year follow-up, most caregivers had stopped actively caring for the relative with cancer because the relative was either in remission (66.2%) or had died (21.2%). However, because cancer survivors face increased morbidity and mortality as they age, the quality of life of their family members after 8 years still depends to some extent on the survivor's prognosis at that time [25, 78].

Just as cancer survivors face increased morbidity and mortality as they age, the quality of life of their caregiving family members at the 8-year mark depends to some extent on the prognosis of survivors at that point. Findings suggest that programs focused primarily on reducing family members' psychological distress can lead to improvements in their overall quality of life 8 years after the family's first cancer diagnosis [25]. Increased uncertainty and concern about disease recurrence remained a significant source of anxiety for caregiving family members, even though patients recovered physically and were free of cancer-related symptoms [74]. In a recent study, family caregivers expressed, on average, a moderate level of anxiety about cancer recurrence in their survivors take [79]. However, the most significant unmet needs of family caregivers were coping with fears of cancer recurrence and transitioning to the "new normal," as this influential group of family caregivers of patients who no longer require cancer treatment remain "lost" in the health care system [3]. These data suggest that years of active involvement in cancer care or resumption of such a caregiver role after initial diagnosis are most likely associated with overall more significant caregiving needs [3]. However, recent findings show that 11% of respondents returned to actively caring for patients several years after being recruited [80]. At this point, we must emphasize that there is compelling evidence that psychosocial support should be prioritized throughout the long-term survival trajectory for family caregivers of patients with recurrent or chronic illness, as well as for higher caregiver depression symptoms [30]. In addition, they are pertinent indicators of vulnerability variables associated with caring for cancer patients.

2.5   Bereavement Burden

Recent evidence suggests that the death of the care recipient places additional stress on cancer caregivers who are already psychologically and socially exhausted by performing the role of the family caregiver. This supports the attrition model of caregiving [25], in contrast to the stress reduction model of grief, which assumes that the care recipient's death alleviates caregiving stress [81, 82]. Due to stress and lack of social support for caregiving spouses, they are less likely to benefit from bereavement [83]. With this in mind, early identification of those at risk for poor grief outcomes and programs to help caregivers make sense of their loss would help engage or retain these caregivers and protect them as they go through care transitions [83–85].

The psycho-oncology literature on the grief phase, which for some caregivers begins with the death of the care recipient, found that 13% of caregivers of advanced cancer patients met the criteria for a psychiatric disorder; 24% and 18% of caregivers met criteria for complicated and persistent grief, respectively; and 37% and 44% met criteria for a clinical level of depressive symptoms, approximately 3 and 5 years [17, 74, 82]. In addition, 19–24% of bereaved family members reported experiencing grief-specific stress, such as difficulty accepting the death, avoiding reminders of the loss, or having an increased physiological response when reminded of the loss, and 11–50% of bereaved family members reported experiencing increased levels of general stress, such as depression, sadness, loss of interest, fatigue, anxiety, and the inability to relax [86–89]. In a longitudinal study, pre-loss spirituality predicts post-loss distress in bereaved cancer caregivers [50].

Recently, the first prospective study to examine a cohort of primary caregivers of cancer patients in the last stage of life, collecting pre-loss mental health data and systematically following up the cohort for up to 3 years after the loss, found that 20% of caregivers exhibited symptoms of persistent grief disorder for 37 months after the loss [90]. In addition, studies have shown that family caregivers who are no longer involved in the cancer patient's care reported that many of their needs remained unmet. In addition, unmet needs for coping with loss were a significant predictor of acute emotional response to loss, persistent complex grief, and post-traumatic stress disorder-like symptoms related to loss that occurred years, not months, after death [3].

Caregiving stress, which was shown to be strongly associated with unmet needs during grief, was not the objective assessment of the severity of the index patient's cancer but the subjective assessment of caregivers who found caring for the index patient stressful [91]. Resuming daily and social activities benefits caregivers by alleviating the anxiety associated with grief years after the loss [17]. By improving their ability to care for themselves, informal caregivers can optimize care for their loved ones, reducing the likelihood of hospital readmissions and the associated costs to the medical services providing care [38, 92, 93].

All of these findings suggest that cancer caregiver programs should include information on how to manage caregiver-related stress in the early survivorship phase and how best to identify and recruit effective social programs to improve caregivers' personal and social resources in early survivorship, as depression is a long-term problem for this population [78]. In addition, the different characteristics of cancer care and the psychological factors of individuals participating in cancer care at various stages of survivorship are critical to improving the effectiveness of care and maximizing the quality of life of survivors and caregivers [94].

3   Interventions for the Management of Caregivers' Burden

Family caregivers report high levels of discomfort, highlighting the need to screen caregivers and identify individuals who might benefit from psychological interventions and support [95]. In addition, the literature states that given a choice between a social support system intervention and a reduction in caregiver burden, the latter may be better suited to reduce the intensity of depressive symptoms in spousal caregivers of cancer patients [54]. These insecure caregivers would benefit from educational programs that would improve their caregiving skills and encourage them to seek help from other family members or community members [23].

3.1   Good Examples

The reality is that stress management, family-based interventions, and programs for family members are needed throughout the disease course [74, 91]. Findings imply that cancer survivorship programs should engage family members and provide regular psychological treatment beyond the initial survivorship phase. In addition, persistent psychological distress and difficulties with role adjustment have been documented in spousal caregivers approximately 1 year after the completion of cancer treatment, with scores significantly higher than healthy controls [74].

Patients' spouses, siblings, children, parents, and friends are considered family caregivers. Family caregivers bear a significant burden in providing informal and supportive care to cancer patients throughout cancer treatment, as they must cope with suffering at a considerable physical distance from their support networks, give up their jobs to be within reach of services, or struggle to incorporate religious and cultural requirements into caregiving [40]. The psychological adjustment of cancer caregivers who perform multiple roles, particularly those employed and care for children, depends on the availability of community-based services. Intervention programs targeting informal cancer caregivers who fulfill multiple social functions should be developed to help them adjust to their new caregiving roles and improve their quality of life [96]. In addition, couples may benefit from interventions that will enhance their ability to cope with psychological distress, especially their spouse. This may support both couples' mental and physical health coping with cancer [97]. Research shows that cancer survivors and their caregivers are inextricably linked. Therefore, caregiver quality of life initiatives should focus on caregivers and caregiver-survivor couples [98]. While our knowledge of the caregiving process is improving, there is an urgent need to pay more attention to the barriers families experience during the disease process [44]. Identifying the unmet needs of family caregivers should be the first step in developing initiatives to improve caregivers' quality of life [99].

We have established a solid foundation for establishing successful programs over the past two decades as various research efforts have identified the needs of cancer patient caregivers [44]. Despite the decreasing stigma associated with seeking psychological support in the modern era, some research indicates that informal caregivers of patients with terminal cancer are rarely offered psychosocial support [100]. Studies examining the effectiveness of psychosocial interventions to reduce psychological distress in cancer caregivers found that psychosocial interventions successfully reduced depression and anxiety in cancer caregivers compared with usual care [101]. Psychological interventions may help reduce the burden on informal caregivers of cancer patients. However, more careful, multicenter randomized controlled trials and examining the long-term effects of psychosocial interventions on caregivers are needed [102]. Caregivers' needs may vary at different stages of the care pathway, and support should be tailored to meet those needs accordingly. There is still considerable range and inconsistency in the content and quality of research examining the function of psychological support for caregivers. Psychoeducational programs to support family caregivers are widely used [21], but cognitive-behavioral interventions for informal caregivers of cancer patients and survivors have had a modest overall impact [75]. Although cognitive-behavioral therapy components such as coping skills training, problem-solving, cognitive restructuring, structured homework, and relaxation were found to be marginally more effective for younger, female caregivers, the effect of cognitive-behavioral interventions was not statistically significant compared to a control group in randomized designs [75]. Caregiver stress can be managed with emotion regulation therapy and life review therapy, which may also have a protective effect on informal caregivers' self-esteem [84, 103, 104].

In addition, findings suggest that both survivors and caregivers may benefit from interventions that increase their capacity for meaning and peace in the cancer experience, which may be associated with improved mental and physical health for themselves and their partners as they engage with cancer beyond the early stages of the disease process [52]. In addition, informal caregivers may benefit from interventions that strengthen their ability to accept their circumstances and find meaning in their caregiving experience, resulting in overall satisfaction with life and decreasing depressive symptoms [105].

The needs of informal caregivers in cancer are primarily unmet, as studies have shown that informal caregiving for a relative or friend who has cancer or advanced terminal illness can lead to a variety of problems, including insomnia, deterioration in overall health, exhaustion, and anxiety/depression [106]. Here, there is a particular need to identify the unmet needs of family caregivers during the long-term survivorship phase and establish programs to assist them in psychosocial and spiritual adjustment to cancer in the family [78]. In the long-term survivorship phase, interventions for caregivers must take into account caregivers' fear of recurrence of their patient's cancer [3]. In addition, cancer survivors and their family caregivers may benefit from interventions that improve their ability to control the fear of recurrence, improving their mental and physical health later in life, such as during the long-term survival phase [107].

As the number of older cancer patients continues to increase, the growing number of caregivers of older cancer patients has expanded the caregiving work to include the unique issues associated with the needs of oncology, palliative, and end-of-life care [18, 108]. Although caregivers are essential partners in promoting the health and well-being of older cancer patients, they are often excluded from patient education initiatives before discharge [53]. A recent review examining the impact of various support programs focusing on psychoeducational needs through face-to-face sessions, and counseling indicates that support programs aimed at addressing disparities must be effective and sustainable if they are to go beyond addressing a specific health disparity and help affected groups empower themselves through systemic change [109].

3.2   eHealth Options

Information and communication technology has become increasingly important in recent decades in facilitating information delivery and data sharing, overcoming physical barriers, and addressing human needs. eHealth refers to disseminating information about diseases or health care and supporting patients and informal caregivers through computers or related technologies. eHealth interventions are increasingly used in cancer care, for example, to help patients and informal caregivers manage everyday symptoms and problems [110].

In addition, eHealth systems can enable collaboration among numerous hospital settings to improve health services, patient engagement, monitoring, and management and provide rapid access to expert advice and patient information regardless of where patients are located or where data are collected. For example, interventions that use phone calls or eHealth technologies aim to improve caregivers' physical and emotional well-being to meet various user needs [14]. Although studies indicated substantial benefits in some of the caregiver categories studied, they often had tiny effect sizes [69]. While systematic research found an impact of eHealth on cancer patients' knowledge, information literacy, and perceptions of the help they received, very few systematic reviews examined eHealth for informal caregivers of cancer patients [110]. Caregivers will benefit from tailored programs based on their early survivorship demographic characteristics (younger caregivers, e.g., reported high levels of unmet needs), which will ensure their long-term quality of life after diagnosis, as gender was significantly associated with unmet psychosocial needs at 2 years [98]. From the perspective of the post-cancer, survivorship period, caregivers' baseline demographic characteristics, and perceived caregiver stress must be examined earlier. This will help identify subgroups of caregivers whose different needs are less likely to be met after their patients die [77]. Caregivers' ethnicity, income, and marital status should be considered when developing programs to help subgroups of caregivers meet their needs related to cancer care [98].

Future studies are essential to examine whether video-based instructional interventions are feasible and helpful as a support tool for caregivers, mainly when YouTube is used for pain management [111]. To this point, evaluations have suggested that nurses and helping professionals could more effectively support home-based caregivers by providing the knowledge and feedback needed to perform practical caregiving tasks. By meeting the suitable needs of informal caregivers, health professionals working at the interface of home and palliative care may assist informal caregivers more effectively [112].

3.3 Policy Action Needed

Family caregivers of cancer patients may benefit from social, health, and service policies that uniquely address their emotional and physical distress [113]. Because informal caregivers make a significant contribution to cancer care, cancer policy increasingly focuses on and recognizes the importance of providing effective and appropriate support to informal caregivers in managing the impact of their caregiving responsibilities in addition to their regular job or other caregiving responsibilities [21]. For example, employers may provide early support and assistance to employees caring for cancer patients, such as 45 sick leave days per year [114]. The importance of this issue may reflect a widespread recognition of the tasks caregivers undertake and the associated expenses [72].

Because of the complexity of the caregiving experience, known characteristics that contribute to caregiver burdens, such as physical health, mental health issues, socioeconomic status, social isolation, and family or social support, will persist and often be exacerbated by new cancer therapies. However, given the essential role informal caregivers play in complementing formal care, creative solutions are needed to address these new issues and needs on care throughout the cancer trajectory [115]. This requires the development of appropriate care plans for family caregivers of cancer survivors as long-term survival progresses [77]. While key family caregiver organizations are fighting for "caregiver-friendly" legislation and programs at the national level, advocating for the unique needs of family caregivers of cancer patients may be most successful at the state and local level, where legislators are most accessible [44]. Given the significant burden and distress associated with cancer caregiving, greater emphasis should be placed on improving social service policies and practices [113].

4 Conclusion and Outlook

Most of us will be affected by cancer at some point in our lives. Given the increasing investment in psychosocial cancer care research [72] and the fact that cancer caregivers face the simultaneous stress of significant role transitions and additional responsibility for patient needs, often resulting in caregiver burden, there is acknowledgment that informal caregivers of chronically ill patients also require care and support [75]. However, despite the rapid increase in cancer caregivers, there remain significant gaps in knowledge regarding the variables that lead to individual differences in the cancer care experience [23].

The COVID-19 pandemic directly impacted informal caregiving and increased the burden of family caregivers [116]. The need to maintain a social distance and take extra measures to avoid COVID-19 viral transmission almost certainly significantly impacted the experience of formal and informal cancer care [117]. Family caregivers of community-dwelling elders have faced significant caregiving challenges due to the breakdown of institutional and informal support networks during the COVID-19 epidemic [118]. Nonverbal information cannot always be sent or received, making it difficult to offer and receive care in delicate situations [119]. Increased stress, pain, depression, sleep problems, and irritability are frequently reported health outcomes [116]. Informal caregivers, in particular, may need treatments to promote sleep duration and quality during COVID-19 [120]. Therefore, immediate action is required to alleviate the increasing burden of cancer caregiving and continue supporting caregivers.

Acknowledgments Chapter preparation was supported by a grant from the Ministry of Research, Innovation and Digitization, CNCS/CCCDI—UEFISCDI, project number PN-III-P1-1.1-TE-2019-0097, within PNCDI III.

References

1. Hunt G, Whiting C, Longacre M, Kent E, Weber-Raley L, Popham L (2016) Cancer caregiving in the US–An intense, episodic, and challenging care experience. National alliance for caregiving. National Cancer Institute, and Cancer Support Community
2. Ganz P (1990) Abolishing the myths: the facts about cancer. An almanac of practical resources for cancer survivors Mount Vernon (NY): Consumers Union, pp 7–30
3. Kim Y, Carver CS, Ting A (2019) Family caregivers' unmet needs in long-term cancer survivorship. Semin Oncol Nurs 35(4):380–383
4. Reinhard SC, Ryan E (2017) From home alone to the CARE act: collaboration for family caregivers. Public Policy Institute Retrieved from https://www.aarp.org/ppi/info-2017/from-home-alone-to-the-care-act.html
5. Thompson T, Ketcher D, Gray TF, Kent EE (2021) The dyadic cancer outcomes framework: a general framework of the effects of cancer on patients and informal caregivers. Soc Sci Med 287:9
6. Liu B, Kent EE, Dionne-Odom JN, Alpert N, Ornstein KA (2021) A national profile of health-focused caregiving activities prior to a new cancer diagnosis. J Geriatric Oncol S1879-4068(21):00256–00253
7. Borsky AE, Zuvekas SH, Kent EE, de Moor JS, Ngo-Metzger Q, Soni A (2021) Understanding the characteristics of US cancer survivors with informal caregivers. Cancer 127(15):2752–2761
8. Ornstein KA, Liu B, Schwartz RM, Smith CB, Alpert N, Taioli E (2020) Cancer in the context of aging: health characteristics, function and caregiving needs prior to a new cancer diagnosis in a national sample of older adults. J Geriatric Oncol 11(1):75–81
9. Silva AR, Petry S (2021) As experiências de cuidadores informais de pacientes em tratamento oncológico paliativo: uma revisão integrativa. Cuidado e Saúde, Ciência, p 20

10. Gardiner C, Robinson J, Connolly M, Hulme C, Kang K, Rowland C et al (2020) Equity and the financial costs of informal caregiving in palliative care: a critical debate. BMC Palliat Care 19(1):7

11. Sun V, Raz DJ, Kim JY (2019) Caring for the informal cancer caregiver. Curr Opin Support Palliat Car. 13(3):238–242

12. Tranberg M, Andersson M, Nilbert M, Rasmussen BH (2019) Co-afflicted but invisible: a qualitative study of perceptions among informal caregivers in cancer care. J Health Psychol 26(11):1850–1859

13. Colgrove LA, Kim Y, Thompson N (2007) The effect of spirituality and gender on the quality of life of spousal caregivers of cancer survivors. Ann Behav Med 33(1):90–98

14. Kent EE, Mollica MA, Buckenmaier S, Smith AW (2019) The characteristics of informal cancer caregivers in the United States. Semin Oncol Nurs 35(4):328–332

15. Kroenke CH (2018) A conceptual model of social networks and mechanisms of cancer mortality, and potential strategies to improve survival. Transl Behav Med 8(4):629–642

16. Fry R (2017) The share of Americans living without a partner has increased, especially among young adults

17. Schildmann EK, Higginson IJ (2011) Evaluating psycho-educational interventions for informal carers of patients receiving cancer care or palliative care: strengths and limitations of different study designs. Palliat Med 25(4):345–356

18. Baider L, Goldzweig G, Jacobs JM, Ghrayeb IM, Sapir E, Rottenberg Y (2021) Informal caregivers of older Muslims diagnosed with cancer: a portrait of depression, social support, and faith. Palliat Support Care 19(5):598–604

19. Jansen L, Dauphin S, van den Akker M, De Burghgraeve T, Schoenmakers B, Buntinx F (2018) Prevalence and predictors of psychosocial problems in informal caregivers of older cancer survivors – a systematic review: still major gaps in current research. Eur J Cancer Care 27(6):13

20. Bevans M, Sternberg EM (2012) Caregiving burden, stress, and health effects among family caregivers of adult cancer patients. JAMA 307(4):398–403

21. Treanor CJ (2020) Psychosocial support interventions for cancer caregivers: reducing caregiver burden. Curr Opin Support Palliat Car 14(3):247–262

22. Treanor CJ, Santin O, Prue G, Coleman H, Cardwell CR, O'Halloran P et al (2019) Psychosocial interventions for informal caregivers of people living with cancer. Cochrane Database Syst Rev 6:140

23. Kim Y, Carver CS (2007) Frequency and difficulty in caregiving among spouses of individuals with cancer: effects of adult attachment and gender. Psycho-Oncology 16(8):714–723

24. Pristavec T, Luth EA (2020) Informal caregiver burden, benefits, and older adult mortality: a survival analysis. J Gerontol 75(10):2193–2206

25. Kim Y, Shaffer KM, Carver CS, Cannady RS (2016) Quality of life of family caregivers 8 years after a relative's cancer diagnosis: follow-up of the national quality of life survey for caregivers. Psycho-Oncology 25(3):266–274

26. Kim Y, Carver CS, Shaffer KM, Gansler T, Cannady RS (2015) Cancer caregiving predicts physical impairments: roles of earlier caregiving stress and being a spousal caregiver. Cancer 121(2):302–310

27. Teixeira RJ, Remondes-Costa S, Pereira MG, Brandao T (2019) The impact of informal cancer caregiving: a literature review on psychophysiological studies. Eur J Cancer Care 28(4):10

28. Zhou ES, Kim Y, Rasheed M, Benedict C, Bustillo NE, Soloway M et al (2011) Marital satisfaction of advanced prostate cancer survivors and their spousal caregivers: the dyadic effects of physical and mental health. Psycho-Oncology 20(12):1353–1357

29. Shaffer KM, Kim Y, Carver CS (2016) Physical and mental health trajectories of cancer patients and caregivers across the year post-diagnosis: a dyadic investigation. Psychol Health 31(6):655–674

30. Shaffer KM, Kim Y, Carver CS, Cannady RS (2017) Depressive symptoms predict cancer caregivers' physical health decline. Cancer 123(21):4277–4285

31. Wang T, Molassiotis A, Chung BPM, Tan JY (2018) Unmet care needs of advanced cancer patients and their informal caregivers: a systematic review. BMC Palliat Care 17:29

32. Kotronoulas G, Wengstrom Y, Kearney N (2013) Sleep patterns and sleep-impairing factors of persons providing informal care for people with cancer: a critical review of the literature. Cancer Nurs 36(1):E1–E15

33. Maltby KF, Sanderson CR, Lobb EA, Phillips JL (2017) Sleep disturbances in caregivers of patients with advanced cancer: a systematic review. Palliat Support Care 15(1):125–140

34. Bhattacharjee A, Ananya Mondal M, Tanima Chatterjee PS, Mukhopadhyay P (2015) Informal caregivers' psychological distress and coping style during cancer care. Scholars J Arts Human Soc Sci 3(1):144–152

35. Kotronoulas G, Wengstrom Y, Kearney N (2013) Sleep and sleep-wake disturbances in care recipient-caregiver dyads in the context of a chronic illness: a critical review of the literature. J Pain Symptom Manag 45(3):579–594

36. Kim Y, Carver CS (2012) Recognizing the value and needs of the caregiver in oncology. Curr Opin Support Palliat Car 6(2):280–288

37. Kornblith AB, Regan MM, Kim YM, Greer G, Parker B, Bennett S et al (2006) Cancer-related communication between female patients and male partners scale: a pilot study. Psycho-Oncology 15(9):780–794

38. Pössel P, Mitchell A, Harbison B, Fernandez-Botran G (2022) Association of cancer caregiver stress and negative attribution style with depressive symptoms and cortisol: a cross-sectional study. Support Care Cancer 30(6):4945–4952

39. Shaffer KM, Kim Y, Llabre MM, Carver CS (2016) Dyadic associations between cancer-related stress and fruit and vegetable consumption among colorectal cancer patients and their family caregivers. J Behav Med 39(1):75–84

40. Harrison R, Raman M, Walpola RL, Chauhan A, Sansom-Daly UM (2021) Preparing for partnerships in cancer care: an explorative analysis of the role of family-based caregivers. BMC Health Serv Res 21(1):10

41. Kim Y, Wellisch DK, Spillers RL (2008) Effects of psychological distress on quality of life of adult daughters and their mothers with cancer. Psycho-Oncology 17(11):1129–1136

42. Kim Y, Wellisch DK, Spillers RL, Crammer C (2007) Psychological distress of female cancer caregivers: effects of type of cancer and caregivers' spirituality. Support Care Cancer 15(12):1367–1374

43. Kim Y, Baker F, Spillers RL (2007) Cancer caregivers' quality of life: effects of gender, relationship, and appraisal. J Pain Symptom Manag 34(3):294–304

44. Talley RC, McCorkle R, Baile WF (2012) Cancer caregiving in the United States: research, practice, policy. Springer Science & Business Media

45. Kim Y, Baker F, Spillers RL, Wellisch DK (2006) Psychological adjustment of cancer caregivers with multiple roles. Psycho-Oncology 15(9):795–804

46. McElfresh J, Badger T, Segrin C, Thomson C (2021) Exploring spirituality, loneliness and HRQoL in hispanic cancer caregivers. Innov Aging 5(Suppl 1):690–691

47. Ramasamy T, Veeraiah S, Balakrishnan K (2021) Psychosocial issues among primary caregivers of patients with advanced head and neck cancer-a mixed-method study. Indian J Palliat Care 27(4):503

48. Wang T, Mazanec SR, Voss JG (eds) (2021) Needs of informal caregivers of patients with head and neck cancer: a systematic review. Oncology nursing forum. Oncology Nursing Society

49. Kim Y, Van Ryn M, Jensen RE, Griffin JM, Potosky A, Rowland J (2015) Effects of gender and depressive symptoms on quality of life among colorectal and lung cancer patients and their family caregivers. Psycho-Oncology 24(1):95–105

50. Ting A, Lucette A, Carver CS, Cannady RS, Kim Y (2019) Preloss spirituality predicts postloss distress of bereaved cancer caregivers. Ann Behav Med 53(2):150–157

51. Adams RN, Mosher CE, Cannady RS, Lucette A, Kim Y (2014) Caregiving experiences predict changes in spiritual well-being among family caregivers of cancer patients. Psycho-Oncology 23(10):1178–1184

52. Kim Y, Carver CS, Spillers RL, Crammer C, Zhou ES (2011) Individual and dyadic relations between spiritual well-being and quality of life among cancer survivors and their spousal caregivers. Psycho-Oncology 20(7):762–770
53. Hekman D, Mueller A, Fields B (2021) How frequently are caregivers included in patient education for oncology patients? Innov Aging 5(Suppl 1):802
54. Kim Y, Duberstein PR, Sörensen S, Larson MR (2005) Levels of depressive symptoms in spouses of people with lung cancer: effects of personality, social support, and caregiving burden. Psychosomatics 46(2):123–130
55. Kim Y, Kashy DA, Evans TV (2007) Age and attachment style impact stress and depressive symptoms among caregivers: a prospective investigation. J Cancer Survivorship 1(1):35–43
56. Lippiett KA, Richardson A, Myall M, Cummings A, May CR (2019) Patients and informal caregivers' experiences of burden of treatment in lung cancer and chronic obstructive pulmonary disease (COPD): a systematic review and synthesis of qualitative research. BMJ Open 9(2):17
57. Kim Y, Carver CS, Cannady RS (2015) Caregiving motivation predicts long-term spirituality and quality of life of the caregivers. Ann Behav Med 49(4):500–509
58. Sadigh G, Switchenko J, Weaver KE, Elchoufi D, Meisel J, Bilen MA et al (2022) Correlates of financial toxicity in adult cancer patients and their informal caregivers. Support Care Cancer 30(1):217–225
59. Yabroff KR, Kim Y (2009) Time costs associated with informal caregiving for cancer survivors. Cancer 115(18):4362–4373
60. Round J, Jones L, Morris S (2015) Estimating the cost of caring for people with cancer at the end of life: a modelling study. Palliat Med 29(10):899–907
61. Coumoundouros C, Brahim LO, Lambert SD, McCusker J (2019) The direct and indirect financial costs of informal cancer care: a scoping review. Health Soc Care Community 27(5):E622–EE36
62. Olson RE (2016) Towards a sociology of cancer caregiving: time to feel. Routledge
63. Longo CJ, Fitch MI, Loree JM, Carlson LE, Turner D, Cheung WY et al (2021) Patient and family financial burden associated with cancer treatment in Canada: a national study. Support Care Cancer 29(6):3377–3386
64. Mitchell HR, Kim Y, Carver CS, Llabre MM, Ting A, Mendez AJ (2021) Roles of age and sources of cancer caregiving stress in self-reported health and neuroendocrine biomarkers. Psychol Health 36(8):952–966
65. Bernard LL, Guarnaccia CA (2003) Two models of caregiver strain and bereavement adjustment: a comparison of husband and daughter caregivers of breast cancer hospice patients. The Gerontologist 43(6):808–816
66. Spillers RL, Wellisch DK, Kim Y, Matthews A, Baker F (2008) Family caregivers and guilt in the context of cancer care. Psychosomatics 49(6):511–519
67. Ferszt G, Yun S, Weber K, Qualls S (2021) The relationship between burden and financial factors for help-seeking older adult caregivers. Innov Aging 5(Suppl 1):813–814
68. Elbert NJ, van Os-Medendorp H, van Renselaar W, Ekeland AG, Hakkaart-van Roijen L, Raat H et al (2014) Effectiveness and cost-effectiveness of eHealth interventions in somatic diseases: a systematic review of systematic reviews and meta-analyses. J Med Internet Res 16(4):182–204
69. Marzorati C, Renzi C, Russell-Edu SW, Pravettoni G (2018) Telemedicine use among caregivers of cancer patients: systematic review. J Med Internet Res 20(6):15
70. Chai H, Guerriere DN, Zagorski B, Coyte PC (2014) The magnitude, share and determinants of unpaid care costs for home-based palliative care service provision in Toronto, Canada. Health Soc Care Community 22(1):30–39
71. EUROSTAT. Earnings statistics 2022. Available from: https://ec.europa.eu/eurostat/statistics-explained/index.php/Earnings_statistics
72. Lambert SD, Ould Brahim L, Morrison M, Girgis A, Yaffe M, Belzile E et al (2019) Priorities for caregiver research in cancer care: an international Delphi survey of caregivers, clinicians, managers, and researchers. Support Care Cancer 27(3):805–817

73. Kim Y, Shaffer KM, Carver CS, Cannady RS (2014) Prevalence and predictors of depressive symptoms among cancer caregivers 5 years after the relative's cancer diagnosis. J Consult Clin Psychol 82(1):1

74. Kim Y, Given BA (2008) Quality of life of family caregivers of cancer survivors: across the trajectory of the illness. Cancer 112(S11):2556–2568

75. O'Toole MS, Zachariae R, Renna ME, Mennin DS, Applebaum A (2017) Cognitive behavioral therapies for informal caregivers of patients with cancer and cancer survivors: a systematic review and meta-analysis. Psycho-Oncology 26(4):428–437

76. Shaffer KM, Kim Y, Carver CS, Cannady RS (2017) Effects of caregiving status and changes in depressive symptoms on development of physical morbidity among long-term cancer caregivers. Health Psychol 36(8):770–778

77. Kim Y, Carver CS (2019) Unmet needs of family cancer caregivers predict quality of life in long-term cancer survivorship. J Cancer Surviv 13(5):749–758

78. Kim Y, Spillers RL, Hall DL (2012) Quality of life of family caregivers 5 years after a relative's cancer diagnosis: follow-up of the national quality of life survey for caregivers. Psycho-Oncology 21(3):273–281

79. Takeuchi E, Kim Y, Shaffer KM, Cannady RS, Carver CS (2020) Fear of cancer recurrence promotes cancer screening behaviors among family caregivers of cancer survivors. Cancer 126(8):1784–1792

80. Kim Y, Carver CS, Ting A, Cannady RS (2020) Passages of cancer caregivers' unmet needs across 8 years. Cancer 126(20):4593–4601

81. Bass DM, Bowman K (1990) The transition from caregiving to bereavement: the relationship of care-related strain and adjustment to death. The Gerontologist 30(1):35–42

82. Kim Y, Carver CS, Spiegel D, Mitchell HR, Cannady RS (2017) Role of family caregivers' self-perceived preparedness for the death of the cancer patient in long-term adjustment to bereavement. Psycho-Oncology 26(4):484–492

83. Kim Y, Carver CS, Schulz R, Lucette A, Cannady RS (2013) Finding benefit in bereavement among family cancer caregivers. J Palliat Med 16(9):1040–1047

84. Applebaum AJ, Panjwani AA, Buda K, O'Toole MS, Hoyt MA, Garcia A et al (2020) Emotion regulation therapy for cancer caregivers-an open trial of a mechanism-targeted approach to addressing caregiver distress. Transl Behav Med 10(2):413–422

85. Applebaum AJ (2017) Survival of the fittest… caregiver? Palliat Support Care 15(1):1–2

86. Allen JY, Haley WE, Small BJ, Schonwetter RS, McMillan SC (2013) Bereavement among hospice caregivers of cancer patients one year following loss: predictors of grief, complicated grief, and symptoms of depression. J Palliat Med 16(7):745–751

87. Bradley EH, Prigerson H, Carlson MD, Cherlin E, Johnson-Hurzeler R, Kasl SV (2004) Depression among surviving caregivers: does length of hospice enrollment matter? Am J Psychiatr 161(12):2257–2262

88. Chiu Y-W, Huang C-T, Yin S-M, Huang Y-C, Chien C-h, Chuang H-Y (2010) Determinants of complicated grief in caregivers who cared for terminal cancer patients. Support Care Cancer 18(10):1321–1327

89. Ling S-F, Chang W-C, Shen WC (eds) (2013) Trajectory and influencing factors of depressive symptoms in family caregivers before and after the death of terminally ill patients with cancer. Oncology Nursing Forum. Oncology Nursing Society

90. Zordan RD, Bell ML, Price M, Remedios C, Lobb E, Hall C et al (2019) Long-term prevalence and predictors of prolonged grief disorder amongst bereaved cancer caregivers: a cohort study. Palliat Support Care 17(5):507–514

91. Kim Y, Carver CS, Cannady RS (2020) Bereaved family cancer caregivers' unmet needs: measure development and validation. Ann Behav Med 54(3):164–175

92. Burke RE, Coleman EA (2013) Interventions to decrease hospital readmissions: keys for cost-effectiveness. JAMA Intern Med 173(8):695–698

93. Harding R, Higginson IJ (2003) What is the best way to help caregivers in cancer and palliative care? A systematic literature review of interventions and their effectiveness. Palliat Med 17(1):63–74

94. Kim Y, Kashy DA, Kaw CK, Smith T, Spillers RL (2009) Sampling in population-based cancer caregivers research. Qual Life Res 18(8):981–989
95. Cochrane A, Reid O, Woods S, Gallagher P, Dunne S (2021) Variables associated with distress amongst informal caregivers of people with lung cancer: a systematic review of the literature. Psycho-Oncology 30(8):1246–1261
96. Kim Y, Loscalzo MJ, Wellisch DK, Spillers RL (2006) Gender differences in caregiving stress among caregivers of cancer survivors. Psycho-Oncology 15(12):1086–1092
97. Kim Y, Kashy DA, Wellisch DK, Spillers RL, Kaw CK, Smith TG (2008) Quality of life of couples dealing with cancer: dyadic and individual adjustment among breast and prostate cancer survivors and their spousal caregivers. Ann Behav Med 35(2):230–238
98. Kim Y, Spillers RL (2010) Quality of life of family caregivers at 2 years after a relative's cancer diagnosis. Psycho-Oncology 19(4):431–440
99. Kim Y, Kashy DA, Spillers RL, Evans TV (2010) Needs assessment of family caregivers of cancer survivors: three cohorts comparison. Psycho-Oncology 19(6):573–582
100. van Roij J, de Zeeuw B, Zijlstra M, Claessens N, Raijmakers N, de Poll-Franse LV et al (2021) Shared perspectives of patients with advanced cancer and their informal caregivers on essential aspects of health care: a qualitative study. J Palliative Care 0825859721989524
101. Zhang Z, Wang S, Liu Z, Li Z (2020) Psychosocial interventions to improve psychological distress of informal caregivers of cancer patients: a meta-analysis of randomized controlled trial. Am J Nurs 9(6):459–465
102. Frambes D, Given B, Lehto R, Sikorskii A, Wyatt G (2018) Informal caregivers of cancer patients: review of interventions, care activities, and outcomes. West J Nurs Res 40(7):1069–1097
103. Kleijn G, Lissenberg-Witte BI, Bohlmeijer ET, Steunenberg B, Knipscheer-Kuijpers K, Willemsen V et al (2018) The efficacy of life review therapy combined with memory specificity training (LRT-MST) targeting cancer patients in palliative care: a randomized controlled trial. PLoS One 13(5):e0197277
104. Kleijn G, Lissenberg-Witte BI, Bohlmeijer ET, Willemsen V, Becker-Commissaris A, Eeltink CM et al (2021) A randomized controlled trial on the efficacy of life review therapy targeting incurably ill cancer patients: do their informal caregivers benefit? Support Care Cancer 29(3):1257–1264
105. Kim Y, Schulz R, Carver CS (2007) Benefit finding in the cancer caregiving experience. Psychosom Med 69(3):283–291
106. Harding R, List S, Epiphaniou E, Jones H (2012) How can informal caregivers in cancer and palliative care be supported? An updated systematic literature review of interventions and their effectiveness. Palliat Med 26(1):7–22
107. Kim Y, Carver CS, Spillers RL, Love-Ghaffari M, Kaw C-K (2012) Dyadic effects of fear of recurrence on the quality of life of cancer survivors and their caregivers. Qual Life Res 21(3):517–525
108. Adashek JJ, Subbiah IM (2020) Caring for the caregiver: a systematic review characterising the experience of caregivers of older adults with advanced cancers. ESMO Open 5(5):7
109. Papadakos J, Samoil D, Umakanthan B, Charow R, Jones JM, Matthew A et al (2021) What are we doing to support informal caregivers? A scoping review of caregiver education programs in cancer care. Patient Educ Couns
110. Slev VN, Mistiaen P, Pasman HRW, Verdonck-de Leeuw IM, van Uden-Kraan CF, Francke AL (2016) Effects of eHealth for patients and informal caregivers confronted with cancer: a meta-review. Int J Med Inform 87:54–67
111. Wittenberg-Lyles E, Oliver DP, Demiris G, Swarz J, Rendo M (2014) YouTube as a tool for pain management with informal caregivers of cancer patients: a systematic review. J Pain Symptom Manag 48(6):1200–1210
112. Bee PE, Barnes P, Luker KA (2009) A systematic review of informal caregivers' needs in providing home-based end-of-life care to people with cancer. J Clin Nurs 18(10):1379–1393
113. Kim Y, Schulz R (2008) Family caregivers' strains: comparative analysis of cancer caregiving with dementia, diabetes, and frail elderly caregiving. J Aging Health 20(5):483–503

114. Ochoa CY, Lunsford NB, Smith JL (2020) Impact of informal cancer caregiving across the cancer experience: a systematic literature review of quality of life. Palliat Support Care 18(2):220–240

115. Thana K, Lehto R, Sikorskii A, Wyatt G (2021) Informal caregiver burden for solid tumour cancer patients: a review and future directions. Psychol Health 36(12):1514–1535

116. MacLeod S (2021) The growing burden of informal caregivers during COVID-19. Innov Aging 5(Suppl 1):962–963

117. Balmuth A (2021) Caregiving through the pandemic: exploring the impacts of COVID-19 on caregivers and their caregiving experiences. Innov Aging 5(Suppl 1):185

118. Marnfeldt K, Estenson L, Rowan J, Wilber K (2021) Caregiving and COVID-19: perspectives from a care coach. Innov Aging 5(Suppl 1):937

119. Thiessen M, Soriano AM, Loewen HJ, Decker KM (2020) Impact of telemedicine use by oncology physicians on the patient and informal caregiver experience of receiving care: protocol for a scoping review in the context of COVID-19. JMIR Res Protoc 9(12):e25501

120. Greaney ML, Kunicki ZJ, Drohan MM, Nash CC, Cohen SA (2022) Sleep quality among informal caregivers during the COVID-19 pandemic: a cross-sectional study. Gerontol Geriatr Med 8:10

Caregiving Within the Context of Elder Care

Deborah Boyle

1   Introduction

Societal aging is a global phenomenon. It refers to the proportion of older people (age 65 or above) relative to the rest of the population. Worldwide, an estimated 703 million persons are age 65 or older [1]. By 2050, this number will total over 1.6 billion people, with 1.3 billion (75%) residing in developing regions [2, 3]. The twenty-first century has the unique distinction of being the first era when older adults outnumber children [4–6].

There are several origins of this aging evolution. First is the significant escalation in life expectancy, second is the aging of the "baby boomer" generation, and third is the increase in the world's older populace, commonly referred to as the "Silver Tsunami."

2   Origins of Global Aging

2.1   Extension of Life Expectancy

Since the mid-twentieth century, longevity projections have doubled in most developed nations [7]. Currently, 34 countries have life expectancies over age 80 years (Table 1). The ability to live longer is associated with enhancements in three major areas:

1. Socioeconomic development (i.e., quality of water and food supply, improved hygiene, housing expansion, enculturation of safety prototypes)

D. Boyle (✉)
Clinical Nurse Specialist/Oncology and Geriatrics, Advanced Oncology Nursing Resources, Phoenix, AZ, USA

Table 1 Top country rankings with the highest life expectancy[a] (>age 80)

Rank	Country	Life expectancy (both sexes)
1	Hong Kong	85.29
2	Japan	85.03
3	Macao	84.68
4	Switzerland	84.25
5	Singapore	84.07
6	Italy	84.01
7	Spain	83.99
8	Australia	83.94
9	Channel Islands	83.60
10	Iceland	83.52
11	South Korea	83.50
12	Israel	83.49
13	Sweden	83.33
14	France	83.13
	Martinique	
15	Malta	83.06
16	Canada	82.96
17	Norway	82.94
18	Ireland	82.81
19	New Zealand	82.80
	Greece	
20	Netherlands	82.78
21	Guadeloupe	82.74
22	Portugal	82.65
23	Finland	82.48
24	Belgium	82.17
25	Austria	82.05
26	Germany	81.88
27	Slovenia	81.85
28	United Kingdom	81.77
29	Cyprus	81.51
30	Denmark	81.40
31	US Virgin Isles	81.17
32	Taiwan	81.04

Source: worldometers.info.demographics/life-expectancy/# counttries-ranked-bylife-expectancy; retrieved 1/20/2022
[a]Of note are life expectancies in the world's largest countries: Russia 72 years, China 77 years, US 79 years

2. Advent of public health initiatives (i.e., illness screening potential, vaccination availability, improved sanitation, expanded community-based health education, and outreach to rural settings)
3. Growing sophistication of medical expertise; examples of which includes:
   - *Scientific discoveries in drug development* (i.e., antibiotics, pharmacotherapies to manage chronic illness, supportive care medications)

- *Technological innovation* (i.e., radiological capacity and availability, critical care monitoring)
- *Evolution of medical sub-specialization expertise* (i.e., condition or illness-specific knowledge for a select patient population)

Yet, while these considerable improvements have positively influenced the likelihood of living longer, they have also elicited a global burden of late-life disease, which most healthcare systems have not anticipated nor prepared for [4, 7–9]. Aging is challenging the maintenance and viability of existing health systems, particularly in developed countries [10].

2.2   The "Baby Boomer" Generation

The cohort of those born between 1946 and 1964 are referred to as "baby boomers" [11]. They characterize the outcome of the significant birthrate escalation following the end of World War II. Baby boomers represent the largest developmental subset in many developed nations. Their aging has significant implications for healthcare service utilization in later life and caregiving requirements associated with age-related dependency. The year 2011 was a key milestone in the genesis of the baby boomers as this marked the first year that the initial cohort (born in 1946) reached age 65 and officially became older adults. Their full transition into old age will culminate in 2029 when all the baby boomers will be elderly (between the ages of 65 and 83 years).

2.3   The "Silver Tsunami"

The worldwide escalation of older adults within population demographics has been termed the "Silver Tsunami" [8, 12, 13]. Table 2 depicts this global growth. Asia and Europe are home to the world's largest elderly populations. Countries with the highest percentage (at least one in five) of older adults are listed in Table 3. Southern Europe represents the oldest region in the world with an average of 21% of the population being elderly. Six countries have both large percentages of elderly and extended life expectancies, namely, Japan (85 years), Italy (84 years), Croatia, Portugal and Greece (each with 83 years), and Finland (82 years) (www.prb.org/resources/countries-with-the-oldest-populations-in-the-word). As a result, many European countries are facing serious limitations within their national public health welfare systems. Of note is that this current dilemma precedes the full contingent of baby boomers reaching old age.

A declining global birthrate has also influenced the predominance of the elder majority [20]. This has resulted in an altered dependency ratio, namely, a disproportionate number of older adults requiring care, in tandem with a reduction in the availability of lay family caregivers to render needed care [2, 19, 21, 22]. Additionally, the presence of home-based female caregivers has declined mostly

Table 2 General global implications of the 'Silver Tsunami'

Country/region	Current and future projections
Asia	• Among developing countries, China is the fastest growing aging country where the older population will account for 25% of the country's population by 2050 • 70–85% of those aged 60 or older live with their children • Within southeast Asia in particular, a faster rate of aging is occurring compared to other regions
Europe	• Europe is aging faster than any other region in the world and will remain the oldest global site for the remainder of the twenty-first century • 25% (one in four) of the collective population is over age 60 years, and this population will reach 35% by 2050 • 35–40% of elders who reside in Sweden, the United Kingdom, Finland, and Denmark live alone • Over 82 million people of migrant origin live in European countries of which 14.4% are older than age 65; these numbers are expected to increase in the coming decades
United States	• Between 2015 and 2030, the US population aged 65 and older will escalate by 55% with 10,000 individuals turning 65 years old daily
Combined metrics	• By 2030, the elderly in Asia, Latin America, and the Caribbean will double

Source: [14–19]; DesRoches, Chang, Kim, Mukunda, Norman, Dittus, Donelan (2022); Monsees J, Schmachtenberg T & Thyrian J (2022); Zubiashvili & Zubiashvili, 2021; Bachman; Sambasivam, R, Liu J, Vaingankar et al. (2019); Jakovljevic; Marois

Table 3 Countries with the largest % older adults

Country	% Elderly
Japan	28.2
Italy	22.8
Finland	21.9
Portugal	21.8
Greece	
Germany	21.4
Bulgaria	21.3
Croatia	20.4
France	20.3
Latvia	
Serbia	20.2

Source: United Nations; Population Division, World Population Prospects, 2019; https://population.un.org/wpp/download/standard/population

due to the increased integration of women into the workplace. High rates of divorce and greater geographic relocation of adult children also have limited on-site caregiver availability and heightened numbers of elders potentially requiring care (i.e., step-parents, step-grandparents).

3   Prominent Themes in Elder Caregiving

In 1990, the term "informal caregiver" first appeared in the literature [23]. The role characterized the provision of free, home-based support by a lay family member or friend [24]. In the United States, it paralleled the increasing exodus of healthcare delivery rendered outside of the acute care setting. Unfortunately, an absence of an equivocal transition of healthcare professionals to ambulatory and home settings did not occur. Thus, this gap was filled by unprofessional, untrained family caregivers.

Globally, the largest cohort of informal caregivers are older adults. The ill family member's condition largely dictates caregiving responsibilities. However, there are additional considerations that influence caregiving capacity. These include the phenomena of caregiver burden, the prominence of co-morbidity, problems navigating the healthcare system, and the presence of ageism.

3.1   Caregiver Burden

Research into the nature of older adults rendering care to an older spouse, sibling, or adult child has depicted generally negative consequences. Examples of such include the prominence of poor sleep, increased fatigue, inadequate diet, absence of self-care, and overall declining physical and mental health [25]. The concept of caregiver burden has been conceptualized as the extent to which caregivers perceive their assistance has had an adverse effect on their emotional, social, financial, physical, and spiritual functioning [26]. Given and Given [27] characterized it as an imbalance between demands (objective and subjective) and caregiver coping resources.

Globally, geography and socioeconomic status best correlate with the provision and availability of caregiver support to counter burden. In developing nations, the expectation to care for an ill loved one usually remains with the family unit, often with little or no assistance from government or other external agencies. Service procurement within developed countries (i.e., European nations, Canada, Australia) vary greatly. Even with support availability, it may be episodic, time-limited, and problem-focused (vs comprehensive) and may engender added cost. In this regard, two extremes typify the varied nature of caregiving assistance across countries.

The US healthcare system has the least consistency of service options. Cost and availability are largely dependent on health insurance type, employment type and status, and geographic residency. Shift-specific and around-the-clock support at home are always an out-of-pocket expense. Long-term care requires added insurance supplements, and that which is provided via federal subsidy (i.e., Medicaid) is continually scrutinized for need justification. On the other hand, municipalities in Sweden are required by law to render needed healthcare services in the home setting for their residents [28].

Whether with or without the provision of external aide, the overall orchestration of care remains with the primary caregiver. This course of action involves scheduling appointments, managing transportation needs, navigating the healthcare system, managing finances, and acting as an intermediary [29]. Van Houten and colleagues [30] enumerated varied caregiver overarching roles of manager and gatekeeper as well as direct care provider, which all require knowledge, organizational, tactical, and recruiting skills on behalf of the ill family member. Other categories of expected caregiver competencies are depicted in Table 4. The number of tasks, their complexity, and the time required to plan and perform them directly correlate with caregiver

Table 4 Multidimensional components of care mastery expected of informal cancer caregivers

Care coordination	*Informational*
• Schedule medical care appointments • Accompany and navigate the healthcare system: parking, waiting, accessing wheelchair • Understand varied roles of providers (i.e., who to ask for what) • Coordinate visitation • Shop for and order supplies, medications, equipment • Mobilize resources • Determine delegation of tasks (i.e., which and to who) • Anticipate and troubleshoot gaps in care • Plan transition to new care sites	• Prepare questions relative to appropriate care provider • Chronicle progress to providers • Liaison with professional network to determine next steps • Manage information exchange • Participate in problem-solving and decision-making • Provide medical updates about patient status to social and employment network • Liaison with family network to inform nature of patient status • Explain rational for treatment decisions to family members
Psychosocial	*Functional*
• Respond to negative emotions • Provide encouragement to patient • Offer reassurance to family • Plan opportunities for socializing • Manage personal emotions • Manage frustration related to system fragmentation • Contain anxiety about the unknown • Assume responsibility for self-care	• Assist with ADLs, IADLs • Assume responsibilities for doing or delegating domestic tasks (i.e., meal shopping and preparation, cleaning, home upkeep) • Assist with adherence to care recommendations (i.e., exercise) • Troubleshoot medical equipment malfunction • Arrange or provide for transportation
Nursing care	*Pharmaceutical*
• Assist with toileting, mobility • Monitor weight loss, sleep, pain, mood, fatigue, and other symptoms • Assess intensity and pattern of toxicity • Manage symptom distress • Advocate for medication titration • Describe the nature of potentially emergent symptoms and scenarios • Modify patient care based on condition changes • Perform drain, port, wound care, and dressing changes • Determine environmental safety • Advocate on patient's behalf • Assess nature of patient and family coping • Make referrals when indicated • Ensure advance care planning paperwork is available	• Oversee drug utilization • Organize, supervise, request refill orders • Ensure dose/schedule accuracy • Fill pill reminder devices • Monitor level of adherence • Consider strategies to improve adherence • Monitor symptoms associated with new medication • Respond to and/or research suggestions advocating use of complementary substances
	Financial
	• Maintain/file of medical paperwork • Oversee bill payment • Lobby with insurers • Track paperwork documenting discrepancies or problems • Establish location of will

stress. This influences the perception of burden which directly correlates with the degree of caregiver well-being. While each caregiver has their own threshold of what can be accommodated, generally, the higher the number of responsibilities, the more difficult they are, and the amount of time required to complete them influences the magnitude of caregiver distress.

Of critical importance is the fact that lay family caregivers, usually with no background in a medical field, are expected to assume numerous caregiving duties, which are often complex and multifaceted and must be learned quickly [21, 31]. These expectations are proxy professional duties that nurses, physical therapists, physicians, pharmacists, dieticians, and social workers enact that require years of study to master [32].

Foundational to the experience of burden is the critical absence of caregiver education [33]. This lack of preparatory training engenders anxiety about the caregiver's assumption of new responsibilities, especially those customarily performed by professional healthcare providers [32, 34, 35]. Caregivers are expected to be overnight "pseudo clinicians" and "learn on the job." In tandem with this is the absence of ongoing support by the healthcare team to assist with problem-solving and offer counsel over time. If the ill person's needs are complex and extensive and when considerable caregiver strain is likely (such as in the case of end-of-life care), this gap in professional service availability becomes particularly relevant [36, 37]. As a result, caregiver worry, fear, and feelings of alienation and abandonment prevail and are likely intensified by the uncertainty, unpredictability, and uncontrollability of the care situation [38, 39].

The magnitude of caregiving competency expected of lay family members is greatly underappreciated by healthcare professionals. An excellent example of this relates to medication management, which is a care expectation that many lay caregivers worry most about. Table 5 delineates numerous components of proficiency required to assist the patient with drug administration and adherence.

3.2   Co-morbidity

The traditional medical care model has focused on the treatment of one disease [42]. This orientation is not appropriate within the context of aged care due to the common prominence of multiple chronic illnesses co-occurring. This condition is referred to as co-morbidity and most distinguishes the elderly from the young.

Common co-morbid illnesses include ischemic heart disease, hypertension, hyperlipidemia, diabetes, and arthritis [43, 44]. The likelihood of having two or three concomitant diagnoses increases with age and a history of negative lifestyle behaviors (i.e., smoking, obesity). In the United States, nearly 70% of Medicare beneficiaries have two or more chronic illnesses [45]. Hence, with increasing longevity comes the potential for living years with disability.

Associated with co-morbidity is the corollary of polypharmacy, which refers the prescription of five or more drugs for routine use. Generally, one to two medications are ordered per illness; hence, polypharmacy is common in older adults with

Table 5 Expected elements of medication management by informal family caregivers

Need	Specific indication
Administering	• Assist with device use when needed • Perform injections (i.e., anticoagulants, growth factors, sub-cutaneous pain medications)
Communicating	• Interface with provider and pharmacy to ensure correct medication and dosage • Follow-up with PCP, pharma with questions and/or delay issues • Provide information for pharma assistance with medication purchase • Document dosing • Relay perceptions with PCP about adherence issues • Reiterate/lobby/persuade drug need with patient • Lobby for drug change with data
Handling	• Cut tablets • Check/assess consumption (by route) • Ensure proper use of waste containment (when indicated)
Organizing	• Pill box (or related device) ongoing/repeated nature • Documentation log to track use
Procuring	• Order and oversee medication availability in home • Pick up medications • Purchase supplies (pill box or system), gloves, alcohol wipes, bandaids, miscellaneous devices (inhaler, nasal spray, BP machine, diabetic testing strips, anticoagulant monitoring); special waste receptacle (antineoplastics)
Understanding	• Gather information (nature of toxicity) • Evaluate response • Make dose/schedule adjustments for PRN dosing • Correlate toxicity with potential drug source

Sources: [40, 41]

multiple chronic conditions [46]. Concerns when this prevails are increased toxicity due to age-related changes in pharmacokinetics and pharmacodynamics, which alter drug metabolism. Drug-drug interactions may occur. Non-adherence, falls, and acute confusion are also likely but are potentially avoidable.

When multiple healthcare providers focus singularly on one ailment, often a coordinated effort to oversee drug therapies does not occur. For older adults under the care of three or more providers, patients may be prescribed more than a dozen medications routinely usually with some type of negative sequelae occurring. The SHARE (Survey of Health, Aging and Retirement in Europe) database has been used to determine the prevalence of polypharmacy in 17 European countries [47]. This research revealed that Switzerland, Croatia, and Slovenia had the lowest rate of polypharmacy (i.e., 25.0–27.4%), while Portugal, Israel, and the Czech Republic had the highest (37.5–39.9%). De-prescribing, or the purposeful discontinuation of unnecessary drugs or those with toxicity potential, is a contemporary approach to medication reconciliation that can reduce the negative sequelae of multiple drug therapy prescribing.

While considering the challenges co-morbidity poses for patients, the older caregivers' health status must also be taken into account as they too may have multiple illnesses requiring ongoing management. The combined implications of dual caregiving (for spouse and self) may be overwhelming for the elder caregiver. In these instances, the caregiver often prioritizes the needs of their ill family member and neglects their own health. Thus, elder caregiving may occur at the expense of their own physical and emotional health, which in turn can also impact the quality of caregiving [48]. Hence, the caregiver may be an "invisible" or "hidden" patient. When this occurs, the dyad, not just the patient, becomes in need of professional care [49–52]. Further investigation is needed into concerns about heightened mortality rates in older caregivers due to these dual demands of caregiving [53, 54].

3.3   Problematic Healthcare Navigation

Whether it be the office, clinic, hospital, or care home, healthcare environments represent foreign domiciles to older adults. These locations are generally associated with illness, bad news, pain, suffering, and the unknown. Thus, anxiety often prevails when older adults enter these care settings.

The presence of age-related neurosensory alterations can compromise sight, hearing, memory, and gait and thus require accommodation in new environments. Also, visits are traditionally short, not allowing for discussion and questions. This is particularly important as information often requires reiteration due to hearing and sight impairment. Hence, acknowledging signage, reading consents, hearing instructions (and remembering them), and making adjustments to small, cluttered spaces present a plethora of navigation obstacles for many older adults within healthcare settings.[1]

3.4   Ageism

Most Asian and indigenous cultures revere their elders and respect them for their wisdom emanating from life experiences [55, 56]. Many older matriarchs and patriarchs serve critical roles as decision-makers within their family constellation. Filial piety, the duty and responsibility for adult children to care for aged parents, is embedded in many of these customs [57]. Being disrespectful, perceiving older family members as burdens, and undermining or dismissing elders needs are never tolerated. Yet, in other parts of the world, these negative attitudes and behaviors are the norm.

Ageism refers to prejudice against people of older age. Similar to racial, gender, and ethnic discrimination, it is based on negative stereotypes that marginalize and oppress [58]. Contemporary ageism prevails in a world that idealizes youth over old

---

[1] Traversing these settings has been recognized as so stressful for older adults that some elder-centric hospitals employ valets to help with reading signage, using stairs and elevators, locating designated areas within the hospital, and even having font size enlarged on patient education materials so it can be read without the use of a magnifying glass. These are examples of age-friendly environments especially designed with older adults needs prioritized.

age. It transcends the boundaries of the healthcare environment where inequities can be manifested and takes many forms. Ageism creates assumptions that all older adults are homogeneous, namely, frail, dependent, cognitively impaired, asexual, and intolerant of treatment, and are uninterested in wellness [59, 60]. A major example of ageism in clinical practice is the absence of differentiating subsets of older adults.

In health care, all older adults over age 65 are assumed to be the same. Yet, with increasing age, there is a biophysiological decline that differentiates a 65 years old from an 85 years old. Changes based on progressing age influence clinical assessment, treatment decision-making, and psychosocial adjustment. This is comparable to how children are appraised by developmental subset. To that end, geriatric specialists recommend utilizing comparable age-specific subsets of older adults. This representation commonly distinguishes "young-old," as being age 65–75 years; "middle-old," as being age 75–84 years; "old-old," as being age 85 years and above; and "elite old," being age 100 and over [61].

3.4.1 Choosing Geriatrics as a Specialty

There is a critical component of ageism that has global implications for the future of health care. Despite forecasts warning that a heightened demand for a workforce focusing on the needs of older adults is required, this has not resulted in an expanding cohort of students and clinicians entering the field of gerontology [8, 14].

Numerous etiologies of this dilemma include the presence of ageism, which likens care of older adults as less exciting and research-driven than other high-tech specialties. The absence of required education in gerontology within professional training curricula diminishes aged care's importance as compared to other specialty foci. The predominance and challenges of ethical concerns embedded in clinical practice may also be a factor [62]. Finally, difficult work conditions, inadequate pay, and lack of social recognition of geriatric health specialists also contribute to the lack of appeal as a career choice [9].

Now and in the immediate future, there is a pressing disconnect between demand and availability of a geriatrically trained healthcare workforce [63]. Building specialty labor capacity requires the support of many stakeholders and necessitates considerable educational effort to heighten awareness [64]. Thus, there is a pressing need to expose the reality of ageism's prominence throughout all of health care before elder-sensitive positive change can occur.

4   Major Illnesses in the Elderly

Advanced age is a well-known risk factor for cancer, dementia, heart failure, and stroke. The caregiving expectations associated with these four illnesses relate to the disease itself, the acute or chronic nature of the condition, the point in time which it occurs across the disease continuum, and the type(s) of treatment employed. To elucidate family caregiving requirements, select characteristics of each illness are highlighted.

4.1   Cancer

Cancer is responsible for an overwhelming disease burden globally. Consider the following:

- Between 2006 and 2016, worldwide cancer incidence increased by 28%.
- Currently, one in five men and one in six women will develop cancer in their lifetimes; one in eight men and one in 11 women will die from it.
- Contemporary death rates in men are 43% higher than in women.
- Half of all new cases and more than half of cancer deaths occur in Asia in part due to the continent's home to nearly 60% of the world's populations.
- By 2040:
  - Global cancer incidence will exceed 27 million new cancer cases.
    While an estimated increase in cancer incidence will occur in all countries, there will be proportionately greatest increase in low- and middle-income countries.[2]
  - Cancer will increase by 21% in Europe [65–69].

These societal trends are expected to continue due in large part to increases in life expectancy.

4.1.1   Distinguishing Characteristics

Cancer is a unique illness in that it encompasses over 100 subtypes, each characterized by its tissue of origin, pathological features, illness trajectory, treatment options, and prognostic indicators. Yet despite these distinctions, malignancies share the common feature of an overproduction of abnormal cells, with no purpose other than to usurp nutrients from normal structures and interfere with customary bodily function. Ultimately, the cancer cells' viability is maintained to the detriment of normal tissue.

Cancer is a disease of aging. Nearly two-thirds of all cancer diagnoses occur in adults over age 65 years and one's risk for developing cancer increases with age [70]. The most frequent cancers globally vary depending upon the region's economic development status and associated socio-behavioral norms [71]. However, four malignancies—breast, prostate, lung, and colorectal—make up nearly one-half of all cancer incidence worldwide, and these cancers occur predominantly in the elderly [72, 73].

---

[2] The World Bank classifies global economies into four groups based on gross national income per capita: high income (>$12,695.00; exs = Australia, Canada, Finland, Germany, United States), upper middle income ($4096.00–12,695.00; exs = Angola, Brazil, China, Libya, South Africa), lower middle income ($1046–$4.095; exs. = Congo, Egypt, India, Nigeria, Sudan), and low income (<$1046; exs. = Afghanistan, Ethiopia, Honduras, Nepal, Uganda)
   Source: https://www.worldbank.org; www.blogs.worldbank.org

4.1.2   Themes in Elder Cancer Caregiving

There are two prevalent content domains in cancer caregiver coping that require elucidation. They include reactions to the most universally feared illness and engaging in complex caregiving.

Fear

While contemporary advances in early detection and treatment have resulted in significant improvements for numerous malignancies, cancer remains the most feared illness globally. The common perception of cancer as an automatic death sentence is foundational to understanding family caregiving. Anticipating a premature death prompts ongoing, and at times unrelenting, anxiety that interferes with the patient/ family dyads' ability to comprehend and adjust to the many new demands imposed upon the family unit. Contributing to this fear is the common occurrence of toxicity related to therapeutic interventions. When caregivers observe their loved one struggling to manage multiple side effects, they often feel helpless to reduce what they consider to be "suffering."

Also, there is lack of understanding about the heterogeneity of cancer. Not all cancer diagnoses are alike. Cancer is an umbrella term with many subtypes, each having caregiving responsibilities highly dependent on the type of malignancy, the treatment employed, and stage of disease. Thus, expectations to care for an elderly spouse with advanced prostate cancer with bone metastases are very different than those required by an elderly widower upon hospital discharge with newly diagnosed acute myeloid leukemia. This fact needs to be emphasized as many caregivers have expectations based on hearsay, conjecture, and past experience that influence their coping. Educating the caregiver about the unique aspects of the malignancy can reduce emotional distress through the provision of accurate information and negate the worry associated with false assumptions.

New Caregiving Expectations

Older informal caregivers often find themselves assuming and balancing a plethora of new roles [2]. These responsibilities may occur overnight and without notice [32, 74]. In instances where long-term marriage or partnership is the norm, it is difficult to assume new responsibilities when roles have been enacted over decades. Additionally, patient needs often fluctuate across the cancer continuum necessitating caregivers to be in a perpetual learning mode. Given and Given [27] identified three timeframes when caregiver involvement is most intense: during active cancer treatment, the first 2 years following diagnosis, and during end-of-life care. These points in caregiving require different skill sets and thus competency enhancements.

Stress may also stem from financial concerns. When living on a fixed income, the presence of added cancer-related expenses can strain a relationship. The number of hours of caregiving required and the degree of lifestyle disruption that ensues are other important parameters of stress. The majority of older cancer caregivers render support to their spouse/partner for an average of 40 h per week [75]. In addition to worry about financial insecurity, the cumulative outcomes of ongoing stress may include a reduction in quality of life, an increase in depression, and incidence of new health issues, even early death in lay caregivers [29, 33].

4.2 Dementia

Dementia is one of the greatest healthcare challenges of the twenty-first century [76]. Globally, more than 50 million people are living with dementia, and this estimate is expected to triple, reaching 152 million by 2050 [77]. Additionally, in the past two decades, dementia-related deaths have increased by more than 145% [78]. Pervasive stigma about the disease prevails due to a global lack of understanding and its association with mental health challenges [79]. Limited resources to diagnose and manage dementia, a low level of awareness of the disease, and an absence of supportive health services position low- and middle-income countries (LMIC) to struggle most with the provision of dementia care [80–82].

Dementia is an age-related neurodegenerative illness characterized by an insidious downward trajectory of progressive deterioration often evolving over a decade [83, 84]. Existing therapies attempt to alter dementia's course and manage disease-related neuropsychiatric symptoms (NPS) [76]. However, it remains an irreversible, terminal illness with no cure. Alzheimer's disease is the most common cause of dementia and is staged using mild, moderate, and advanced severity ratings.

4.2.1 Caregiver Characteristics

Dementia is a family illness that affects the well-being of all its members [80]. The initial diagnosis confirms their official transition into a caregiving mode, which impacts interpersonal dynamics [85]. Dementia is often depicted as the most burdensome disease for caregivers, two-thirds of which are women and one-third are over age 65 [78, 79]. In the United States alone, this represents 15.3 billion hours of unpaid help annually, an average of 26.3 h of caregiver care rendered per week.

Caregiving requirements directly relate to the stage of the patient's dementia. Table 6 outlines patient characteristics within distinct disease phases and their associated caregiving implications. As the disease progresses, caregiver

Table 6 Dementia stage and related caregiving corollaries

Stage	Patient characteristics	Caregiver implications
Early	Few visible symptoms of dementia; cognitive testing confirms evidence of neurological change	Minimal assistance required with basic activities of daily living (i.e., bathing, toileting); proactive decision-making regarding advance care planning is in order before cognitive decline evolves
Middle	Assistance required with instrumental activities of daily living (i.e., finances, housekeeping, food preparation, phone); occurrence of neuropsychiatric symptoms evolves (i.e., agitation, wandering, repetition)	Increasing need for caregiver interface begins; supportive services and help from secondary family and friends of benefit; family caregivers aided by professional support to help manage NPSs nonpharmacologically
Late	Escalating care demands may require relocation to alternative care setting; drastic compromise in ability to communicate	Guilt and depression related to placement need; palliative care predominates

Sources: [85, 86]

interventions evolve from oversight and assistance, to the provision of basic daily care [87]. It is not unusual for "hands-on" caregiving to extend for years without a break, pay, vacation, recognition, help, or periodic backup. In addition to stage-associated factors affecting caregiving burden, other variables such as the patient's level of cognitive function, hours of direct caregiving required, evidence of financial difficulties, and caregiver health status impact caregiving capability [81].

4.2.2 Emotional Sequelae

The changing nature of the patient/caregiver dyad relationship is a major source of caregiver distress, which often evolves in tandem with disease progression [83, 88]. The presence and severity of NPS (i.e., agitation, aggression, disinhibition, delusions, hallucinations, irritability, apathy, aberrant motor behavior) develop from ongoing brain degeneration. They often present as symptom clusters rather than single entities [89]. Caregiver distress is frequently associated with misunderstanding about the nature of NPS, in particular, failing to recognize that these problem behaviors are not under the patient's control. Additionally, caregivers feel ill-equipped with the necessary knowledge and skill to respond to a loved ones changing communication abilities and needs [90]. The presence of NPS is more associated with caregiver depression than the degree of the patient's cognitive impairment [87, 91]. Of note is that depression occurs in at least one in three female dementia caregivers [79, 85, 87, 92]. Other negative caregiver sequelae are reports of high anxiety, worse subjective well-being and physical health as compared to controls, and a prevailing sense of loneliness [84, 93, 94].

The most pressing needs of caregivers have been identified as their well-being and learning how to cope with difficult feelings and emotions [95]. Caregivers often report feeling ignored, undervalued, and reaching a "tipping point" when their loved one's care is less than ideal [52, 96]. Service fragmentation results in poor coordination of services, interagency communication, and information sharing [97]. A lack of proactive care planning can result in emergent scenarios where caregivers must make decisions without professional decision support. Discussions about admission to a residential care facility are particularly problematic [98]. They represent changes in the patient's condition indicative of worsening disease. Re-surfacing of guilt is a common corollary related to the caregivers' inability to keep the patient in the home setting. Of note is that caregivers have reported less burdensome emotional distress and fewer depressive symptoms when the presence of a secondary supportive relative or friend is available [83].

Ambiguous loss is a term typifying a unique corollary of grief that has been applied to dementia caregivers' experiences. It portrays chronic sadness associated with the duality of being simultaneously absent and present [99]. The loved one with dementia remains physically present, but their persona has been lost to their illness. This coexistence complicates the grieving process. Because death has not occurred, there is no enactment of mourning rituals, and the caregiver's bereavement is deprived.

4.3   Heart Failure

Heart failure is both a progressive and symptom-intensive illness characterized by diminished quality of life for both caregivers and patients. A disease of aging more commonly diagnosed in socioeconomically deprived regions, heart failure, affects more than 40 million people worldwide [100–102]. Currently, 15 million Europeans and seven million Americans (the majority of which are over age 70 years) live with the debility secondary to reduced cardiac function [103–105]. In the United States, deaths from heart failure have recently increased by 5% representing its most significant escalation since 2012 [106]. By 2035, incidence is expected to rise by 40% [107, 108].

4.3.1   The Female Caregiver Imperative

The physiological burden imposed by heart failure is often multifocal and includes dyspnea, fatigue, pedal edema, chest pain, insomnia, and depression, which impacts family life [109, 110]. The common presence of co-morbidity adds to symptom distress and the complexity of heart failure management (Fig. 1). This cumulative effect of debility results in dependency on caregivers to assist with many activities of daily living.

Since heart failure predominates in men, women are frequently the primary informal caregiver. They assist with personal care needs, plan, and oversee meals (including preparation, managing diet and fluid restrictions), orchestrate transportation, offer emotional support, manage medications, advocate on behalf of the patient, and navigate the complex healthcare system [89, 111, 112]. As a result of these added demands on time and labor, caregivers often report feelings of social

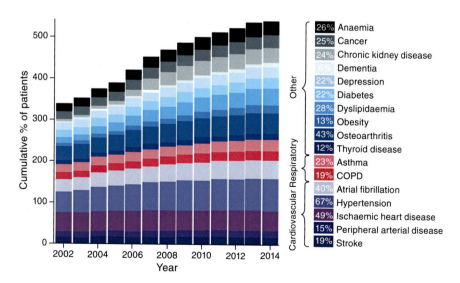

Fig. 1 Individual co-morbidities among patients diagnosed with incident heart failure from 2002 to 2014. Source: [102], with permission

isolation, experiencing identity loss, changes in work performance, financial strain, anxiety, depression, fatigue, sleep disruption, hypervigilance, and neglect of their personal healthcare needs [112, 113].

4.3.2 Demands Over Time

The protracted nature of the heart failure trajectory is characterized by worsening symptom distress and an increase in care needs (Fig. 2). Frequent exacerbations result in emergency department visits and hospitalizations [105]. These status fluctuations between illness stability and instability make the disease course unpredictable and highly stressful.

Patients have identified that medication oversight and engaging in self-care are emotionally challenging [110]. Both of these entities are cornerstones of heart failure management [114]. While the patient is expected to assume primary accountability for these entities, many caregivers assume supervisory roles. Medication adherence, diet, exercise, weight scrutiny, and abstinence from smoking may be monitored by the caregiver and result in strain when self-care practices are less than ideal. Other sources of distress occur when the patient minimizes their symptoms to their provider or appear passive about needs to make lifestyle adaptations to avoid further decline [115, 116]. Of recent note were two interesting findings relative to heart failure caregiver support needs.

First was the revelation that greater use of hospital services was an independent predictor of worsening quality of life in heart failure caregivers [117]. This likely was associated with hospital admission being proxy for a deteriorating health status and an increased need for the caregiver to intervene in their loved one's care. Second was the finding that while the patient/caregiver dyad appeared to understand general

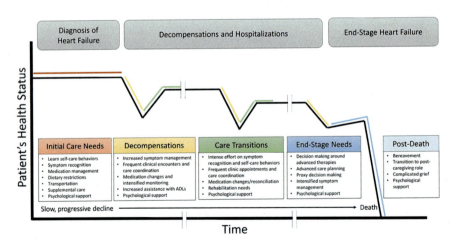

Care Needs Based on Phases of Illness

Fig. 2 Source: [112], with permission

principles of heart failure's management, they were unable to make the association between the progressing nature of the illness with a closer proximity to the end of life [118]. Of note is the increasing introduction of palliative care services within the context of early heart failure management due to the prominence of symptom distress, progressive debility, dyadic coping challenges, and impaired quality of life over time [119]. Assisting with advance care planning is also a benefit of palliative care's collaboration.

4.4   Stroke

Stroke is one of the most debilitating neurological conditions responsible for acute and chronic incapacity globally. Consider the following:
Worldwide

- Stroke is the
  - Main cause of neurologic disability
  - Third leading cause of death
- 15 million people who experience a stroke annually account for 116 million days of health life lost.
- One in three will die following a stroke; 10% will die within 30 days.
- By 90 days post-stroke, new disability of at least moderate severity develops in one-third of adults > age 65 years [120–124].

In the European Union

- Stroke
  - Is the second most common cause of death.
  - Affects 1.1 million people annually.
  - In 2019, 17.1 million people were living with a history of stroke across the 57 EU countries[3] [3, 125, 126].

Despite these grim statistics, it is important to acknowledge that 90% of stroke risk is accounted for by modifiable risk factors (i.e., smoking/tobacco use, sedentary behaviors, obesity, substandard diet, hyperlipidemia, hypertension, diabetes) [127, 128].

---

[3] In reviewing change in countries causes of death attributed to stroke over the past two decades, the majority experienced an increase in death rates of <10%. However, South Korea (22%) and Albania (22%) had an >20% increase in male deaths. For females, seven countries experienced >20% increase: South Korea (29%), Japan (26%), Macedonia (24%), Portugal (22%), Bosnia & Herzegovina (22%), Montenegro (22%), Taiwan (21%) (Cheng).

Following a stroke, patients rely significantly on family caregiver support. The majority of stroke survivors are discharged home under the supervision of their families [129, 130]. Care requirements are most intense within the first 6 months post-stroke and are compounded by the presence of co-morbidity. Both the patient and caregiver often co-manage these post-stroke sequelae (Table 7).

Patient deficits can include losses in cognition (altered memory and concentration), motor deficits limiting physical mobility, visual impairment, headaches, loss of bodily coordination (i.e., incontinence, sexual dysfunction), and speech and language aphasia [131]. Personality changes can include emotional lability and anger [132]. Depression is highly prevalent and can prevail for years. Recovery can take years to achieve maximal return to function and often involves a long course of transition and adaptation for both the patient and their caregiver [80, 133].

Complications during recovery include bone fractures, cognitive impairment, contractures, falling, fatigue, hemiplegic shoulder pain, osteoporosis, pressure ulcers, seizures, spasticity, and thromboembolism. Transitions in care such as from the home to hospital, hospital to admission to the acute rehabilitation setting, and returning home following in-patient rehabilitation with new functional deficits are transition triggers for stressors for both the patient and family caregivers. Table 8

Table 7 Post-stroke sequelae requiring dyad co-management

Behaviors
• 84% of patients struggle to maintain smoking abstinence
• Only 17% of patients achieve healthy weight status
• Less than half of patients exercise according to recommendations
Co-morbidity
• 50–80% of patients have hypertension
• 20–30% of patients have diabetes
• Depression prevails in up to 25% of patients 2 years post stroke
• Other common illnesses
– Anxiety
– Arthritis
– Pulmonary disease
– Renal disease
Home-based care
• Hospital re-admission most common within 30 days post-stroke
• Issues remaining prevalent
– Communication
– Mobility
– Pain control
Medications
• Non-adherence
• First year post-stroke, 97% of patients remain on anti-coagulants
Source: [5]

delineates examples of the range of ongoing sequelae that require the dyad's co-management to maximize recovery.

Since stroke is primarily a male illness, female caregiver burden predominates and is multidimensional in nature. Adversity resulting from caregiving has physical, financial, social, and psychological consequences [134]. In a qualitative investigation of interpersonal relationship challenges among stroke survivors and their family caregivers, McCarthy and colleagues [132] identified seven themes that predominated (Table 9).

Home-based around-the-clock caregiving can increase social isolation and relationship changes (i.e., marital and others) and reduce quality of life (i.e., poor sleep, depression, new evidence of back pain). Supporting a depressed spouse over time can be one of the most challenging aspects of caregiving and can ultimately be associated with the onset of caregiver depression [135]. For older female caregivers, patient support needs that require considerable strength and agility (i.e., patient transfer, toileting) can be especially overwhelming. All these stroke-related alterations and adaptations affecting the health and well-being of stroke caregivers can culminate in the perception that "caregiving is a full-time job" [123].

Table 8 Themes of interpersonal relationship challenges amongst stroke survivors and their family caregivers

Theme	Specific type	Example
Coping with the direct effects of the stroke	Impairments in survivor communication	Aphasia prompts frustration, tension, arguments stemming from dyad's inability to communicate with one another
	Impairments in survivor physical functioning or mobility	Distress associated with dependence on caregiver for help
	Impairments in survivor memory and thinking	Caregiver frustration with fluctuating nature of patient's memory impairment; cognitive impairment promotes limitations in resolving differences
Incongruence in perceptions between survivors and caregivers	Incongruence about the survivor's or caregiver's abilities	Differences between dyads' perception of abilities (i.e., such as driving)
	Incongruence about the value of effectiveness of rehabilitation	Differences in opinion of perceived need for recovery-oriented services
	Incongruence about what the future holds	Related to setting of care discussions
Strained communication		Addressing the provision of practical and emotional support and caregiver needs for personal space and juggling competing time demands
Managing worries		Triggered by financial concerns and caregiver angst over future potential stroke-related disability

(continued)

Table 8 (continued)

Theme	Specific type	Example
Adjusting to changing roles	Adjusting to new roles as survivor and caregiver	Evolution to role of care recipient vs care provider; caregiver questioning ability to provide needed care in the home setting
	Adjusting to new household responsibilities or leadership	Negotiations related to assumption of household duties
	Inability to resume pre-stroke activities together	Functional changes preclude resumption of pre-stroke norm prompting dyad's sense of isolation
	Adjusting to changed level of intimacy	Mostly reduction in physical contact; little communication about issue
Amplification of existing relationship issues	Partners behaviors	Pre-stroke struggles (i.e., substance abuse or other mental health issues) may be exacerbated
	Partners personality characteristics	Pre-stroke characteristics (i.e., frequent negativity, irritability, discomfort with sharing feelings) impacts post-stroke relationship building
Lack of support from other family members and friends		Absence of help created tension in the dyad relationship and prompted feelings of isolation and abandonment

Source: [132]

Table 9 Caregiving assessment considerations

Caregiver variables
• Sex
• Age/developmental stage
• Relationship to ill loved one
• Work status
• Co-occurring responsibility to care for others
• Living status
• Degree of social isolation
• Degree of financial insecurity
• Presence of secondary support for primary caregiver
• Communication adequacy with healthcare providers
• Past integration of self-care practices
• Degree of competency/experience to provide care
Patient-specific characteristics
• Physical care requirements
• Stage of illness
• Presence of anxiety, depression, existential distress
• Pre-morbid history of psychiatric diagnosis
• Hours of care required
• Communication style with family network

5   10 Intervention Caveats and Advocacy Targets

Common identifiers of older caregivers augment the planning of assistive approaches on their behalf. In general, these commonalities include the likelihood that older caregivers are rendering care to a spouse/partner, spend more than 20 h per week caregiving, question their ability to provide quality care, have at least one chronic illness of their own to manage, and are least likely to have secondary support to assist with caregiving [75]. With this background in mind, some overarching interventions include the following:

1. Undertake an *assessment* at the onset of care, which provides a baseline understanding of caregiver and patient variables (Table 9). In particular, consider the nature of patient debility requiring caregiver support. Gather information about specific caregiving expectations and needs [136]. Identify individuals in the family constellation, and specifically, who is willing and available to provide assistance with caregiving. Data gathering includes pre-existing norms and stressors and the nature of family relationships.
2. Expect a *dual focus of professional support* will be needed, namely, address caregiver needs, which historically have not been solicited [21, 29, 137–139]. Practical discussion prompts to solicit caregivers' perspectives are outlined in Table 10.
3. Encourage the primary caregiver to identify and request/accept the support of secondary caregivers and *use of available resources*. The presence and involvement of "caregivers of the primary caregiver" reduces stress [140]. Take an inventory of the caregiving tasks as primary caregivers are responsible for and their complexity. Assist the caregiver with determining what could be delegated to a support team. Inform the caregiver of community, educational, and emotional support opportunities [32].
4. Predict caregivers will not consider *self-care a priority*. They will require encouragement and coaching to routinely engage them in health promoting practices. Sharing the message, *"You need to care for yourself to take the best care of your loved one"* often helps in this regard. The need to *"re-charge your battery"* and *"have gas in the tank to run"* are other analogies that speak to the need for self-care.
5. Anticipate *caregiver stress* will prevail despite their lack of acknowledgement of such. The hard work of caregiving needs to be validated and normalized by the healthcare team. Share the fact that you expect stress rather than the absence of such. Help the caregiver prioritize the most difficult tasks they are encountering and then assist with problem-solving [32].
6. Make intervention *planning a group process*. Purposeful inclusivity of the patient and caregiver increases the likelihood that interventions will be both tailored and meaningful to the dyad. Caregiver-directed interventions usually require a multifocal approach [37]. Include the delineation of strengths in planning. Jointly discuss what a good outcome would be and make a realistic goal specific to that. This provides a tangible target that depicts improvement and progress [32].

Table 10 Discussion prompts for engaging family caregivers

Caregiver health
• To provide the very best patient care, I find I need to also pay attention to my patients' caregivers. Can you tell me a bit about how you are feeling/doing?
• We know that care givers often neglect their own health. When was the last time you saw your physician?
• Do you have your own physician? Is she or he aware of your caregiving situation? What has she or he advised about it?
Quality of Life
• I know that many family caregivers find the role to be stressful. How are you coping with these responsibilities?
• How would you describe your quality of life these days?
• How often do you get out?
• What do you do for fun?
Support
• Many caregivers don't want to burden others—especially their children. Are there times when you really need help but don't ask for fear of being a burden?
• Who gives you support? How helpful is it?
• Caregiving is a very hard job. Taking advantage of available resources can help. Are you using any resources? Do you want help knowing about them?
In case of emergency
• If anything should happen to you, have you made arrangements for someone to take care of (name here)?

Adapted from: [50]

7. In building a formal program of education and support, determine *caregivers' perspectives* on priority problem areas and those where their confidence is lacking. Disease knowledge can be shared via a didactic format. In cases where "hands-on" caregiving skill is required, interactive skill building is imperative to facilitate biophysiological (i.e., dexterity, strength, body mechanics, positioning, manipulation of dressings, flushing protocols) mastery. Similarly, if communication skill building is the target of the intervention, role playing provides practical competence and enhances confidence when assuming new approaches.

8. Consider *technological platforms* to facilitate caregiving. These contemporary strategies to augment care via virtual methodologies have been established post- COVID. These options should be further evaluated and employed in the future repertoire of elder caregiver supportive care. Benefits include providing "as needed" support, do not require transportation access, can reach distance caregivers, and reduce caregivers' sense of isolation.

9. Presume *drug therapies are problematic* and will require ongoing assessment. Determine the nature of non-adherence and plan interventions according to problem (i.e., manage toxicity, reduce confusing schedule, implement strategies to reduce forgetfulness).

10. Ready oneself for the need of *cultural sensitivity and competency* will be increasingly important in the future as global immigration continues. This necessitates translation of materials,, careful attention to norms about informa-

tion disclosure, use of complementary approaches, the role of the family in decision-making, and sensitivity to older adult reliance on cultural norms from their country of origin [109, 141–144].

6 Elder Caregiving Research

There is a plethora of opportunity within the realm of caregiving that warrant consideration for future investigation. Table 11 identifies potential foci based on gaps in the existing evidence base.

Table 11 Potential research targets in elder caregiving

Theme	Examples of foci
Chronology of caregiving	• Identify nature of caregiving over time and by stage of illness • Investigate longitudinal psychological distress screening in caregivers (vs one point in time assessment)
Co-morbidity	• Explore the relationship between number of caregiving tasks and their complexity with caregiver self-care practices • Examine the relationship between caregiver co-morbidity and the extent of dyad emotional distress • Describe drug management expectations by degree of polypharmacy. Drug classification and toxicity prevalence
Diversity	• Target samples other than Caucasian, non-Hispanic highly educated caregivers across research topics • Identify unique caregiving issues of elder immigrant dyads • Depict the results of culturally-prescribed, dyad-focused program planning originating from a co-design methodology
Ethical implications	• Delineate the nature and scope of specific ethical dilemmas (i.e., paternalism vs. autonomy, longevity versus quality of life, veracity/truth-telling) encountered in critical care units by older dyads • Describe the benefits of generating an automatic ethical consult with all primary caregivers of the oldest old admitted to medical-surgical inpatient units
End-of-life	• Examine the relationship between regularly scheduled family meetings in extended care facilities on the prominence of caregiver's complicated grief • Illustrate examples of illness uncertainty in caregivers with and without the presence of a secondary caregiver
Stress exacerbation	• Describe the nature of caregiver support needs during times of setting of care transition • Compare the nature and intensity of reported stress by caregiver gender
Technology	• Investigate enhancers to the integration of novel technology in the home setting (i.e., remote tracking devices, communication platforms, virtual care monitoring) • Report the benefits of a graduate, sequential learning approach to older caregiver adoption of communication technology
Well-being	• Investigate the efficacy of a designated coach model (lay navigator vs nurse navigator) in fostering caregiver well-being • Delineate caregiver and patient factors associated with caregiver burnout

7   The Healthy Aging Agenda

The potential is limitless for health professionals to engage in efforts to maximize a core element of elder care that to date has largely remains untapped—namely, healthy aging. This represents yet another example of ageism, the perception that older adults would not benefit from efforts that foster their well-being. Recognizing this gap, both the United Nations (UN) and World Health Organization (WHO) have taken steps to leverage this focus [145, 146].

Targeting health promotion in older adults does not imply striving for the absence of illness and disability [147]. Rather, it refers to developing, maintaining, and maximizing physical, mental, emotional, and social wellness that fosters enhanced capability in older adults [148]. Potential outcomes include reducing co-morbidity due to the elimination of risk factors and unhealthy behaviors (i.e., diet modification to eliminate hyperlipidemia and diabetes, create novel support programs to stop smoking) and increasing functional status (i.e., physical therapy interventions and exercise clubs incentivized with lowering biologic markers (i.e., hypertension, blood sugar levels). Figure 3 depicts the common causes of death, the most salient of which have potential reversible etiologies. It has been estimated that efforts to reduce obesity, stop smoking, minimize alcohol consumption, and increase physical activity could ultimately prevent one in five deaths across Europe [126].

Health-promoting efforts can reduce frailty, the biological state of vulnerability emanating from progressive and cumulative reduction in reserve capacity and overall fitness [10]. A significant reduction in those deemed frail could reduce costly hospitalizations and emergency department use with parallel financial savings [149]. However, workforce enhancement is needed to add prevention and health promotion knowledge and skill to the existing repertoire of expertise that focuses on disease management.

The WHO identified 2020–2030 as the "Decade of Healthy Aging." They created a framework for countries to engage in cultivating an infrastructure that promotes well-being in older adults. Primarily, this targeted the creation of age friendly communities where elder's quality of life could be improved in a number of sectors (i.e., housing, transportation, social participation, communication and information dissemination, community-based support, and health service availability) [150]. Singapore, Australia, and New Zealand have been recognized as leaders in implementing these initiatives. Non-siloed, country-specific, interdisciplinary, and comprehensive planning is required to integrate this healthy aging agenda globally.

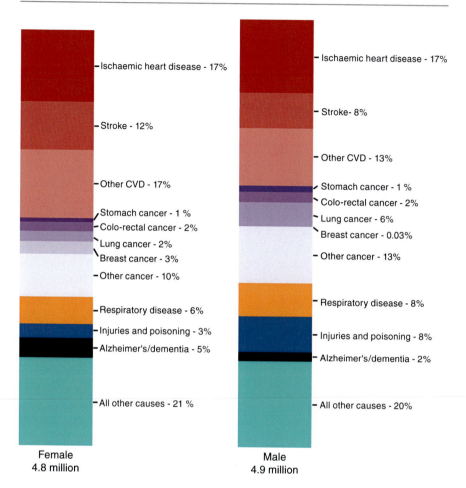

Fig. 3 National causes of death in females and males in European Society of Cardiology Member Countries. Source: [112], with permission

8 Conclusion

The immediate future portends a predominantly elderly society worldwide. Four global illnesses common in older adults—stroke, heart failure, cancer, and dementia—will predominate. Also of note will be the heightened potential for the co-occurrence of these major illnesses. For example, a male with an initial diagnosis of heart failure at age 60 could be diagnosed with prostate cancer at age 67, followed by a subsequent diagnosis of dementia at age 75 years [151].

Regardless of geography, informal family caregivers are generally expected to assume responsibility for the care required by an elder loved one. Yet needed caregiving skills are not taught, remain uncompensated, and often exceed in complexity what a lay family caregiver can confidently provide. It is the absence of tailored family-focused instruction individualized to the explicit needs of the patient, and caregivers are relegated to an ongoing position of vulnerability. Major country-specific policies are needed to support regional and local efforts [152].

Nurses and midwives are the largest group of health professionals globally [153]. It is imperative that they embrace care of the elderly with rigor and intensity unlike that which has been observed to date [60]. In particular, efforts to build nursing workforce capacity to care for older adults in low- and middle-income countries are of utmost importance now and for the future.

A major opportunity to enhance our elder care requires us to re-frame our opinions about caregivers. They should be perceived and utilized as partners in care delivery, namely, formal members of the team planning and rendering care [32, 35, 49, 50, 154]. After all, they know the patient best and can share invaluable insight into strategies and interventions with the greatest likelihood of benefit.

Foundational to the global improvement of care elders is the dismantling of pervasive ageism [155]. This social discrimination negates the possibility of healthy aging and coexists with racism, sexism, gender, and religious discrimination. Aging is rooted in the negative, biomedically prejudiced view of long life as a spiraling downward continuum. This encompasses loss and deprivation that is characterized by a state of decline and vulnerability. Directly correlated is the absence of required training of healthcare professionals, the paucity of research in medical specialties where the care of older adults predominates, and the nonexistence of clinical approaches addressing the special needs of older adults (i.e., vision, hearing, memory compromise). Also, it is important to note that ageism is not only directed toward individuals in the later years of their lives; it also affects nurses who choose to care for them [155].

As nurses and global citizens, perhaps re-considering our current reality would formulate the aging imperative in a more personal context. The work we engage in now to address deficits in care during later life will be personally critical to ourselves and our families. None of us can afford to think of growing old as a distant event [60]. We all are aging and will require the provision of a highly enhanced version of today's eldercare in our later years.

References

1. United Nations (2019) World population ageing, 2019. https://www.un.org/en/development/desa/population/publications/pdf/ageing/WorldPopulationAgeing2019-Highlights.pdf
2. Zubiashvivi T, Zubiashvili. (2021) Population aging – a global challenge. Ecoforum 10:2(25)

3. Cheng X, Yanf Y, Schwebel D, Liu Z, Li L, Cheng P et al (2020) Population aging and mortality during 1990–2017: a global decompensation analysis. PLoS Med 17(6):e1003138. https://doi.org/10.1371/journal.pmed.1003138

4. Dixon A (2021) The United Nations decade of healthy aging requires concrete global action. Nat Aging 1. https://doi.org/10.1038/S43587-020-00011-5

5. Kahn H (2019) Population aging in a globalized world: risks and dilemmas. J Eval Clin Pract 25:754–760. https://doi.org/10.1111/jep.13071

6. Rudnicka E, Napierala P, Podfigurna A, Meczekalski B, Smolarczyk R, Grymowicz M (2020) The World Health Organization (WHO) approach to healthy aging. Maturitas 139:6–11. https://doi.org/10.1016/j.maturitas.2020.05.018

7. Partridge L, Deelen J, Slagboom P (2018) Facing up to the global challenges of ageing. Nature 561(7221):45–56. https://doi.org/10.1038/s41586-018-0457-8

8. Rowe J, Fulmer T, Fried L (2016) Preparing for better health and health care for an aging population. J Am Med Assoc 316(16):1643–1644. https://doi.org/10.1001/jama.2016.12335

9. Michel J, Ecarnot F (2020) The shortage of skilled workers in Europe: its impact on geriatric medicine. Eur Geriatr Med 11(3):345–347. https://doi.org/10.1007/s41999-020-0032300

10. Ilinca S, Calciolari S (2015) The patterns of health care utilization by elderly Europeans: frailty and its implications for health systems. Health Serv Res 50(1):305–320. https://doi.org/10.1111/1475-6773.12211

11. Miyawaki C, Bouldin E, Taylor C, McGuire L (2021) Baby Boomers who provide informal care for people living with dementia in the community. Int J Environ Res Public Health 18(18):9694. https://doi.org/10.3390/ijerph18189694

12. Ogura S, Jakovljevic M (2018) Global population aging – health care, social, and economic consequences. Front Pub Health 6:335. https://doi.org/10.3389/fpubh.2018.00335

13. Anderson J, Rose K (2019) Family-focused care of older adults: contemporary issues and challenges. J Fam Nurs 25(4):499–505. https://doi.org/10.1177/1074840719885337

14. DesRoches C, Chang Y, Kim J, Mukunda S, Norman L, Dittus R et al (2022) Who wants to work in geriatrics: findings from a national survey of physicians and nurse practitioners. Nurs Outlook 70:309–314. https://doi.org/10.1016/j.outlook.2021.10.004

15. Monsees J, Schmachtenberg T, Thyrian J (2022) Intercultural care for people of migrant origin with dementia: a literature analysis. Dementia 21(5):1753–1770. https://doi.org/10.1177/14713012221086702

16. Bachman P (2020) Caregivers' experience of caring for a family member with Alzheimer's disease: a content analysis of longitudinal social media communication. Int J Envir Res Pub Health 17:4412. https://doi.org/10.3390/ijerph17124412

17. Sambasivam R, Liu J, Vaingankar J, Ong H, Tan M, Fauziana R, Picco L, Chong S, Subramaniam M (2019) The hidden patient: chronic physical morbidity, psychological distress, and quality of life in caregiver of older adults. Psychogeriatrics 19:65–72. https://doi.org/10.1111/psyg.12365

18. Jakovljevic M, Netz Y, Buttigieg S, Adany R, Laaser U, Varjacic M (2018) Population aging and migration – history and UN forecasts in the EU-28 and its east and south near neighborhood – one century perspective 1950-2050. 2018. Glob Health 14:30. https://doi.org/10.1186/s12992-018-0348-7

19. Marois G, Belanger A, Lutz W (2020) Population aging, migration, and productivity in Europe. PNAS 117(14):7690–7695. https://doi.org/10.1073/pnas.1918988117

20. Wolff J, Mulcahy J, Huang J, Roth D, Covinsky K, Kasper J (2018) Family caregivers of older adults, 1999-2015: trends in characteristics, circumstances, and role-related appraisal. Gerontol 58(6):1021–1032. https://doi.org/10.1093/geront/gnx093

21. Michaels J, Chen C, Meeker M (2022) Navigating the caregiving abyss: a metasynthesis of how family caregivers manage end-of-life care for older adults at home. Pallia Med 36(1):81–94. https://doi.org/10.1177/02692163211042999

22. Bell J, Whitney R, Young H (2019) Family caregiving in serious illness in the United States: recommendations to support an invisible workforce. J Am Geriatr Soc 67:S5451–S5456. https://doi.org/10.1111/jgs.15820

23. Ferreira B, Diz A, Silva P, Sousa L, Pinho L, Fonseca C et al (2022) Bibiometric analysis of the informal caregiver's scientific production. J Person Med 12:61. https://doi.org/10.3390/jpm12010061
24. Wasmani A, Rahnama M, Abdollahimohohammad A, Badakhsh M, Hashemi Z (2022) The effect of family centered education on the care burden of family caregivers of the elderly with cancer: a quasi-experimental study. Asian Pac J Canc Prev 23(3):1077–1082. https://doi.org/10.31557/APJCP.2022.23.3.1077
25. National Academy of Science, Engineering, and Medicine (2016) Families caring for an aging America. National Academies Press, Washington, DC
26. Zarit S, Todd P, Zarit J (1986) Subjective burden of husbands and wives as caregivers: a longitudinal study. Gerontol 26(3):260–266. https://doi.org/10.1043/gerontol/26.3.260
27. Given B, Given C (2019) The burden of cancer caregivers. In: Applebaum A (ed) Cancer caregivers. Oxford University Press, New York, pp 20–33
28. Wranker L, Elmstahl S, Cecilia F (2021) The health of older family caregivers – a 6-year follow-up. J Gerontol Soc Work 64(2):190–207. https://doi.org/10.1080/01634372.2020.1843098
29. Berry L, Del Wade S, Jacobson J (2017) Supporting the supporters: what family caregivers need to care for a loved one with cancer. J Oncol Pr 13(1):35–41. https://doi.org/10.1200/JOP.2016.017913
30. Van Houten C, Volis C, Weinberger M (2011) An organizing framework for informal caregiver interventions: detailing caregiving activities and caregiver and care recipient outcomes to optimize evaluation efforts. BMC Geriatr 11:77. https://doi.org/10.1186/1471-23318-11-17
31. Bierhals C, Low G, Paskulin L (2019) Quality of life perceptions of family caregivers of older adult stroke survivors: a longitudinal study. Appl Nurs Res 47:57–62. https://doi.org/10.1016/j.apnr.2019.05.003
32. Boyle D (2020) The caregiver's companion. Oncology Nursing Society, Pittsburgh, PA
33. Kent E, Longacre M, Chou W, Mollica M (2019) Who are informal cancer caregivers? In: Applebaum A (ed) Cancer caregivers. Oxford University Press, New York, pp 3–19
34. Crist J, Steinheiser M (2020) Caring for the family/lay caregiver of older adults. J Infus Nurs 43(5):255–261. https://doi.org/10.1097/NAN.0000000000000384
35. Messecar D (2021) Family caregiving. In: Boltz M, Capezuti E, Zwicker D, Fulmer T (eds) Evidence-based geriatric nursing protocols for best practice, 6th edn. Springer Publishing, New York, pp 191–221
36. Wachterman M, Luth E, Semco R, Weissman J (2022) Where Americans die – is there really 'no place like home?'. N Engl J Med 386:11. https://doi.org/10.1056/NEJMp2112297
37. Marco D, Thomas K, Ivynian S, Wilding H, Parker D, Tiernan J, Hudson P (2021) Family carer needs in advanced disease: systematic review of reviews. BMJ Supp Pallia Care. https://doi.org/10.1136//bmjspcare-2021-003299
38. Assa A, Umberger R (2021) A concept analysis of family caregivers' uncertainty of patient's illness. Nurs Forum 57:121–126. https://doi.org/10.1111/nuf.12645
39. Schulz R, Sherwood P (2008) Physical and mental health effects of family caregiving. Am J Nurs. 108(Suppl 9):23–27. https://doi.org/10.1016/j.jagp.2017.06.023oi.org/10
40. Look K, Stone J (2018) Medication management activities performed by informal caregivers of older adults. Res Social Adm Pharm 14(5):418–426. https://doi.org/10.1016/j.sapharm.2017.05.005
41. National Alliance for Caregiving, AARP. Caregiving in the U.S., 2015 Report. https://www.caregiving.org/wp-content/uploads/2020/05/2015_CaregivingintheUS_Final-Report-June-4_WEB.pdf
42. Smith A, Micco G (2018) Serving the very sick, very frail, and very old. Perspect Biol Med 60(4):503–518. https://doi.org/10.1353/pbm.2017.0039
43. Quinones A, Markwardts S, Botoseneanu A (2016) Multimorbidity combinations and disability in older adults. J Gerontol Biol Med 71(6):823–830. https://doi.org/10.1093/Gerona/glw035

44. Crouch A, Champion V, Von Ah D (2022) Co-morbidity, cognitive dysfunction, physical functioning and quality of life in older breast cancer survivors. Supp Care Cancer 30(1):359–366. https://doi.org/10.1007/s00520-021-06427-y

45. Powers B, Yan J, Zhu J, Linn K, Jain S et al (2019) Subgroups of high-cost medicare advantage patients: an observational study. J Gen Int Med 34(2):218–225. https://doi.org/10.1007/s11606-018-4759-1

46. Magnuson A, Sattar S, Nightingale G, Saracino R, Skonecki E, Trevino K (2019) A practical guide to geriatric syndromes in older adults with cancer: a focus on falls, cognition, polypharmacy, and depression. ASCO Education Book 39:e96–e109. https://doi.org/10.1200/EDBK_237641

47. Midao L, Giardini A, Menditto E, Kardas P, Costa E (2018) Polypharmacy prevalence among older adults based on survey of health, ageing, and retirement in Europe. Arch Gerontol Geriat 78:213–220. https://doi.org/10.1016/j.archger.2018.06.018

48. Goldzweig G, Schapira L, Baider L, Jacobs J, Andritsch E, Rottenberg Y (2019) Who will care for the caregiver? Distress and depression among spousal caregivers of older patients undergoing treatment for cancer. Supp Care Cancer 27(11):4221–4227. https://doi.org/10.1007/s00520-019-04711-6

49. Nemati S, Rassouli M, Ilkhani M, Baghestani A (2018) Perceptions of family caregivers of cancer patients about the challenges of caregiving: a qualitative study. Scan J Caring Sci 32(1):309–316. https://doi.org/10.1111/scs.12463

50. Adelman R, Timanova L, Delgado D, Dion S, Lachs M (2014) Caregiver burden: a clinical review. JAMA 311(10):1052–1059. https://doi.org/10.1001/jama.2014.304

51. Savela R, Nykanen I, Schwab U, Valmaki T (2021) Social and environmental determinants of health among family caregivers of older adults. Nurs Res 71(1):3–11. https://doi.org/10.1097/NNR.0000000000000559

52. Samsi K, Cole L, Manthorpe J (2021) 'The time has come': reflections on the 'tipping point' in deciding on a care home move. Aging Ment Health. https://doi.org/10.1080/136078632021.1947963

53. Pristavec T, Luth E (2020) Informal caregiver burden, benefits, and older adult mortality: a survival analysis. J Gerontol Soc Serv 75(10):2193–2206. https://doi.org/10.1093/geronb/gbaa001

54. Tseilou F, Rosato M, Maguire A, Wright D, O'Reilly D (2018) Variation of caregiver health and mortality risks by age: a census-based record linkage study. Am J Epidemiol 187(7):1401–1410. https://doi.org/10.1093/aje/Kwx384

55. Howell B, Peterson J (2020) "With age comes wisdom": a qualitative review of elder perspectives on healthy aging in the Circumpolar North. J Cross Cult Gerontol 35(2):113–131. https://doi.org/10.1007/s10823-020-09399-4

56. Hossain Z, Eisberg G, Schwalb D (2018) Grandparents' social identities in cultural context. Contemp Soc Sci 13(2):275–287. https://doi.org/10.1080/21582041.2018.1433315

57. Pan Y, Chen R, Yang D (2022) The relationship between filial piety and caregiver burden among adult children: a systematic review and meta-analysis. Geriatr Nurs 43:113–123. https://doi.org/10.1016/j.gerinurse.2021.10.024

58. Gendron T (2022) Ageism unmasked. Steer Forth Press, Lebanon, NH

59. Jose J, Amado C, Ilinca S, Buttigieg S, Larsson A (2019) Ageism in health care: a systematic review of operational definitions and inductive conceptualizations. Gerontol 59(2):e98–e108. https://doi.org/10.1093/geront/gnx020

60. Baumbusch J, Blakey E, Carapellotti A, Dohmen M, Fick D, Kagan S et al (2022) Nurses and the decade of healthy aging: an unprecedented opportunity. Geriatr Nurs 47:A1. https://doi.org/10.1016/j.gerinurse.2022.04.015

61. Tabloski P (2022) Gerontological nursing review and resource manual, 4th edn. American Nurses Association, Silver Spring, MD

62. Podgorica N, Flatscher-Thoni M, Deufert D, Siebert U, Ganner M (2021) A systematic review of ethical and legal issues in elder care. Nurs Ethics 28(6):895–910. https://doi.org/10.1177/0969733020921488

63. Li Y, Cimiotti J, Evans K, Clevenger C (2022) The characteristics and practice proficiency of nurse practitioners who care for older adults. Geriatr Nurs 46:213. https://doi.org/10.1016/j.gerinurse.2022.01.1016

64. Yates P, Charalambous A, Fennimore L, Nevidjon B, So W et al (2020) Cancer nursing's potential to reduce the growing burden of cancer across the world. Oncol Nurs Forum 47(6):625–627. https://doi.org/10.1016/j.ejon.2020.101891

65. GBD Cancer Collaborators. Global, regional, and national cancer incidence, mortality, years of life lost, years lived with disability, and disability-adjusted life-years for 29 cancer groups, 1990-2016: a systematic analysis for the GBD study. JAMA Oncol 4(11):1553–1568. https://doi.org/10.1001/jamaoncol.2018.2706

66. Tranberg M, Andersson M, Nilbert M, Rasmussen B (2021) Co-afflicted but invisible: a qualitative study of perceptions among informal caregivers in cancer care. J Health Psychol 26(11):1850–1859. https://doi.org/10.1177/1359105319890407

67. Bray F, Ferlay J, Soerjomataram I, Siegel R, Torre L et al (2018) Global cancer statistics 2018: GLOBOCAN estimates of incidence and mortality worldwide for 36 cancers in 185 countries. CA Cancer J Clin 68(6):394–424. https://doi.org/10.3322/caac.21492

68. Sung H, Ferlay J, Siegel R, Laversanne M, SoerjomataramI JA et al (2020) GLOBOCAN estimates, of incidence and mortality worldwide for 36 cancers in 185 countries. CA-A Cancer J Clin 71(3):209–249. https://doi.org/10.3322/caac.21660

69. Fidler-Benaoudia M, Bray F (2020) Transitions in human development and the global cancer burden. In: Wild C, Widerpass E, Stewart B (eds) World cancer report: cancer research for cancer prevention. International Agency for Research on Cancer, Lyon

70. Bluethmann S, Mariotto A, Rowland J (2016) Anticipating the "Silver Tsunami": prevalence trajectories and co-morbidity burden among older cancer survivors in the United States. Cancer Epidemiol Biomark Prev 25(7):1029–1036. https://doi.org/10.1158/1055-9965.EPI-16-0133

71. Hulvat M (2020) Cancer incidence and trends. Surg Clin N Am 100(3):469–481. https://doi.org/10.1016/j.suc.2020.01.002

72. Miller K, Nogueira L, Devasia T, Mariotto A, Yabroff K, Jemal A et al (2022) Cancer treatment and survival statistics. CA Cancer J Clin 72:409. https://doi.org/10.3322/caac.21731

73. Ferlay J, Colombet M, Soerjomataram I, Dyba T, Randi G et al (2018) Cancer incidence and mortality patterns in Europe: estimates for 40 countries and 25 major cancers in 2018. Eur J Ca 103:356–387. https://doi.org/10.1016/j.ejca.2018.07.005

74. Peh C, Liu J, Mahendran R (2020) Quality of life and emotional distress among caregivers of patients with newly diagnosed with cancer: understanding trajectories across the first year post diagnosis. J Psych Oncol 38(5):557–572. https://doi.org/10.1080/07347332.2020.1760994

75. Litzelman K (2019) The unique experience of caregivers based on their life stage and relationship to the patient. In: Applebaum A (ed) Cancer caregivers. Oxford University Press, New York, pp 34–49

76. Scheltens P, De Strooper B, Kivipelto B, Holstege H, Chetalat G et al (2021) Alzheimer's disease. Lancet 397(10284):1577–1590. https://doi.org/10.1016/S0140-6736(20)32205-4

77. Alzheimer's Dementia International World Report (2021). https://www.alzint.org/resource/world-alzheimer-report-2021

78. Alzheimer's Association (2022) Alzheimers disease facts and figures. Alzheimer's Dementia 18(4):700–789. https://doi.org/10.1002/alz.12638

79. Queluz F, Kervin E, Wozney L, Fancey P, McGrath P, Keefe J (2020) Understanding the needs of caregivers of persons with dementia: a scoping review. Int Psychogeriatr 32(1):35–52. https://doi.org/10.1017/S10416/0219000243

80. Wu Q, Yamaguchi Y, Greiner C (2022) Factors associated with the well-being of family care-givers of people with dementia. Psychogeriatrics 22:218. https://doi.org/10.1111/psyg/12805

81. Yu H, Wang X, He R, Liang R, Znow L (2015) Measuring caregiver burden of caring for community-residing people with Alzheimer's dementia. PLoS One 10(7):e0132168. https://doi.org/10.1371/journal.pone.0132168

82. Jeste D, Mausbach B, Lee E (2021) Caring for caregivers/care partners of persons with dementia. Int Psychogeriatr 33(4):307–310. https://doi.org/10.1017/S1041610221000557

83. Davis L, Gilliss C, Deshefy-Longhi T, Chestnutt D, Molloy M (2011) The nature and scope of stressful spousal caregiving relationships. J Fam Nurs 17(2):224. https://doi.org/10.1177/1074840711405666

84. Mayo A, Siegle K, Savell E, Bullock B, Preston G, Peavy G (2020) Lay caregivers experi-ences with caring for persons with dementia: a phenomenological study. J Gerontol Nurs 46(8):17–27. https://doi.org/10.3928/00989134-20200527-02

85. Lee K, Puga F, Pickering C, Masoud S, White C (2019) Transitioning into the caregiving role following a diagnosis of Alzheimer's dementia or related dementia: a scoping review. Int J Nurs Stud 96:119–136. https://doi.org/10.1016/j.ijnurstu.2019.02.007

86. Whitlach C, Orsulis-Jeras S (2018) Meeting informational, educational, and psychosocial support needs of persons living with dementia and their family caregivers. Gerontol 58(Suppl 1):558–573. https://doi.org/10.1093/geront/gux162

87. Ying J, Yap P, Ghandhi M, Liew T (2019) Validity and utility of the center for epidemiologi-cal studies depression scale for determining depression in family caregivers of persons with dementia. Demen Geriatr Cogn Disord 47(4–6):323–334. https://doi.org/10.1159/000500440

88. Hazzan A, Dauenhauer J, Follansbee P, Hazzan J, Allen K, Omobepade J (2022) Family care-giver quality of life and the care provided to older people living with dementia: quality analy-ses of caregiver interviews. BMC Geriatr 22:86. https://doi.org/10.1186/s12877-022-02787-0

89. Kim B, Noh G, Kim K (2021) Behavioural and psychological symptoms of dementia in patients with Alzheimer's dementia and family caregiving burden: a pathological analysis. BMC Geriatr 21(2):160. https://doi.org/10.1186/s12877-021-02109-w

90. Nguyen H, Eccleston C, Doherty K, Jang S, McInerney F (2022) Communication in dementia care: experiences and needs of carers. Dementia 21(4):1381–1398. https://doi.org/10.1177/14713012221080003

91. Hiyoshi-Taniguchi K, Becker C, Konoshita A (2018) What behavioral and psychological symptoms effect caregiver burnout? Clin Gerontol 41(3):249–254. https://doi.org/10.1080/07317115.2017.1398797

92. Huang S (2022) Depression among caregivers of patients with dementia: association of fac-tors and management approaches. World J Psychiatry 12(1):59–76. https://doi.org/10.5498/wjp.v12159

93. Brini S, Hodkinson A, Davies A, Hirani S, Gathercole R, Howard R, Newman S (2022) In-home dementia caregiving is associated with greater psychological burden and poorer mental health than out-of-home caregiving: a cross-sectional study. Aging Ment Health 26(4):709–715. https://doi.org/10.1080/13607863.2021.1881758

94. Peavy G, Mayo A, Avalos C, Rodriguez A, Shifflett B, Edland S (2022) Perceived stress in older dementia caregivers: mediation by loneliness and depression. Am J Alz Dis Other Demen 370:1–8. https://doi.org/10.1177/15333175211064756

95. Mansfield E, Cameron E, Boyes A, Carey M, Nair B, Hall A et al (2022) Prevalence and type of unmet needs experienced by carers of people living with dementia. Aging Ment Health:1. https://doi.org/10.1080/13607863.20222053833

96. Brooks D, Beattie E, Fielding E, Wyles K, Edwards H (2022) Long-term care placement: the transitional support needs and preferences of spousal dementia caregivers. Dementia 21(3):794–809. https://doi.org/10.1177/14713012211056461

97. Martin A, O'Connor S, Jackson C (2018) A scoping review of gaps and priorities in dementia care in Europe. Dementia 19(7):2135–2151. https://doi.org/10.1177/1471301218816250

98. Saragosa M, Jetts L, Okrainec K, Kuluski K (2022) Using meta-ethnography to understand the care transition experience of people with dementia and their caregivers. Dementia 21(1):153–180. https://doi.org/10.1177/14713012211031779

99. Boss P (2011) Loss, trauma and resilience: therapeutic work with ambiguous loss. Norton, New York

100. Fonseca A, Lahoz R, Proudfoot C, Corda S, Loefroth E, Jackson J et al (2021) Burden and quality of life among female and male patients with heart failure in Europe: a real-world cross-sectional study. Patient Pref Adher 15:1693–1706

101. Gorodeski E, Goyal P, Hummel S (2018) Domain management approach to heart failure in the geriatric patient: present and future. J Am Coll Cardiol 71:1921–1936. https://doi.org/10.1016/j.jacc.2018.02.059

102. Conrad N, Judge A, Tran J, Mohseni H, Hedgecott D, Crespillo A et al (2018) Temporal trends and patterns of heart failure incidence: a population-based study of 4 million individuals. Lancet 391:572–580. https://doi.org/10.1016/S0140-6736(17)3250-5

103. Westinbrink B, Brugts J, McDonagh T, Filippatos G, Ruschitzka F, van Laake L (2016) Heart failure specialization in Europe. Eur J Heart Fail 18(4):347–349. https://doi.org/10.1002/ejhf.506

104. Testa M, Cappuccio A, Latella M, Napolitano S, Milli M, Volpe M et al (2020) The emotional and social burden of heart failure: integrating physicians and caregivers perspectives through narrative medicine. BMC Cardiovasc Disord 20:522. https://doi.org/10.1186/s12872-020-01809-2

105. Kobulnik J, Wang I, Bell C, Moayedi Y, Troung N, Sinha S (2021) Management of frail and older homebound patients with heart failure: a contemporary virtual ambulatory model. CJC Open 4(1):47–55. https://doi.org/10.1016/j.cjco.2021.08.015

106. Ahmad F, Anderson R (2021) The leading causes of death in the U.S. for 2020. JAMA 325(18):1829–1830. https://doi.org/10.1001/jama.2021.5469

107. Redfoot D, Feinberg L, Hauser A (2013) The aging of the baby boomers and the growing care gap: a look at future declines in the availability of family caregivers. AARP Public Policy Institute, Washington, DC

108. Savarese G, Lung L (2017) Global public health burden of heart failure. Card Fail Rev 3:7–11. https://doi.org/10.15420/cfr.2016:25-2

109. Shamali M, Ostergaard B, Konradsen H (2020) Living with heart failure: perspectives of ethnic minority families. Open Heart 7:e001289. https://doi.org/10.1136/openhrt-2020-001289

110. Nordfonn O, Morken I, Bru L, Husebe A (2019) Patients' experience with heart failure treatment and self-care – a qualitative study exploring the burden of treatment. J Clin Nurs 28(9–10):1782–1793. https://doi.org/10.1111/joen.14799

111. Alonso W, Kitko L (2018) Intergenerational caregivers of parents with end-stage heart failure. Res Theory Nurs Pract 32(4):413–435. https://doi.org/10.1891/1541-6577.32.4.413

112. Kitko L, McIlvennan C, Bidwell J, Dionne-Odom J, Dunlay S et al (2020) Family caregiving for individuals with heart failure: a scientific statement from the American Heart Association. Circulation 141:e864–e878. https://doi.org/10.1161/CIR.0000000000000768

113. Kim E, Oh S, Son Y (2020) Caring experiences of family caregivers of patients with heart failure: a meta-ethnographic review of the past 10 years. Eur J Cardiovasc Nurs 19(6):473–485. https://doi.org/10.1177/1474515120915040

114. Prochota B, Szwamel K, Uchmanowicz I (2019) Socio-cultural variables affecting the level of self-care in elderly patients with heart failure. Eur J Cardiovasc Nurs 18(7):628–636. https://doi.org/10.1177/1474515119855600

115. Checa C, Medina-Perucha L, Munoz M, Verdu-Rotellar M, Berenguera A. Living with advanced heart failure: a qualitative study. PLoS One 15(12):e0243974. https://doi.org/10.1371/journal.pone.0243974

116. Bidwell J, Hostinar C, Higgins M, Abshire M, Cothran F, Butts B et al (2021) Caregiver subjective and physiological markers of stress and patient heart failure severity in family care dyads. Psychoneuroendocrinol 133:105399. https://doi.org/10.1016/j.psyneuen.2021.105399

117. Timonet-Andreu E, Morales-Ascensio J, Gutierrez P, Alvarez C, Lopez-Moyano G, Banderas A et al (2020) Health-related quality of life and use of hospital services by patients with heart failure and their family caregivers: a multi-center case-controlled study. J Nurs Scholar 52(2):217–228. https://doi.org/10.1111/jnu.12545

118. Im J, Mak S, Upshur R, Steinberg L, Kuluski K (2019) 'The future is probably now': Understanding of illness uncertainty and end of life discussions in older adults with heart failure and family caregivers. Health Expect 22(6):1331–1340. https://doi.org/10.1111/hex.12980

119. Bierle R, Vuckovic K, Ryan C (2021) Integrating palliative care into heart failure management. Crit Care Nurse 41(3):e9–e18. https://doi.org/10.4037/ccn2021877

120. Caro C, Costa J, DaCruz D (2018) Burden and quality of life of family caregivers of stroke patients. Occ Ther Health Care 32(2):154–171. https://doi.org/10.1080/0738057 7.2018.1449046

121. Feigin V, Brainin M, Norrving B, Martins S, Sacco R et al (2022) World Stroke Organization (WSO): Global stroke factsheet 2022. Int J Stroke 17(1):18–29. https://doi.org/10.1177/17474930211065917

122. Roth G, Mensah G, Johnson C, Addolorato G, Ammirati E et al (2020) Global burden of cardiovascular disease and risk factors, 1990–2019: Update for the GBD 2019 study. J Am Coll Cardio 76(25):2982–3021. https://doi.org/10.1016/j.jacc.2020.11.010

123. Kokorelias K, Lu F, Santos J, Xu Y, Leung R, Cameron J (2020) "Caregiving is a full time job" impacting stroke caregivers' health and well-being: a qualitative meta-synthesis. Health Soc Care Community 28:325–340. https://doi.org/10.1111/hsc.12895

124. GBD 2019 Diseases and Injuries Collaborators (2020) Global burden of 369 diseases and injuries in 204 countries and territories, 1990–2019: A systematic analysis for the Global Burden of Disease Study, 2019. Lancet 396(10258):1204–1222. https://doi.org/10.1016/S0140-6736(2030925-9

125. Wafa H, Wolfe C, Emmett E, Roth G, Johnson C, Wang Y (2020) Burden of stroke in Europe. Stroke 51:2418–2427. https://doi.org/10.1161/STROKEHA.120.029606

126. Timmis A, Vardas P, Townsend N, Torbica A, Katus H et al (2022) European society of cardiology: cardiovascular disease statistics. Eur Health J 43:716–799. https://doi.org/10.1093/eurheartj/ehab892

127. GBD Stroke Collaborators (2021) Global, regional and national burden of stroke and its risk factors, 1990-2019: a systematic analysis for the Global Burden of Disease Study. Lancet Neurol 20. https://doi.org/10.1016/S1474-4422(21)00252-0

128. Tsao C, Aday A, Almarzooq Z, Alonso A, Beaton A (2022) Heart disease and stroke statistics – 2022 update: a report from the American Heart Association. Circulation 145(8):e153–e639. https://doi.org/10.1161/CIR0000000000001052

129. Bakas T, McCarthy M, Israel J et al (2022) Adapting the telephone assessment and skill-building kit (TASK III) to the telehealth technology preferences of stroke family caregivers. Res Nurs Health 44(1):81–91. https://doi.org/10.1002/nur.22075

130. Virani S, Alvaro A, Benjamin E, Bittencourt M, Callaway C, Carson A et al (2020) On behalf of the American Heart Association Council on Epidemiology and Prevention Statistics Committee and Stroke Statistics Committee. Heart diseases and stroke statistics – 2020. Update: A report from the American Heart Association. Circulation 141:e139–e596. https://doi.org/10.1161/CIR.0000000000000757

131. Felix M, Le T, Wei M, Puspitasari D (2020) Scoping review: health needs of the family caregivers of elderly stroke survivors. Health Soc Care Community 29:1683–1594. https://doi.org/10.1111/hsc.13371

132. McCarthy M, Lyons K, Schellinger J, Stapleton K, Bakas T (2020) Interpersonal relationship challenges among stroke survivors and family caregivers. Soc Work Health Care 59(2):91–107. https://doi.org/10.1080/00981389.2020.1714827

133. Kernan W, Viera A, Billinger S, Bravata D, Stark S et al (2021) Palliative care of adult patients after stroke: a scientific statement from the American Heart Association/American Stroke Association. Stroke 52(9):e558–e571. https://doi.org/10.1161/STR.0000000000000382

134. Freytes I, Sullivan M, Schmitzberger M, LeLaurin J, Orozco T, Eliazar-Macke N et al (2021) Types of stroke-related deficits and their impact on family caregivers depressive symptoms, burden and quality of life. Disabil Health J 14:101109. https://doi.org/10.1016/j.dhjo.2020.101019

135. Pierce L, Steiner V, Hicks B, Holzaepfel A (2006) Problems on new caregivers of persons with stroke. Rehabil Nurs 31(4):166–172. https://doi.org/10.1002/j.2048-7940.2006.tb00382.x

136. Swartz K, Collins L (2019) Caregiver care. Am Fam Phys 99(11):699–706

137. Sabo K, Chin E, Sethares K, Revell S, Nicholas P (2022) Knowledge, attitudes, and practices of primary healthcare providers with assessing and supporting older informal caregivers. Geriatr Nurs 44:150–166. https://doi.org/10.1016/j.gerinurse.2022.02.004

138. Riffin C, Wolff J, Estill M, Prabhu S, Pillemerk K (2020) Caregiver needs assessment in primary care: views of clinicians, staff, patients, and caregivers. J Am Geriatr Soc 68(6):1262–1270. https://doi.org/10.1111/jgs.16401

139. Sherman D (2019) A review of the complex role of family caregivers as health team members and second-order patients. Healthcare 7(2):63. https://doi.org/10.3390/healthcare.7020063

140. Mayo A, Siegle K, Savell E, Bullock B, Preston G et al (2020) Lay caregivers experiences with caring for persons with dementia: a phenomenological study. J Gerontol Nurs 46(8):17–27. https://doi.org/10.3928/00989134-2020527-02

141. Menkin J, Guan S, Araiza D, Reyes C, Trejo L, Choi S et al (2017) Racial/ethnic differences in expectations regarding aging among older adults. Gerontologist 57(S2):S138–S148. https://doi.org/10.1093/geront/gnx078

142. Vonneilich N, Bremer D, von dem Knesebeck O, Ludecke D (2021) Health patterns among migrant and non-migrant middle- and older-aged individuals in Europe – analyses based on Share 2004-2017. Int J Environ Res Public Health 18:12047. https://doi.org/10.3390/ijerph182212047

143. Trinh N, Bernard-Negron R, Ahmed I (2019) Mental health issues in racial and ethnic minority elderly. Curr Psychiatr Rep 21:102. https://doi.org/10.1007/s11920-01901082-4

144. Brandt M, Kaschowitz J, Quashie N (2021) Socioeconomic inequalities in the well-being of informal caregivers across Europe. Aging Ment Health 26:1589. https://doi.org/10.1080/13607863.2021.1926425

145. United Nations (2020) The decade of healthy aging. https://www.who.int/initiatives/decade-of-healthy-aging

146. World Health Organization. World Health Organization Global Campaign to Combat Ageism. http://www.who.int/teams/social-determinants-of-health/demographic-change-and-healthy-ageing/combatting-ageism

147. De Biasi A, Wolfe M, Carmody J, Fulmer T, Auerbach J (2020) Creating an age-friendly pubic health system. Innov Aging 4(1):1–11. https://doi.org/10.1093/geroni/igz044

148. Fallon C, Karlawish J (2019) Is the WHO definition of healthy aging well? Frameworks for "Health" after three score and ten. Am J Public Health 109(8):1104–1106. https://doi.org/10.2105/AJPH.2019.305177

149. Macinko J, Andrade F, de Andrade F, Lima-Costa M (2020) Universal health coverage: are older adults being left behind? Evidence from aging cohorts in twenty-three countries. Health Aff 39(11):1951–1960. https://doi.org/10.1377/hlthaff.2019.01570

150. Emery-Tiburcio E, Mack L, Zonsius M, Carbonelli E, Newman M (2021) The 4Ms of an age-friendly health system. Am J Nurs 121(11):44–49. https://doi.org/10.1097/01.NAJ.0000799016.07144.0d

151. Gilstrap L, Gorodeski E, Goyal P (2022) Heart failure and cognitive impairment: complexity that requires a new approach. J Am Geri Soc 70(S1):1652. https://doi.org/10.1111/jgs.17779

152. Khayatzadeh-Mahani A, Leslie M (2018) Policies supporting informal caregivers across Canada: a scoping review protocol. BMJ Open 8:e019220. https://doi.org/10.1136//bmjopen-2017-019220

153. Khayatzadeh-Mahani A (2020) The state of nursing and midwifery in the world. Lancet 395(10231):1167. https://doi.org/10.1016/S0140-6736(20)30821-7

154. Matthys O, Dierickx S, Deliens L, Lapeire L, Hudson P, Van Audenhove C (2022) How are family caregivers of people with a serious illness supported by healthcare professionals in their caregiving tasks? A cross-sectional survey of bereaved family caregivers. Palliat Med 36(3):529–539. https://doi.org/10.1177/02692163211070228

155. Resnick B, Young H, Fick D, Kagan S (2022) Making care for older people the choice of nurses today, tomorrow, and forever. Geriatr Nurs 46:A1. https://doi.org/10.1016/j.gerinurse.2022.04.014

Informal Caregivers in Care Efficiency

Andreas Charalambous

1 Introduction

Healthcare systems around the globe are struggling with rising costs, and the lack of economic sustainability of most healthcare systems has contributed to the development of regulation in the health sector. Now more than ever, it has become pivotal that public resources are used in the most efficient and effective way to the best interest of the people in the receiving end of care.

As part of the wider transformation in healthcare, there has been a tendency toward shorter hospital stays, and a growing number of patients (across diseases) are now being cared for by family caregivers at home, rather than in hospitals. The involvement of informal caregivers in the care has increased expediently to include the active treatment phase (either at home or in the hospital) where family caregivers are still required for daily care. Therefore, these informal caregivers are assuming major responsibilities for patients' care, and their essential role is one that can influence the quality of the care provided and the quality of life experienced by the patients. Furthermore, informal caregivers as the natural liaison with the healthcare setting are also taking the responsibility for the continuation of care at the home setting in a way that this is personalized and efficiently organized to achieve the best possible health outcomes. Progressively, as patients become unable to perform activities of daily living, informal caregivers need not only to assume disease-related responsibilities, including treatment management and symptom monitoring, but also to undertake additional assistance in activities of daily living.

A. Charalambous (✉)
Department of Nursing, School of Health Sciences, Cyprus University of Technology, Limassol, Cyprus

Department of Nursing Science, Faculty of Medicine, University of Turku, Turku, Finland
e-mail: andreas.charalambous@cut.ac.cy

The worldwide demographic changes project that the number of people aged 80 and above will triple over the next 30 years. As this age group of people tend to have an increased disease prevalence, there is a growing concern about expanding public expenditure on long-term care services in the future. Consequently, the policies of several countries have encouraged informal caregiving to reduce public healthcare spending, which has resulted in a shift in responsibilities for care away from the state and onto families and individuals. Thus, informal caregivers play a crucial role in supporting the health, well-being, functional independence, and quality of life of persons in long-term care.

2   The Concept of Efficiency

Healthcare is a complex investment that requires a number of direct and indirect stakeholders' contribution to produce the desired health outcomes. In addition to its complex nature, imperfect market in the field and limited/scarce resources for providing healthcare for population poses a number of questions for policy makers [1]. A report released by OECD in 2017 provides estimations on the wasteful expenditures within healthcare [2]. Based on the report, it is estimated that about one fifth of health spending across the OECD is wasted across three distinct types: wasteful clinical care, operational waste, and governance-related waste [3].

The impact of wasteful spending extends beyond that on the healthcare systems to include considerable and unnecessary costs for patients and their families in terms of lost time, anxiety and fear, impact on quality of life, and financial burden. Potentially, any ineffective interventions may also increase risk of harm and ultimately lead to poorer outcomes for patients [4].

The concept of efficiency is not new in the literature, and it refers to the relation between resource inputs (costs, in the form of labor, capital, or equipment) and either intermediate outputs (numbers treated, waiting time, etc.) or final health outcomes (lives saved, life years gained, quality-adjusted life years (QALYs)) [2]. Efficiency of organizations with multiple inputs and outputs such as hospitals can be calculated by weighed cost approach by dividing the weighed sum outputs with the weighed sum of inputs [3, 4]. Although many evaluations use intermediate outputs as a measure of effectiveness, this can lead to suboptimal recommendations. Ideally, economic evaluations should focus on final health outcomes [2].

There are two basic measures of efficiency: allocative and technical efficiency. Allocative efficiency (an economic concept) is about whether to do something, or how much of it to do, rather than how to do it. Allocative efficiency in healthcare is achieved when it is not possible to increase the overall benefits produced by the health system by reallocating resources between programs. This occurs where the ratio of marginal benefits to marginal costs is equal across all health care programs in the system [5]. Technical efficiency is about how best to achieve objectives. Strictly, technical efficiency is about ensuring the production of the same level of output with less of one input and no more of other inputs or, equivalently, maximizing the output that one gets from given quantities of inputs. Technical efficiency is linked to cost-effectiveness. The combination of technically efficient inputs that minimizes the cost of achieving a given level of output is that which is cost-effective [5].

In the context of efficiency within healthcare, the concept of productive efficiency should also be considered. Productive efficiency refers to the maximization of health outcome for a given cost, or the minimization of cost for a given outcome. In healthcare, productive efficiency enables assessment of the relative value for money of interventions with directly comparable outcomes [2].

3   Efficiency in the Context of Cancer

Although greater efficiency is needed across all disease areas, in cancer, this need is increasing becoming more urgent. This can be attributed partly to the growing prevalence of cancer, which in turn results in high expenditure. The economic burden that cancer poses on our society is staggering—25 million years of healthy life lost, at cost of 126 billion euros including 52 billion euros in lost productivity—and continues to grow with the aging of the population. It is imperative, in light of growing financial pressures on our healthcare systems, that we find ways to make the best use of available resources to deliver high-quality cancer care to patients [6]. In this context, decision-makers are increasingly faced with the challenge of reconciling growing demand for healthcare services with available funds, whereas economists argue that the achievement of efficiency from scarce resources should be a major criterion for priority setting [7]. However, other issues such as the significant variations in outcomes of care, the growing inequalities in access to care, and the financial toxicity for patients and their families should also be acknowledged as sources of concerns in the context of efficiency.

Based on the report "Towards sustainable cancer care: Reducing inefficiencies, improving outcomes" published by All.Can [8] efficient cancer care delivers the best possible health outcomes using the human, financial, infrastructural, and technological resources available, with a focus on what really matters to patients and society. Achieving greater efficiency requires putting patients at the center, promoting an evidence-based and data-driven learning system, investing in technology, breaking down silos, scaling up good practices, and implementing appropriate policies and incentives [8]. Compared to the definitions presented earlier, emphasis is now placed not only on costs but also on outcomes stressing the need for comprehensive data on outcomes as well as costs across the entire care pathway to underpin any efficiency effort and to guide decisions.

4   Informal Caregivers as Means of Efficiency

Taking as a point of reference the cancer efficiency definition provided by All.Can and utilizing the cancer paradigm as an exemplar, the role of the informal caregiver as a tool to promote efficiency will be demonstrated and discussed. The informal caregiver role has been extensively studied across various diseases and settings, demonstrating its potential, for example, in the care of community-dwelling dementia patients [9], in institutionalized long-term care-ILTC [10], older adults [11], and cancer patients [12, 13] in an effort to balance the detrimental effects of chronic illness on families. Even though the role of the informal caregiver (e.g., needs, preferences, tasks) has been studied across the disease continuum, there is scarcity of studies who explored the commonalities and the disparities of the role depending on the varying needs of the persons at the receiving end of the care (i.e., between diseases). Papastavrou et al. [14] in a cross-sectional, descriptive, and correlational study with 410 caregivers of patients with cancer, Alzheimer's disease, or schizophrenia explored the role across these three groups. The results indicated a high level of burden and depression among all informal caregivers. Significant differences ($P < 0.001$, $F = 26.11$) between the three caregiving groups were detected in terms of burden, with the highest reported for Alzheimer's disease caregivers. One-way analysis of variance showed significant differences ($P = 0.008$, $F = 4.85$) between the three caregiving groups in terms of depression, with the highest depression levels being for cancer caregivers. The study highlighted that the tasks that informal caregivers are assuming in varying disease diagnoses have significant commonalities although the level and the intensity of their efforts to accomplish these might vary. This is a finding that was also reflected in the differing levels of caregiver burden and depression reported by the authors.

However, systematically, it has been reported that the caregiving role (i.e., irrelevant of disease diagnoses and setting where care is provided) often entails assuming the responsibility for medical, physical, financial, and emotional needs of the care recipient [15]. These tasks often correlate to communicating with healthcare professionals, managing symptoms, administering medications, performing medical or nursing treatments, and handling patient behavioral problems and emotional reactions [16]. Additional tasks assumed by informal caregivers include the prioritization of home care demands, the reprioritization of responsibilities related to child care and employment, and the negotiation and renegotiation of factors related to familial and generational relationships [17, 18].

4.1   Putting Patients at the Centre of the Care…and Delivering Care That Really Matters to Patients

The literature includes several definitions of person-centeredness, but a universally agreed one is lacking [19]. The Institute of Medicine (IOM) defines patient-centered care as providing care that is respectful of, and responsive to, individual patient preferences, needs, and values and ensuring that patient values guide all clinical decisions [20]. Research by the Picker Institute has delineated eight dimensions of patient-centered care, including: (a) respect for the patient's values, preferences, and expressed needs; (b) information and education; (c) access to care; (d) emotional support to relieve fear and anxiety; (e) involvement of family and friends; (f) continuity and secure transition between healthcare settings; (g) physical comfort; and (h) coordination of care [21]. Despite the many definitions proposed in the literature, there is a set of common elements that can be identified, which include: (a) empowering and facilitating the person's participation in decision-making processes about their own care, and/or to manage their own health and care; (b) establishing an ongoing relationship between the professional, the person receiving care, and the informal caregiver, which is based on respectful communication and active listening; (c) having an understanding of the specific (health) concerns of the person and their individual needs and preferences; (d) addressing the physical, cognitive, psychological, and social domains of the person's life; and (e) providing coordinated care to achieve continuity and coherence of care and support [22, 23].

Based on what has been presented in chapter "Caregiving and Caregivers: Concepts, Caregiving Models and Systems" and the previous section on the type of tasks that informal caregivers assume across the disease continuum, there are a number of areas where these can support and facilitate the provision of person-centered care. A prominent area includes the activities supporting communication and information exchange between informal caregivers and professionals through various channels (e.g., home visits, phone calls, or e-mail contact). This communication is essential in conveying valuable information to professionals on the specific preferences and needs of the person in need for the care [24]. This can facilitate the provision of care that is tailored according to these needs and preferences and assure the continuation of the care when an institutional admission is required at times of disease exacerbations or disease-related complications. Similarly, informal caregivers being in a position of better knowing the person and having a trusting relationship, they have the potential to adjust the recommendations (i.e., health information) by professionals to best suit the needs of the person maintain and respecting his or her independence and facilitating their participation in decision-making [25].

Despite the potential of such professional and informal caregiver communication, this is not without its challenges. Blanck [26], in a qualitative study in Sweden, concluded that informal caregivers sought more contact with healthcare personnel and they wanted to receive information without repeatedly reminding the staff. Furthermore, the informal caregivers were also disconcerted because they did not receive timely and clear answers to their questions. Preceding studies identified further challenges including the difficulties in initiating the communication between professionals and informal caregivers as well as the presence of uncertainties about responsibility in collaborating and communicating with the informal caregiver [24]. Toscan et al. [27], Boros [28], and Buscher et al. [29] described a lack of communication in general between professionals and informal caregivers, which was insufficient and irregular. Smith [25] argued that improved communication between caregivers, their care recipients, and healthcare professionals has the potential to reduce confusion about care plans, decrease errors during the process of care, and reduce caregiver burden.

4.2   Efficient Cancer Care Delivers the Best Possible Health Outcomes (e.g. Continuation of Care)

Care transitions are described as the transfer of a patient between different settings and healthcare providers during the course of an acute or chronic illness. Care transitions are significant as they can often lead to fragmented care, decreased quality of care, and an increase in adverse events. These "vulnerable exchange points" may also contribute to high rates of health services and healthcare costs, which is often the case since care transitions from hospital to home continue to be poorly managed and pose a high risk for harm [30].

The caregiving role often entails managing symptoms, administering medications, assessing the response to therapeutic interventions, recognizing possible deteriorations in physical status, and performing medical or nursing treatments. These tasks demonstrate that the informal caregivers play an essential role in arranging and managing the continuity of care of the dependent person. An empirical qualitative case study by Willemse et al. [31] on informal caregivers in five European countries (Belgium, the Netherlands, Luxembourg, France, and Germany) demonstrated that caregivers to some extent provide personal care or support at home and ensure the continuity of care through coordination of formal care. The findings showed that informal caregivers preferred to do as much as possible without professional help. Finally, the informal caregiver was often the key person to provide care and coordination for the dependent elderly.

Similarly, Backman [30] in a qualitative descriptive study with patients and informal caregivers across selected Canadian provinces explored the role of informal caregivers during transitions from hospital to home. The researched concluded that engaging patients and their informal caregivers is an important strategy for examining care transition practices in order to facilitate the development of innovative solutions for safer care transitions between hospital and home. Specific areas of interest for successful transitions included providing appropriate communication between providers and patients/informal caregivers, providing discharge teaching and access to adequate resources needs, and empowering patients and informal caregivers in their care during the transition from hospital to home.

4.3   Efficient Cancer Care... with a Focus on What Really Matters to (Patients) and Society

Inefficient care in the context of the definition provided by All.Can can be related to the negative outcomes of caregiving, which in term can be the result of poor support provided to caregivers in performing their role. These negative outcomes can include caregiver burden, psychosocial burden, psychiatric morbidity, life changes, lower quality of life, and physical problems (e.g., sleep disturbances, fatigue, vulnerability to infections) to report a few. These outcomes can significantly have a negative impact on the ability of the person to maintain their social connections.

The challenges associated with informal care affect not only informal caregivers themselves but also society at large: intensive informal caregiving can result in higher demand and costs for healthcare as a consequence of its negative impact on the physical and mental health of caregivers, reduced labor market participation, and consequently higher risks of poverty and social exclusion. Social connections are key to maintaining positive emotional and physical health, while social isolation is associated with adverse mental health [32]. Therefore, the threats posed by informal caregiving can weakened or diminish these social connections with devastating consequences (e.g., loneliness and social isolation) for the person and the society. Loneliness and social isolation are increasingly recognized as important societal challenges beyond the context of informal caregiving.

Based on the caregiver stress model introduced by Pearlin et al. [33], caregiving can cover various stressors including caregiver burden. Depending on the coping resources, these stressors can also affect loneliness and social isolation [34]. Preceding studies highlighted the complex manifestations of informal caregiving on the social aspects of the person assuming the role and the wider societal effects including but not limited to loneliness and social isolation [35–37].

Social exclusion comprises a wide range of domains including limited or nonparticipation in economic, educational, political, and leisure or cultural activities and social relationships [37]. In the context of informal caregivers of people with dementia and mental illness, social exclusion can be conceptualized as a form of stigma, or as the result of stigma. Informal caregivers of people with mental health problems suffer social exclusion due to stigma by association [38], whereas others considered marginalization and isolation to be contributed to social exclusion [39].

Rokach et al. [40–42] also stated that the restriction of social contact caused by the provision of informal care can increase feelings of loneliness due to the caregiving burden, the absence of time for social engagement, and various negative feelings (e.g., resentment or guilt). Loneliness has been defined as "a discrepancy between one's desired and achieved levels of social relations" [43, p. 32], and this discrepancy may concern the number of relationships or the intimacy of the relationships [44].

Vasiliou et al. [45] acknowledged that significant life transitions that induce changes in one's existing or desired social relations and interactions as another factor that can precipitate the onset of loneliness. These life transitions within the context of informal caregiving also include the identity transitions that the person who is assuming the role is experiencing. The identity of caregiver is situated in the tacit, internal acknowledgement of the same self-identity—one can only be a caregiver, policies and services will only apply, and the role can only be relinquished if the caregiver identity is accepted and recognized by the caregiver themselves [46]. However, in the absence of external influence, family members might struggle to see their caring role as more than just an extension of their accepted familial position—thus the label of caregiver will be socially and externally constructed and the identity either accepted or rejected. O'Connor [47] considered this self-positioning to have important negative aspects. Once the label of caregiver is applied, previous identity labels of familial position (daughter, son, etc.) begin to wear away:

"caregivers experience the loss of their identity...and other personal and social identities are reduced as the demands of caring dominates their lives" [48, p. 253], raising "existential issues" for caregivers [48, p. 255].

At times of crisis, such as the SARS-CoV-2 pandemic when options of caregiving become somewhat limited, maintaining positive family relationships and social connections may be unattainable leaving caregivers experiencing significant levels of loneliness and social isolation [32]. In a sequential mixed-methods study with 82 informal caregivers, the researchers aimed to examine the effect of the COVID-19 pandemic on family caregivers' social connections. The researchers concluded that the loss of superficial, everyday social interactions negatively impacted mental health and coping as caregiving duties increased. Bristol stressed the high vulnerability of informal caregivers to changes in their social networks due to the emotional and instrumental support provided that previously offset the stresses of long-term caregiving.

5 Conclusion

Healthcare costs in most developed economies have grown dramatically over the last few decades, and it is widely believed that the inefficiency of healthcare institutions, at least in part, has contributed. Future projections foresee that healthcare systems around the world will continue in an increasingly way to emphasize on efficiency in the provided care. As a result of the wider transformation in healthcare, much emphasis has been placed on the care of patients by informal caregivers at the home setting. The role of the caregiver, although at first not believed to be closely related to efficiency in care, serves as a means to establish better efficiency through promoting person-center care, acting as liaison with healthcare providers and minimizing the societal impact of informal caregiving. However, to maximize the positive impact of informal caregiving on efficiency, the complexities of the role, need to be acknowledged, and informal caregivers must be appropriately and systematically supported.

References

1. Sorato MM, Asl AA, Davari M (2020) Improving health care system efficiency for equity, quality and access: does the healthcare decision making involve the concerns of equity? Explan Rev J Health Med Econ 6(1):45
2. OECD (2017) Tackling wasteful spending on health. OECD Publishing, Paris
3. Chalkidou K, Appleby J (2017) Eliminating waste in healthcare spending. Br Med J 356:j570
4. Wait S, Han D, Muthu V, Oliver K, Chrostowski S, Florindi F, de Lorenzo F, Gandouet B, Spurrier G, Ryll B, Wierinck L, Szucs T, Hess R, Rosvall-Puplett T, Roediger A, Arora J, Yared W, Hanna S, Steinmann K, Aapro M (2017) Towards sustainable cancer care: reducing inefficiencies, improving outcomes—a policy report from the All.Can initiative. J Cancer Policy 13:47–64
5. Palmer S, Torgerson DJ (1999) Economic notes: definitions of efficiency. BMJ 318(7191):1136. https://doi.org/10.1136/bmj.318.7191.1136

6. Chisholm DED (2010) Improving health system efficiency as a means of moving towards universal coverage. Background paper for world health report: health systems financing: the path to universal coverage. WHO, Geneva
7. Young J, Hulme C, Smith A, Buckell J, Godfrey M, et al. Health services and delivery research. Measuring and optimising the efficiency of community hospital inpatient care for older people: the MoCHA mixed-methods study. NIHR Journals Library
8. All.Can. Towards sustainable cancer care: Reducing inefficiencies, improving outcomes. Available at file:///C:/Users/andreas.charalambous/Downloads/AllCan-Policy-report_A4_Interactive_desktop.pdf
9. Ribeiro O, Brandão D, Oliveira AF, Teixeira L, Paúl C (2020 Aug) Positive aspects of care in informal caregivers of community-dwelling dementia patients. J Psychiatr Ment Health Nurs 27(4):330–341. https://doi.org/10.1111/jpm.12582
10. Metzelthin SF, Verbakel E, Veenstra MY, van Exel J, Ambergen AW, Kempen GIJM (2017) Positive and negative outcomes of informal caregiving at home and in institutionalised long-term care: a cross-sectional study. BMC Geriatr 17(1):232. https://doi.org/10.1186/s12877-017-0620-3
11. Bom J, Bakx P, Schut F, van Doorslaer E (2019) The impact of informal caregiving for older adults on the health of various types of caregivers: a systematic review. Gerontologist 59(5):e629–e642. https://doi.org/10.1093/geront/gny137
12. Ochoa C, Buchanan Lunsford N, Lee Smith J (2020) Impact of informal cancer caregiving across the cancer experience: a systematic literature review of quality of life. Palliative Supportive Care 18(2):220–240. https://doi.org/10.1017/S1478951519000622
13. Papastavrou E, Charalambous A, Tsangari H (2012) How do informal caregivers of patients with cancer cope: a descriptive study of the coping strategies employed. Eur J Oncol Nurs 16(3):258–263. https://doi.org/10.1016/j.ejon.2011.06.001
14. Papastavrou E, Charalambous A, Tsangari H, Karayiannis G (2012) The burdensome and depressive experience of caring: what cancer, schizophrenia, and Alzheimer's disease caregivers have in common. Cancer Nurs 35(3):187–194. https://doi.org/10.1097/NCC.0b013e31822cb4a0
15. Adejoh SO, Boele F, Akeju D et al (2021) The role, impact, and support of informal caregivers in the delivery of palliative care for patients with advanced cancer: a multi-country qualitative study. Palliat Med 35(3):552–562. https://doi.org/10.1177/0269216320974925
16. Wittenberg Y, Kwekkeboom R, Staaks J, Verhoeff A, de Boer A (2018) Informal caregivers' views on the division of responsibilities between themselves and professionals: a scoping review. Health Soc Care Community 26(4):e460–e473. https://doi.org/10.1111/hsc.12529
17. Cejalvo E, Martí-Vilar M, Merino-Soto C, Aguirre-Morales MT (2021) Caregiving role and psychosocial and individual factors: a systematic review. Healthcare 9:1690. https://doi.org/10.3390/healthcare9121690
18. Albini A. The case of the caregivers. CancerWorld. Available at https://cancerworld.net/the-case-of-the-caregivers/ (Shiell A, Donaldson C, Mitton C, et al. Health economic evaluation. J Epidemiol Commun Health 2002;56:85–88)
19. Scholl I, Zill JM, Härter M, Dirmaier J (2014) An integrative model of patient-centeredness - a systematic review and concept analysis. PLoS One 9(9):e107828
20. A New Health System for the 21st Century. Washington, DC: The National Academies Press; 2001. Committee on Quality of Health Care in America Crossing the Quality Chasm: Institute of Medicine (U.S.)
21. Davis K, Schoenbaum SC, Audet AM (2005) A 2020 vision of patient-centered primary care. J Gen Intern Med 20(10):953–957. https://doi.org/10.1111/j.1525-1497.2005.0178.x
22. Stoop A, Lette M, Ambugo EA et al (2020) Improving person-centredness in integrated care for older people: experiences from thirteen integrated care sites in Europe. Int J Integr Care 20(2):16. https://doi.org/10.5334/ijic.5427
23. Langberg EM, Dyhr L, Davidsen AS (2019) Development of the concept of patient-centredness - a systematic review. Patient Educ Couns 102(7):1228–1236
24. Hengelaar AH, van Hartingsveldt M, Wittenberg Y, van Etten-Jamaludin F, Kwekkeboom R, Satink T (2018 Jul) Exploring the collaboration between formal and informal care from the

professional perspective-a thematic synthesis. Health Soc Care Community 26(4):474–485. https://doi.org/10.1111/hsc.12503

25. Smith PD, Martin B, Chewning B et al (2018) Improving health care communication for caregivers: a pilot study. Gerontol Geriatr Educ 39(4):433–444. https://doi.org/10.1080/0270196 0.2016.1188810

26. Blanck E, Fors A, Ali L, Brännström M, Ekman I (2021) Informal carers in Sweden – striving for partnership. Int J Qual Stud Health Well Being 16:1. https://doi.org/10.1080/1748263 1.2021.1994804

27. Toscan J, Mairs K, Hinton S, Stolee P (2012) Integrated transitional care: patient, informal caregiver and health care provider perspectives on care transitions for older persons with hip fracture. Int J Integr Care 12:13

28. Boros AK (2010) Clinics and home-based care organisations: an interface between the formal and informal health sectors. Afr J AIDS Res 9:315–324

29. Buscher A, Astedt-Kurki P, Paavilainen E, Schnepp W (2011) Negotiations about helpfulness– the relationship between formal and informal care in home care arrangements. Scand J Caring Sci 25(4):706–715

30. Backman C, Cho-Young D (2019) Engaging patients and informal caregivers to improve safety and facilitate person- and family-centered care during transitions from hospital to home – a qualitative descriptive study. Patient Prefer Adherence 13:617–626. https://doi.org/10.2147/PPA.S201054

31. Willemse E, Anthierens S, Farfan-Portet MI et al (2016) Do informal caregivers for elderly in the community use support measures? A qualitative study in five European countries. BMC Health Serv Res 16:270. https://doi.org/10.1186/s12913-016-1487-2

32. Bristol AA, Mata AC, Mickens M et al (2021) "You feel very isolated": effects of COVID-19 pandemic on caregiver social connections. Gerontol Geriatric Med. https://doi.org/10.1177/23337214211060166

33. Pearlin LI, Mullan JT, Semple SJ et al (1990) Caregiving and the stress process: an overview of concepts and their measures. Gerontologist 30:583–594

34. Zwar L, König H-H, Hajek A (2020) Psychosocial consequences of transitioning into informal caregiving in male and female caregivers: findings from a population-based panel study. Soc Sci Med 264:113281

35. Brown RM, Brown SL (2014) Informal caregiving: a reappraisal of effects on caregivers. Soc Issues Policy Rev 8:74–102. https://doi.org/10.1111/sipr.12002

36. Broese van Groenou MI, De Boer A (2016) Providing informal care in a changing society. Eur J Ageing 13:271–279. https://doi.org/10.1007/s10433-016-0370-7

37. Greenwood N, Mezey G, Smith R (2018) Social exclusion in adult informal carers: a systematic narrative review of the experiences of informal carers of people with dementia and mental illness. Maturitas 112:39–45

38. van der Sanden RL, Stutterheim SE, Pryor JB, Kok G, Bos AE (2014) Coping with stigma by association and family burden among family members of people with mental illness. J Nerv Ment Dis 202(10):710–717

39. Daly L, McCarron M, Higgins A, McCallion P (2012) 'Sustaining place'—a grounded theory of how informal carers of people with dementia manage alterations to relationships within their social worlds. J Clin Nurs 22:501–512

40. Rokach A, Miller Y, Schick S, Bercovitch M (2014) Coping with loneliness: caregivers of cancer patients. Clin Nurs Stud 2:42

41. Rokach A, Rosenstreich E, Brill S, Aryeh IG (2016) Caregivers of chronic pain patients: their loneliness and burden. Nurs Palliative Care 1:111–117

42. Rokach A, Rosenstreich E, Brill S, Aryeh IG (2017) People with chronic pain and caregivers: experiencing loneliness and coping with it. Curr Psychol:1–8

43. Perlman D, Peplau LA (1981) Toward a social psychology of loneliness. In: Duck D, Gilmour G (eds) Personal relationships in disorder. Academic Press, London, pp 31–56

44. Dahlberg L, McKee KJ (2014) Correlates of social and emotional loneliness in older people: evidence from an English community study. Aging Ment Health 18(4):504–514. https://doi.org/10.1080/13607863.2013.856863
45. Konstantina V, Julie B, Manuela B, John V, Mark A, Shaun L, Michael W (2017) Experiences of loneliness associated with being an informal caregiver: a qualitative investigation. Front Psychol 8:585
46. Trees R (2019) Caring for the elderly – identity transitions in informal carers. Thesis or dissertation. Business School, The University of Hull
47. O'Connor D (2007) Self-identifying as a caregiver: exploring the positioning process. J Aging Stud 21(2):165–174
48. O'Shaughnessy M, Lee K, Lintern T (2010) Changes in the couple relationship in dementia care: spouse carers' experiences. Dementia 9(2):237–258

Caring for the Informal Carer: Coping in Caregiving

Elizabeth Hanson

1   Introduction

Despite the recent increased spotlight on the situation of informal carers afforded by the COVID 19 pandemic [1], it remains far from the case that informal carers are routinely recognized and supported in their role by health and social care practitioners [2]. Rather, support for carers still tends to be provided at a time of crisis and/or much later on when carers have been caring for an extended period of time, or alternatively not at all. As a result, when support is offered, it is often perceived by carers as being "too little, too late" [3]. The issue is also a complex one because many carers do not always see themselves as informal carers, but view their caring activities simply as a natural part of or extension of their relationship as partner, family member, relative, or friend to the person they are caring for [4]. Consequently, carers tend not to seek help and support at an early stage of their caring. Rather, their primary focus is often the health and well-being of the person they are caring for so that their own needs and goals are not prioritized or are put on hold indefinitely [5, 6].

In this chapter, several strategies for how front-line practitioners and representatives from civil societies can help to support and empower informal carers are presented. In particular, there are ways to enable those carers who wish to care to manage their individual caring situation, while maintaining their own health and well-being and pursuing their personal life goals. Also, to recognise how best to support a person who does not wish to take on board a caring role, or a carer who no longer wishes to continue in their caring role.

E. Hanson (✉)
Department of Health and Caring Sciences, Linnaeus University, Swedish Family Care Competence Centre, Eurocarers, Kalmar, Sweden
e-mail: elizabeth.hanson@lnu.se

© The Author(s), under exclusive license to Springer Nature Switzerland AG 2023
A. Charalambous (ed.), *Informal Caregivers: From Hidden Heroes to Integral Part of Care*, https://doi.org/10.1007/978-3-031-16745-4_5

2   Caring for the Carer: A Comprehensive Approach

As explained in the advocacy and policy perspective chapter (i.e., chapter "Informal Caregivers: The Advocacy and Policy Perspective"), caring for the carer at a societal (macro) level requires a comprehensive approach with a set of legislative rights and carer-friendly policies, which both support and empower people who wish to care for a relative/significant other with a long-lasting health and/or care need or disability. In the chapter "Informal Caregivers: The Advocacy and Policy Perspective", the example of the Eurocarers EU Carers Strategy "Enabling Carers to Care" is presented together with the ten steps required to bring out more carer friendly societies [7]. In the context of this chapter, all the ten steps are important for being able to provide a fully supportive and empowering environment for informal carers (see Table 1).

In the advocacy/policy perspective chapter (i.e., chapter "Informal Caregivers: The Advocacy and Policy Perspective"), the focus was mainly at the macro or societal level. In this current chapter, the focus is mainly at the individual (or micro) level in relation to the practitioner caring for the individual carer (and the care recipient) but also at a meso or organizational level concerning caring for carers as a group (albeit with individual needs and preferences), such as in a municipality, local authority, or health care region.

Table 1 The ten steps to ensuring more carer friendly societies

1. Define and acknowledge carers
2. Identify your carers
3. Assess the needs of your carers
4. Support multisectoral care partnerships for integrated and community-based care services
5. Facilitate carers' access to information and advice about care, caring, and care-life balance
6. Pay attention to carers' health and prevent negative health outcomes
7. Give carers a break
8. Provide carers with access to training and recognize their skills
9. Prevent carers' poverty and allow them to main an active professional/educational life
10. Adopt the carers' perspective in all relevant policies

3 Start by Carrying out a Holistic Carers Assessment

Crucial first steps for professionals and service providers working directly with informal carers are to identify informal carers in their health/social care/school setting/organization/context [8, 9] and to subsequently carry out a comprehensive carers' assessment as early as possible after their first contact with the carer [10]. An essential aspect of any holistic carers assessment is to enable the carer to reflect on their caring situation and to consider how they view their caring role [11, 12]. This can help the carer to better understand their situation and to be able to make a conscious decision (wherever feasible) as to whether or not to take on board a caring role in the first place, or if they genuinely wish to continue in a caring role or not. If they do, it is important for professionals/service providers to discuss with the carer about the type and intensity of the care they may wish to provide and to actively ensure the preferences of their relative/person close to them in need of care are taken into account. Clearly, the decision as to whether to take on board a caring role is not always feasible in situations where the relative/significant other has an acute illness/accident that results in them requiring care overnight, giving little if no time for an informed choice to take place [12]. However, being able to make an informed choice, wherever feasible, as early as possible can help the carer to make a decision about their caring role and subsequently to be offered timely support in their role [13].

As outlined in the introduction section above, when asked about their caring role, it is usual for a carer to reply that they don't consider themselves to be a carer and neither is it something that they generally stop and think about [4]. However, when given the opportunity to reflect on their caring role, some carers reply that they feel it's something perfectly natural and goes without saying to help care for a relative/someone close to them [14]. In this way, they tend to view caring as being a natural part or extension of their relationship as partner/spouse, relative or close friend, "*My Mum has helped me and done things for me all my life and now it's my turn to help her.*" However, it is important to highlight that not all carers feel this way and some carers also openly express that they felt obliged to take on board the role as carer [13], "*I felt I didn't really have any other choice but to care for my wife to be honest.*" Further, for those carers caring for someone with a more chronic, long-standing condition that develops gradually, carers describe their caring role as a gradual process—"*it crept up gradually on me really,*" "*I slipped sideways into caring*" [15].

An earlier study [15] highlighted that carers' personal beliefs about caring influenced their own subjective health and well-being. For example, those carers who felt that they didn't really have any choice but were obliged to care for their relative and that no one else either in their family/informal support network or from formal care providers could give the care that they gave and that they were alone in the care of their relative, appeared to experience poorer subjective health and perceived their caring to be burdensome for them. In contrast, those carers who perceived caring to be meaningful and felt that it gave them an aim in life and who felt that they could share the responsibility with others close to them and/or with formal service providers tended to experience better subjective health and well-being than those carers who perceived caring to be a burden [15].

Clearly, how caring for a relative or someone close is perceived varies from one person to another, and it is important to emphasize that there are no right or wrong beliefs or views. However, being aware of how a person views caring for a relative or someone close to them is an important first step for a carer to learn more about themselves in relation to their potential or actual caring situation and is likely to help them to make a choice about whether or not to take on a caring role or whether to continue in a caring role. It also represents an important aspect for practitioners to explore with potential carers and actual carers as early on as possible [10, 16].

Increasingly, carer research highlights that a comprehensive assessment that focuses on the carer's own goals and preferences both with regards to their caring situation and their life in general, together with those of the person they care for, is preferable to using a standard "tick box" type assessment guide where carers' needs tend to be fitted within existing standard carer support services [17]. Instead, a carer outcome-focused approach is recommended, which advocates for a more open, qualitative approach, which involves having a good conversation with carers about what matters most to them in the context of their whole lives, which subsequently informs the planning and implementation of support and services [18].

There are a wide variety of examples of carer assessment templates and frameworks currently in use by professionals and service providers. The framework by Nicholas [19, 20] has provided the basis for subsequent work that adopts a more carer-oriented outcomes approach. In her work, she identified four key domains for exploring with carers:

- A good quality of life for the care recipient
- A good quality of life for the carer
- Recognition and support in the caring role
- Service process outcomes

Subsequent researchers have used Nicholas' framework as the basis for their research and development work regarding carer assessments, together with carers themselves, professionals, and representatives from civil society (see Hanson et al. and Miller et al.,) [10, 18]. For example, The Carers Outcome Agreement Tool (COAT) [10] originally consisted of four sets of questionnaires and an action/evaluation plan for each of the questionnaires. The four questionnaires addressed the following domains:

- Helping you to care, which considered the type of help, information and skills that carers might need
- Making life better for you, which explored support that might improve the carer's quality of life
- Making life better for your relative, which explored what might improve the quality of life of the care recipient
- Getting good quality help, which considered what carers wanted from a quality service

Following completion of COAT, the carer and practitioner discuss a series of action plans and decide upon the type of support needed, who will provide it and when, the goals of the support, and when/how it will be evaluated [10, 11].

It is important to highlight that COAT can be used both at the individual (micro level) involving the individual carer and practitioner, and it can also be used at an organizational (meso) level to help develop carer support services. Firstly, at an organizational level, carrying out COAT assessments with a larger number of carers in participant municipalities in Sweden, enabled carer advocates (a dedicated role, involving direct support to individual carers and on a strategic level to develop carer support services at the municipality level) to easily identify carers' key preferences for support and thus target support services and further development of services in these specific areas. In some instances, a decision made with regard to carer support services was in direct contrast to the compiled expressed needs of carers who had undertaken a COAT assessment. For example, in one municipality, it was decided that carer benefit would be discontinued as it was seen to be tokenistic and only applied to a specific group of carers (predominantly older, retired spousal, high-intensity carers). However, from the compiled COAT data, financial support for carers was one of the most valued forms of support expressed by carers themselves. Carers explained that the benefit was of symbolic value, signaling that they were recognized and valued in their role, in addition to its economic value. They expressed feeling disappointed and "let down" when they heard that the carer benefit was planning to be discontinued. By presenting the compiled COAT data to decision-makers, the carer advocates were able to argue for the carers benefit to be continued in the municipality concerned.

An essential element of COAT, in keeping with an outcome-focused approach to carer assessment, and more broadly a partnership approach to working with carers, is that it builds on the strengths and resources of carers and importantly helps carers to identify these themselves, while addressing their goals for support. A key finding from our implementation work with COAT in several municipalities across Sweden was that it enabled practitioners to work in genuine partnership with carers [21].

Participant carers identified the following benefits:

- Allowed them to raise issues that were causing concern
- Helped them to discuss such concerns in an open and frank manner
- Provided new insights into their caring situation
- Helped them to focus on issues that they had not previously considered
- Helped to structure their discussions with practitioners
- Helped to validate their experiences as carers

Equally, practitioners also identified a number of benefits:

- All practitioners felt that COAT worked well in promoting a personal and detailed discussion about individual caring situations.
- Despite some practitioners having detailed prior knowledge of the caring situation, completing COAT provided new insights for many of them.

- Practitioners considered that COAT enabled them to get to know the carers well and provided a comprehensive view of the caring situation from the carers' perspective.
- COAT enabled carers to talk openly about their situation and helped them to focus on areas that they had not previously considered, such as their own quality of life and personal goals outside of their caring situation.
- The process of completing COAT allowed practitioners to begin to address some of the carers' concerns, for example, for further information.
- Completing COAT was seen by some as potentially therapeutic in its own right [21].

Carrying out a comprehensive carer assessment that builds on the carer's own outcomes enables the practitioner to sensitively explore with carers their motivations for caring or otherwise as openly as possible within the context of a trusting relationship. In this way, it is possible for the practitioners to identify those carers who genuinely wish to continue caring and discuss together the most appropriate forms of support to enable them to do so, while at the same time maintaining their own health and well-being [10]. Many carers who have been caring for several years have often learnt on a "trial-and-error" basis how best to care for their relative/significant other so that they have learnt how to carry out practical and personal caring tasks, including more complex medical or nursing procedures [12]. However, experienced carers may nevertheless require help with coping strategies and tips for how to best manage their caring situation, which in turn can help to reduce any stress or burden they may be experiencing [12]. In this next section, several coping strategies are highlighted that many carers themselves have expressed are useful to them in their individual caring situation.

4   Self-Care for the Carer

Experienced and former informal carers when they look back over their caring experiences may often express an important lesson learned, namely, no matter how difficult it may seem is the ability to make time to look after themselves as well as the person they are caring for, or as a carer aptly explained it *"putting on your own life vest first before you help your loved one."* As outlined earlier in the introduction section above, it is common for carers to put their own needs and life goals second or even on hold altogether to care for the person close to them, which in the long term can have negative consequences on their own health and well-being, in addition to their social situation, paid work situation (for carers of working age), financial situation, and overall quality of life and life goals [22].

The next section provides a description of the key coping strategies deemed to be useful by carers to enable them to be aware of and to look after their own health and well-being.

5   Coping Strategies

Historically and, even to some extent, to the present day, most of the research that has been carried out in the area of informal carers and caring tends to focus almost exclusively on the burdensome aspects of caring [23, 24]. That is, the negative and stressful aspects of caring. While it is important not to ignore or downplay the negative aspects of caring that are experienced by carers, especially those carers carrying out intensive amounts of caring and for a prolonged period of time, it is nevertheless increasingly acknowledged that having a sole focus on carer burden, in research, policy, and practice, may not necessarily fully address the entire caregiving experience [25, 26]. Furthermore, in practice situations, a sole focus on the burdensome aspects of caring may not be perceived by the carer to be so directly helpful for them either and may cause the carer to experience additional stress or discomfort, as the following carer anecdote highlights. An experienced spousal carer, in the context of a practice development project, was asked to complete a carer burden scale by giving a score from 1 to 10 as to her current level of burden, to which she aptly replied, *"It doesn't matter what number I write here because at the end of the day I still have to go home and look after my husband-just writing a high score just makes me feel more stressed."*

5.1   Maximizing the Positives and Minimizing the Negatives

In keeping with a partnership approach to working with informal carers, as well as exploring what carers perceive to be the difficult aspects of their caring situation, it is also important for practitioners to explore with carers what they perceive to be the satisfying aspects of caring, which help them to feel good about their caring experience and/or to find it meaningful [27]. Grant and Nolan [28] in their work with carers found that a key strategy for practitioners to use with carers who wish to continuing caring is to enable carers to maximize the positive or satisfying aspects of their caring situation. Equally, it is to help carers minimize the negative aspects of their caring situation, such as those activities that they don't enjoy carrying out or that they would prefer not to do at all. Common sources of satisfaction expressed by carers include the following examples:

- Caring has allowed me to develop new skills and abilities.
- Caring has brought me closer to the person I care for.
- I feel that if the situation were reversed, the person I care for would do the same for me.
- It's nice when something I do gives the person I care for pleasure.

Further examples, based on extensive interviews with carers, can be found in the Carers Assessment of Satisfactions Index (CASI) developed by Nolan, Grant, and Keady [16].

Having identified their personal sources of satisfaction in caring for their relative/significant other, a way of maximizing them is to encourage the individual carer to focus on these positive aspects of caring when thinking about their individual caring situation and when carrying out caring activities. It can also help to talk about the positive aspects with family members, friends, and practitioners. Carers often find that doing this helps them to boost their self-esteem and to feel good about their caring role and gives them more energy and helps them to feel well.

However, in some situations, carers may find that it is difficult or simply not possible to think of any positive or satisfying aspects of their caring role whatsoever. This is often a critical signal to the practitioner that the caring situation is most likely becoming burdensome and possibly unsustainable for the carer [12]. Further, they are approaching or are already experiencing a crisis or breaking point. In such situations, it is important for the practitioner to listen to both the carer and the care recipient and actively help with securing a prompt solution to the situation. This can mean for example, urgently securing additional sources of support (such as home help and home care nursing services, and/or from their own family and informal support network as appropriate) or alternative sources of support so that the carer can be relieved of their active caring role as appropriate–either for a shorter period of time (such as the care recipient receiving respite care) [29] or on a permanent basis (such as the care recipient entering residential care/nursing home or being cared for by another family member/significant other as appropriate) [30]. If the carer continues to be unsupported, it may, in extreme situations, lead to abuse of the care recipient by the informal carer [31].

Examples of the negative aspects of caring that carers may need help from practitioners/service providers to help minimize include the following:

– It (caring) can put a strain on family relationships.
– I sometimes feel helpless/not in control of the (caring) situation.
– The person I care for needs a lot of help with personal care.
– I can't have a break or take a holiday.

Further examples can be found in the Carers Assessment of Difficulties Index (CADI) also developed by Nolan et al. [16] and based on interviews with carers.

Discussing the difficulties of caring with someone who they trust and who understands them can often be a useful first step in the carer getting the actual help and support they need and prefer. It can involve talking with someone close to them, or it may involve talking with a practitioner or a member of a carer organization/ NGO. Subsequently, a practical way of helping the carer is for the practitioner or service provider to arrange with help with the aspects of caring the individual carer finds difficult and burdensome so that they can devote their time instead to maintaining their relationship with the person they care for (as a wife/husband, son/ daughter, etc.) and doing the caring activities they enjoy and consider meaningful and to be able to live their lives. This in turn can help the carer to feel well and can help those carers who wish to continue caring to sustain them in their caring role [32].

As can be seen in the above examples, the types of support offered to help minimize the negative aspects of caring vary according to the nature of the identified problem. The first two items above relate more to the emotional and psychological responses of the carer to their caring situation, which in turn is likely to require emotional support. For example, this can involve talking with someone understanding who the carer trusts and who genuinely listens to them; individual counselling and/or a carers support group. As well, it can involve cognitive skills training to help carers learn to re-frame their coping responses to their caring situation and to extend their coping repertoire, which can form part of a broader psychotherapeutic or psychosocial support intervention delivered in a variety of formats (online/face to face, individually/group, peer driven/professionally led) (see for example, González-Fraile et al. and Carretero, Stewart and Centeno) [33, 34]. In contrast, the third and fourth items relate to the need for more practical types of help and support, in the form of, for example, additional home nursing services and respite care services and/or additional help by family members/informal support networks as appropriate. This highlights the importance of tailoring the help and support to the individual carers' and the care recipients' preferences and goals [10].

An additional coping strategy commonly used by carers is to seek and gain reliable and accessible information about a range of supports available to them and the person they care for and to be able to accept help from others as described in the following section.

5.2   Information Seeking and Provision, Accepting Help from Others

Finding out what help and support is available from formal health and social care providers and from the voluntary sector is also a crucial first step for carers as it can help them to make an informed choice, together with the person close to them in need of care, as to whether to take on board a caring role or not and if so to avoid taking on board too onerous caring responsibilities that may negatively affect their own health and well-being and life goals [35]. The most common expressed need among carers irrespective of the health and/or care need of the care recipient is the request for information. Previous research has shown that for carers to know what help is available to them and who to contact in an emergency situation can help them and the person they care for to feel more secure in their caring situation [19].

However, many carers express that they do not always find it so easy or straightforward to access the information they require about the range of supports available to them [36], such as their legal rights (if existing in their particular country/region), financial benefits, "hands-on" skilled support with personal care activities and practical help around the home, the range of assistive devices and adaptations available to make caregiving more safe and secure at home and information about counseling services and education, and support groups available for carers and for the carer dyad, namely, the person with a health and/or care need and their informal carer [37].

In more recent years however, as highlighted in more detail in the chapter "The Use of Information and Communication Technology Among Informal Caregivers" focusing on technical solutions for carers, a growing number of targeted websites, online information hubs and online psycho-educational groups, and support programs have been developed and are available, some of which are dedicated to carers and a number that are directed mainly at the person with a health and/or care need or the carer dyad [38]. Nevertheless, not all carers have access to and/or are equipped with the digital skills necessary to benefit from available information and communication technology (ICT)-based services [39]. Thus, it is important that both formal health and social care providers and the voluntary sector continue to provide information in printed formats and verbally in one-to-one meetings and group sessions to avoid some carers and the person they care for being socially excluded from potentially useful sources of information to help them in their caring situation. Examples of groups of carers that are more likely to be at risk of social exclusion include the oldest old carers and more hard-to-reach groups of carers, such as carers from ethnic minority groups and carers living in rural areas where internet connection may be less than adequate or nonexistent and carers fleeing war and trauma.

It is also relevant to highlight that information giving by practitioners, carer organizations, and other civil societies about available support (among other topics) is not a "one-off" activity but rather is a continuous process where information is regularly updated to ensure it is current and relevant and that the most appropriate information is communicated effectively so that it matches or fits with the carer's own needs and preferences for information and their level of digital literacy [40]. Also, it matches with their particular phase of caring yet, at the same time, also enables them to plan ahead with the person they care for and those close to them for the potential future caregiving situation to reduce feelings of uncertainty or unpredictability among the carer and the person they are caring for [12].

In addition to information seeking by carers and information provision by practitioners and the voluntary sector, an equally relevant strategy highlighted by experienced informal carers is for carers to accept help from others, wherever possible and as soon as possible, to avoid or minimize potential carer fatigue and burden as outlined above in the earlier section above related to personal beliefs about caring [15]. An audit of the support system for carers in Sweden [41], which has a history of a generous welfare state provision for its citizens, highlighted that the best possible support for informal carers is a well-functioning health and social care system. In other words, when gaps exist in the formal health and social care systems, it is much more likely that informal carers, predominantly daughters, but also to some extent sons, step in and compensate, which often results in them reducing their hours of paid work to support and care for an aged parent/s for example. As explained earlier in the introduction to the policy and advocacy chapter (i.e., chapter "Informal Caregivers: The Advocacy and Policy Perspective"), many countries globally are experiencing cut-backs in formal long-term care provision, at the same time as there is an increased focus on integrated, people-centered health and care systems operating in the community. Thus, community-based and home-based long-term care services act as an essential form of support for carers, to prevent them from taking on onerous amounts of caregiving and to prevent carer burden and breakdown and to enable them to have a life outside of caring and for carers of working age to continue in paid work [42].

Indeed, regular, respite care services deemed to be of good quality by both the care recipient and the carer and provided in their own home or in the community (day center, institutional long-term care setting, such as a residential or nursing home) by the local municipality/authority or voluntary sector have long been recognized by carers' themselves as being essential to maintain their well-being [43, 44]. This is highly relevant for those carers providing intensive amounts of care and/or for a prolonged period of time.

In addition to community-based service provision, previous research highlighted that those carers with more extensive informal support networks consisting of wider relatives, friends, neighbors, and work colleagues are less likely to experience social isolation and, as a result, are able to feel well as they are able to share their caring tasks and activities with them, get a short break from caring, and receive emotional support from people they know well and trust [15, 45]. Findings from work with COAT (e.g., Hanson et al.) [21] highlighted that a number of carers when they carried out a COAT assessment found that they had not previously thought about asking a family member or neighbor for help for fear of being seen as a nuisance or potentially burdening them, as one carer expressed it "*I don't want to ask my adult kids as they have their own lives to lead.*" Nevertheless, after a more in-depth discussion with a practitioner, they often identified a person/s in their personal network who they felt they could ask for help and who would potentially genuinely enjoy being able to help. A word of caution is warranted here however as this example of support by the wider informal support network should not be taken to mean that asking a good neighbor or friend for help negates the need for formal support in any way, yet it enables the carer dyad to have a more extensive repertoire of people to draw from and thus avoid being isolated or alone in their caring situation.

Carers carrying out intensive amounts of caring for a prolonged period may express feelings of grief or regret over the fact that they haven't had the time and/or energy to keep up their relationships with those deemed important to them. They may also admit that their social life and social network have dwindled over time or that it is simply nonexistent [46]. Equally, they may express that they no longer have the opportunity to carry out their own favorite leisure activities or keep up their interests that they previously enjoyed doing, either on their own and/or together with the person they care for [47]. Carer research clearly reveals that those carers who can find a balance in providing care to their relative/significant other and find ways to keep up their relationships and interests are often better placed to feel well and maintain their health and well-being [7]. Carers of working age combining paid work with care of someone close to them can find it particularly challenging to find a suitable balance in their lives due to the challenges of combining paid work and caring tasks with possibly raising a family, causing them to have little time over for pursuing their hobbies/leisure activities [48]. Thus, a key task for practitioners and service providers working with carers is to provide or direct carers to both practical and emotional forms of support to enable carers to find a balance in their lives that feels right for them.

In the next section, the strategy of planning ahead in relation to the future caring situation is explained.

5.3   Planning Ahead

As a carer, it is not always at all so easy to be able to plan ahead and predict how their caring situation will look like in the future because they are often preoccupied with managing their current caring situation. However, research has highlighted that, wherever feasible, it can help with both increasing carers' sense of security and the predictability of their caring situation by planning ahead together with the person they care for, with family members and those closest to them, as well as with relevant practitioners [49, 50]. The amount and level of information required by the carer and care recipient in relation to the recipient's illness/disability, condition and prognosis, and treatment outcomes will vary from individual to individual. Nevertheless, the earlier a practitioner can initiate an open dialogue about the future with the patient/client/service user and their informal carer/s and those closest to them, the better the chances are of avoiding an acute situation from occurring without any emergency plans already being in place.

The subject of planning ahead is a topic that the practitioner or service provider may not always find so easy to broach with the carer and care recipient either. Nevertheless, opening up a dialogue about the future caring situation and making plans together can lead to a more in-depth understanding of the carers' and care recipients' needs and preferences, rather than leaving them to any second guessing later on by practitioners [51]. Being able to document about advanced care planning decisions and sharing the records with carers is also recommended as it can help to ensure an open and transparent communication with practitioners and service providers and to build and maintain trusting relationships with each other in keeping with a partnership approach [52]. This is especially the case in situations where the care recipient's cognitive status may progressively deteriorate as in the case of Alzheimer's disease, for example [53].

As outlined above, knowing who to contact in an emergency situation is important for carers. It can be of practical help for carers to make a list with the names and contact details of the relevant contact people/services in the event of an emergency in their mobile or another accessible place. Carers and care recipients expressed that having such a list made them feel more secure should a sudden and unexpected emergency situation occur. In addition, it was found to be useful within future care planning to include plans for what to do in the event that something unexpected should happen to the carer [21, 37]. Further, such future planning has been shown to relieve stress and anxiety, particularly in situations where a parent is caring for an adult son or daughter with a long-term illness or disability and where there is often a fear about what will happen if the parent carer/s should die before their adult child [54].

6 Conclusion

In this chapter, it is explained how practitioners and service providers can work proactively with informal carers, namely, by offering timely information, advice, and support to carers, in order to enable potential carers to make an informed choice about whether or not to take on board a caring role, together with the person close to them in need of care, and to enable those carers who wish to care to continue caring whilst maintaining their own health and well-being. A variety of strategies were highlighted that carers themselves have expressed are useful to enable them to care for the person close to them and, at the same time, to feel well and to pursue their goals in life. As shown in more detail in the chapter "Informal Caregivers: The Advocacy and Policy Perspective" on informal carers and the policy and advocacy perspective, these coping strategies are likely to be most successful when embedded in an integrated framework of support for carers.

References

1. Eurocarers/IRCCS-INRCA (2021) Impact of the Covid-19 outbreak on informal carers across Europe - final report. Eurocarers/IRCCS-INRCA, Brussels/Ancona
2. UNECE (2019) Policy brief: the challenging roles of informal carers. UNECE Policy Brief on Ageing 22
3. Jelley H, Kerpershoek L, Verhey F, Wolfs C, de Vugt M, Bieber A et al (2021) Carers' experiences of timely access to and use of dementia care services in eight European countries. Ageing Soc 41:403–420
4. Andréasson F, Andreasson J, Hanson E (2017) Developing a carer identity and negotiating everyday life through social networking sites: an explorative study on identity constructions in an online Swedish carer community. Ageing Soc 38(11):2304–2324
5. Ambugo E, De Bruin S, Masana L, MacInnes J, Mateu N, Hagen T et al (2021) A cross-European study of informal carers' needs in the context of caring for older people, and their experiences with professionals working in integrated care settings. Int J Integr Care 21(3):2
6. Clemmensen T, Lauridsen H, Andersen-Ranberg K, Kristensen H (2020) 'I know his needs better than my own' – carers' support needs when caring for a person with dementia. Scand J Caring Sci 35(2):586–599
7. Eurocarers. (2018) Enabling carers to care- an EU strategy to support and empower informal carers. Eurocarers, Brussels
8. Trust C (2018) Identification of carers in GP practices – a good practice document. Carers Trust, London
9. Carers Trust and the National Centre for Social Research (NatCen) (2019) Identification practice of young carers in England – review, tips and tools. Carers Trust, London
10. Hanson E, Nolan J, Magnusson L, Sennermark E, Johansson L, Nolan M (2006) COAT: the Carers Outcome Agreement Tool: a new approach to working with family carers: GRIP-report. University of Sheffield, Sheffield

11. Hanson E, Magnusson M, Nolan J (2008) Swedish experiences of a negotiated approach to carer assessment: the carers outcome agreement tool. J Res Nurs 13(5):391–407
12. Nolan M, Grant G, Keady J (1996) Understanding family care: a multidimensional model of caring and coping. Open University Press, Buckingham
13. Al-Janabi H, Carmichael F, Oyebode J (2018) Informal care: choice or constraint? Scand J Caring Sci 32(1):157–167
14. Committee on Family Caregiving for Older Adults. Board on Health Care Services (2016) Who is a family caregiver. In: Schulz R, Eden J, editors. Families caring for an aging America. Washington, DC
15. Erlingsson C, Magnusson L, Hanson E (2012) Family caregivers' health in connection with providing care. Qualitat Health Res J 22(5):640–655
16. Nolan M, Grant G, Keady J (1998) Carer's assessment of satisfaction index. APA PsycTests
17. Miller E, Seddon D, Toms G, Hanson E. Talking about what matters: a scoping review exploring outcome focused conversations with adult carers. Int J Care Caring (forthcoming)
18. Miller E (2011) Good conversations: assessment and planning as the building blocks of an outcomes approach. Joint Improvement Team
19. Nicholas E (2001) Implementing an outcomes approach in carer assessment and review. In: Qureshi H (ed) Outcomes in social care practice. SPRU, University of York, pp 65–119
20. Nicholas E (2003) An outcomes focus in carer assessment and review: values and challenge. Br J Soc Work 33:31–47
21. Hanson E, Magnusson L, Nolan M (2011) Using the ÄldreVäst Sjuhärad model to judge the quality of user involvement work within the COAT (Carers outcome agreement tool) implementation project. In: Rönnmark L (ed) Brukarens roll i välfärdsforskning och utvecklingsarbete, Vetenskap för profession 18:2011. Högskolan i Borås, Borås
22. Yeandle S (2016) Caring for our carers: an international perspective on policy developments in the UK. The Progressive Policy Think Tank
23. Hanson E, Yeandle S, Anderson R (2015) Eurocarers research priorities. Eurocarers, Brussels
24. Purkis M, Ceci C (2014) Problematising care burden research. Ageing Soc 35(7):1–19
25. Joseph S, Sempik J, Leu A, Becker S (2020) Young carers research, practice and policy: an overview and critical perspective on possible future directions. Adolescent Res Rev 5:77–89
26. Roth DL, Fredman L, Haley WE (2015) Informal caregiving and its impact on health: a reappraisal from population-based studies. Gerontologist 55(2):309–319
27. Nolan M, Lundh U, Grant G, Keady J (eds) (2003) Partnerships in family care : understanding the caregiving career. Open University Press, Maidenhead
28. Grant G, Nolan M (2007) Informal carers: sources and concomitants of satisfaction. Health Soc Care Community 1(3):147–159
29. Plöthner M, Schmidt K, de Jong L, Zeidler J, Damm K (2019) Needs and preferences of informal caregivers regarding outpatient care for the elderly: a systematic literature review. BMC Geriatr 19(1):82
30. Wolff JL, Mulcahy J, Huang J, Roth DL, Covinsky K, Kasper JD (2018) Family caregivers of older adults, 1999-2015: trends in characteristics, circumstances, and role-related appraisal. Gerontologist 58(6):1021–1032
31. NVKG (2020) Elder abuse and abuse by informal carers: Nederlandse Vereniging voor Klinische Geriatrie (NVKG)
32. Nolan M, Grant G, Keady J (1998) Assessing the needs of family carers – a guide for practitioners. Pavilion Publishing, Brighton
33. Carretero S, Stewart J, Centeno C (2015) Information and communication technologies for informal carers and paid assistants: benefits from micro-, meso-, and macro-levels. Eur J Ageing 12(2):163–173
34. Gonzalez-Fraile E, Ballesteros J, Rueda JR, Santos-Zorrozua B, Sola I, McCleery J (2021) Remotely delivered information, training and support for informal caregivers of people with dementia. Cochrane Database Syst Rev 1:CD006440
35. NICE (2020) Guideline supporting adult carers 1.1 information and support for carers: overarching principles: NICE National Institute for Health and Care Excellence

36. Meyer K (2017) Carers' experiences accessing information on supports and services: learning the social care "dance". Qual Soc Work 17(6):832–848
37. Magnusson L (2005) Designing a responsive support service for family carers of frail older people using information and communication technology [Doctoral thesis]. Göteborgs Universitet, Göteborg, Studies in educational sciences 231
38. Eurocarers (2016) Information and Communication Technology (ICT) for carers. Eurocarers, Brussels
39. Barbabella F, Poli A, Hanson E, Andréasson F, Salzmann B, Döhner H et al (2018) Usage and usability of a web-based program for family caregivers of older people in three European countries: a mixed-methods evaluation. Comput Inform Nurs 36(5):232–241
40. Efthymiou A, Middleton N, Charalambous A, Papastavrou E (2021) Identifying the carers' profiles of health literacy, eHealth literacy and caregiving concepts. 14th European Public Health Conference; Virtual
41. Swedish National Audit Office SNAO (2014) Support for carers (RiR 2014:9). Summary in english: SNAO
42. Eurocarers. (2017) The impact of caregiving on informal carers' mental and physical health. Eurocarers, Brussels
43. Hanson E, Tetley J, Clarke A (1999) Respite care for frail older people and their family carers: concept analysis and user focus group findings of a pan-European nursing research project. J Adv Nurs 30(6):1396–1407
44. Zarit S (2015) Benefits of respite for carers' health: findings from the DaSH Study. Presented at the 6th International Carers Conference Gothenburg, Sweden, September 2015
45. Ramli A, Zailly F (2013) Extended family, neighbourhood and friends' network in supporting caregivers of older people with mental health problems. J Pembangunan Sosial (JPS) 16:127
46. Hajek A, Kretzler B, Konig HH (2021) Informal caregiving, loneliness and social isolation: a systematic review. Int J Environ Res Public Health 18(22)
47. Andréasson F (2021) Doing informal care: identity, couplehood, social health and information and communication technologies in older people's everyday lives. Linnaeus University Dissertations, Linnaeus University
48. Spann A, Vicente J, Allard C, Hawley M, Spreeuwenberg M, de Witte L (2020) Challenges of combining work and unpaid care, and solutions: a scoping review. Health Soc Care Community 28(3):699–715
49. Archbold PG, Stewart BJ, Miller LL, Harvath TA, Greenlick MR, Van Buren L et al (1995) The PREP system of nursing interventions: a pilot test with families caring for older members. Preparedness (PR), enrichment (E) and predictability (P). Res Nurs Health 18(1):3–16
50. McIlfatrick S, Doherty LC, Murphy M, Dixon L, Donnelly P, McDonald K et al (2018) The importance of planning for the future': burden and unmet needs of caregivers' in advanced heart failure: a mixed methods study. Palliat Med 32(4):881–890
51. Wendrich-van Dael A, Bunn F, Lynch J, Pivodic L, Van den Block L, Goodman C (2020) Advance care planning for people living with dementia: an umbrella review of effectiveness and experiences. Int J Nurs Stud 107:103576
52. Brazil K, Carter G, Cardwell C, Clarke M, Hudson P, Froggatt K et al (2018) Effectiveness of advance care planning with family carers in dementia nursing homes: a paired cluster randomized controlled trial. Palliat Med 32(3):603–612
53. Dening K, Sampson EL, De Vries K (2019) Advance care planning in dementia: recommendations for healthcare professionals. Palliat Care 12:1178224219826579
54. Greenwood N, Pound C, Brearley S (2019) 'What happens when I can no longer care?' Informal carers' concerns about facing their own illness or death: a qualitative focus group study. BMJ Open 9(8):e030590

Informal Caregivers and Health Literacy

Areti Efthymiou and Evridiki Papastavrou

1 Introducing Health Literacy and eHealth Literacy

Literacy is defined as an ability to identify, understand, explain, create, and calculate verbally and in written form; is considered a process of learning assisting in the accomplishment of set goals [1]. In 1965, almost 50% of the world population was considered illiterate [2]. More recently, data from the Survey of Adult Skills, part of the Programme of the International Assessment of Adult Competencies, reported that 20% of adults performed in the lowest level of literacy and numeracy [3]. Different types of literacies have been defined in the literature, with all having a common basis, the traditional literacy of being able to read, write, and calculate [4–6]. Health literacy has received many different definitions, over 200, and requires a set of literacies such as traditional, cultural, scientific, and informational [7]. Nutbeam proposed a health promotion model with health literacy as a health promotion outcome and health education as a health promotion action [8]. Three types of literacies were distinguished according to Nutbeam: functional (basic skills of reading and writing), communicative (cognitive, social, and literacy skills facilitating social participation, accessing and interpreting information), and critical literacy (advanced skills promoting critical thinking) [8]. According to a more recent definition by Soerensen et al. [9], health literacy is considered the combination of

A. Efthymiou (✉)
Research fellow, Quality of Life Lab, Hellenic Mediterranean University, Heraklion, Crete, Greece

Department of Nursing, Cyprus University of Technology, Limassol, Cyprus
e-mail: aefthymiou@hmu.gr

E. Papastavrou
Department of Nursing, Cyprus University of Technology, Limassol, Cyprus
e-mail: e.papastavrou@cut.ac.cy

A. Charalambous (ed.), *Informal Caregivers: From Hidden Heroes to Integral Part of Care*, https://doi.org/10.1007/978-3-031-16745-4_6

motivation, knowledge, and skills for accessing, assessing, and applying health-related information and decisions related to all aspects of health (healthcare, disease prevention, and health promotion). This definition was adopted by the World Health Organization in 2013 [2, 10]. In the last 20 years, research in this field has grown, and governments promoted policies to enhance the citizens' health literacy level [3, 11]. The Healthy People 2030, an initiative started in 1979 in the United States, is considered the most recent example of policies promoting health literacy and organizational health literacy, the most recent trend in this field. Health Literate Organizations need to comply with ten core attributes making health services accessible to different populations with different levels of health literacy and cultural and linguistic backgrounds [12]. Health literacy skills do not include only the skills of reading and understanding a medical leaflet or making a doctor's appointment as most people may think. Higher level of health literacy is associated with better medicine adherence, an overall better management of disease, and lower costs for the healthcare system [4, 5]. Limited health literacy is associated with lower socio-economical status, decreased social support, lower level of education, higher use of healthcare services, poorer physical and mental health, longer stay in hospitals, poorer self-care, more hospital admissions, and lower quality of life [13–18].

Many different tools have been developed to assess health literacy levels, objective (functional) and subjective, generic, and condition-specific [19, 20]. The most widely used tools are the Test of Functional Health Literacy in adults (TOFHLA), the S-TOFHLA (short version of TOFHLA), and the Rapid Estimate of Adult Learning in Medicine (REALM), which are available in English and Spanish. TOFHLA is a measure of functional health literacy, which discriminates people in three categories: adequate, marginal, and inadequate literacy [21]. REALM uses health-related words that progressively become harder to pronounce [22]. Another widely used instrument is the Newest Vital Sign (NVS), including six items to assess reading and comprehension of an ice cream nutrition table [23]. These three instruments are considered functional measures as they assess the health literacy skills directly. One of the most widely used subjective measure of health literacy is considered the Health Literacy Survey-Q47 (available in shorter versions of 16, 12, and 6 items) and widely validated to many languages and different populations, including informal caregivers [24, 25]. The HLS-EU-Q47 has four scoring categories: inadequate, problematic, sufficient, and excellent. In the research focusing on informal caregivers of people with dementia, HLS-EU-Q16 was validated extracting five factors (see Fig. 1):

1. Health Promotion. Health promotion included five items regarding risk factors, health screenings, activities for mental well-being, family advice, and everyday behavior related to health. Health promotion could be considered as the means to promote health literacy [18].
2. Media Literacy. Media health literacy was not provided by the HLS-EU framework and included digital and nondigital media. Mistrust of information provided by the media was revealed from this validation [18].

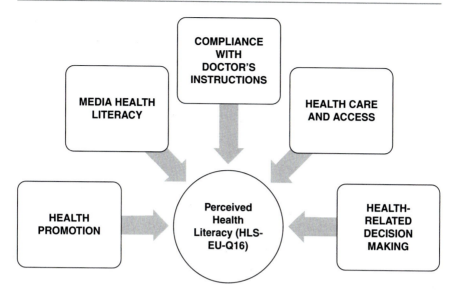

Fig. 1 Five factors of the HLS-EU-Q16 in a sample of informal caregivers of people with dementia (Copyright Efthymiou, A., 2020)

3. Compliance with doctor's instructions. Compliance with doctor's instructions dimension included three items: understanding doctor's spoken and written language, doctor's instructions, and to follow them. The term compliance is an older term used to describe a more paternalistic and passive acceptance of the health professionals' directions and sometimes interchangeably used with the term adherence [18].
4. Health care and access of information. The two first items of the questionnaire, concerning the skills to find information on treatments and the professional help somebody may require, were grouped and included the access component to information regarding health care [18].
5. Health-related decision-making. This domain included three final of deciding to visit a second doctor for a further opinion, making decision on illness based on the information provided by the doctor and finding information to manage mental health problems. Health-related decision-making may be negatively connected with compliance with the doctor's instructions [18].

1.1 eHealth Literacy

With technological advances, another term has gained attention in the last 10 years, the "*e*" dimension of health literacy, integrated in media literacy. eHealth literacy included, based on the lily theory, different types of literacies, traditional, health, informational, scientific, media, and digital [26]. Chan and Kaufman [27] were based on Norman's and Skinner's Lily model and added to the model Bloom's taxonomy of educational objectives forming a model of 36 categories. The use of reading, information, and digital literacy are the most used types when completing a task [27]. Norman's and Skinner's model had limitations that they themselves recognized, focusing on the difficulty to integrate the in-progress technological advances such as web 2.0 [28]. Other researchers expanded the model including the skill to identify and communicate a health issue, the cultural and the moral literacy or focused on specific populations, for example, older adults [29, 30]. eHealth literacy research speeded up the pace during the last 5 years, with researchers focusing on the measurement of this concept and more recently due to the COVID-19 pandemic, focusing on the way that social media is a source of health-related information [31].

There is a lack of eHealth literacy measures. The most frequently used instrument is considered the eHeals by Norman and Skinner [32]. The specific instrument has received critique by other researchers [33] and even by Norman [28]. In a recent review of eHealth literacy measures [34], seven measures were identified: eHeals, eHeals-extended version, eHealth Literacy Scale, eHealth Literacy Questionnaire, and the transactional eHealth literacy instrument. The eHeals was used in many different populations and was adapted for informal caregivers (eHeals-Carers) [35]. The eHeals version for informal caregivers included two core factors: information seeking and information evaluation with internal consistency over 0.77 [35] (Table 1).

Table 1 eHeals-Carers items

	Information seeking
	Information seeking
Q1	"I know what resources/information are available on the Internet concerning the health and caregiving issues of my friend/relative (practical, financial, legal issues, information about the disease and available services)"
Q2	"I know where to find helpful information on the Internet concerning the health and caregiving of my friend/relative (e.g., which websites I will search)"
Q3	"I know how to find helpful information on the internet concerning the health and caregiving of my friend/relative (e.g., concerning the process: Google search)"
Q4	"I know how to use the Internet to answer my questions about the health and caregiving of my friend/relative (e.g., how to ask in order to receive a proper reply to my question)"
Q5	"I know how to use the information about the health and caregiving of my friend/relative I find on the Internet to help me (practical, financial, legal issues, information about the disease and available services)"
	Information evaluation
Q6	"I have the skills I need to evaluate the resources/information I find on the Internet concerning the health and caregiving of my friend/relative"
Q7	"I can tell high-quality resources/information from low-quality resources/information on the Internet concerning the health and caregiving of my friend/relative"
Q8	"I feel confident in using information from the Internet to make decisions concerning the health and caregiving of my friend/relative"

2   Health Literacy Levels Among Informal Caregivers

A caregiver could be defined as a person (family, friend, neighbor), living together, in another household or caring from a distance, mostly providing unpaid care to someone in need [36–38]. More than one person usually cares for a person with dementia. There is a term that we find infrequently in research "secondary informal caregiver," without an agreed definition. In one case, the term is defined as the person who is the second most responsible carer [39] and in other study is defined as the person who provides support to the primary carer [25].

Informal caregivers need to make multiple decisions everyday from the start of their journey on behalf of or in collaboration with their relative in need [40]. They provide care, monitor and manage disease symptoms, communicate with the healthcare professionals, and decide if they trust the healthcare professionals [40]. Caregivers search for information and services available from multiple sources, associations, healthcare professionals, social media, websites, and platforms, and in many cases, the information provided is not tailored and does not cover their needs [41, 42].

Based on the findings of a recent scoping review [43] during the period 2003 to 2015, in half of the studies using levels (6/12) as the scoring method, the low health literacy ranged from 0% to 42.9% for the informal caregivers of adult care-recipients, and in five studies using the average score, informal caregivers reported adequate levels of health literacy [18]. Comparison between formal and informal caregivers is found only in one study with no statistical differences in health literacy scores [44]. High level of health literacy was confirmed in studies with convenient samples of informal caregivers of people with dementia in Greece and Cyprus [25] and in Norway [45]. The level of health literacy was measured in two studies with the use of Health Literacy Survey, 16 items questionnaire (HLS-EU-Q16), and Health Literacy Scale, Norwegian translation of 12 items (HLS-N-12) irrespectively. The methodological issues usually encountered in the studies complicates the interpretation of the results. Informal caregivers' health literacy has been studied among caregivers of older people with memory problems, with heart failure, oncology patients, palliative care patients, and patients with diabetes [46–52]. The studies used different study designs (quantitative or qualitative), different measures, and small samples, making conclusions difficult. Most of the studies found an adequate level of health literacy among informal caregivers with high knowledge of the disease and a different level of health literacy among informal caregivers and patients, with informal caregivers usually reporting a higher level of literacy than the patients [25, 46, 48–50, 53, 54]. Age and informal caregivers' kinship were frequently related to health literacy level, but this is not always the case for education [43]. Memory loss, older age, lower cognitive functioning and working memory, and level of education seem to predict limited health literacy [49].

In the case of informal caregivers of people with dementia, recent literature suggested that informal caregivers had a high level of health literacy and eHealth literacy as it was measured with the HLS-EU-Q16 and eHeals-Carer, with advanced knowledge, understanding of the disease and the procedures of care, and skills to search dementia-specific information [25, 55]. This was confirmed for the informal caregivers of people with schizophrenia, measuring mental health literacy [54]. Most recently, a study on paid caregivers (outpatient caregivers) during the COVID-19 pandemic suggested a sufficient level of health literacy as measured with HLS-EU-Q16 [56].

3 Why Health Literacy Is Important: Health Literacy and Caregiving Variables

Caregiving includes many different dimensions. In this subsection, we will focus on the association of self-efficacy, coping strategies, social support, and health literacy.

3.1 Health Literacy and Self-Efficacy Among Informal Caregivers

In a systematic review [57], self-efficacy among informal caregivers seemed to be associated with the health-related quality of life with a low to medium effect size. Higher self-efficacy was associated with more positive aspects of caring (gain, satisfaction, rewards, mastery) [57]. Higher self-efficacy of controlling upsetting thoughts about caregiving (e.g., thinking about negative aspects of caring, worrying about caregiving) and managing behavioral disorders in dementia (e.g., repeating questions, complaining, anxiety, attachment to informal caregiver) were related to the positive aspects of caregiving. Low self-efficacy of obtaining respite (e.g., asking a friend or family to undertake caring tasks and stay with the patient) was associated with burden and depression [58]. Symptom management self-efficacy acted as a mediator in the relationship between neuropsychiatric symptoms of dementia, burden, and depression and predicted the caregiver's burden and depression [59]. Mastery and self-efficacy mediated in the association of stress levels among a sample of informal caregivers and depression [60].

Higher levels of health literacy and eHealth literacy were associated with higher scores in caregiving self-efficacy for obtaining respite and behavior management in a study with informal caregivers of people with dementia from Greece and Cyprus [25].

Limited health literacy was associated with lower parental self-efficacy [61], and in four studies, the mediating role of self-efficacy was reported; on the association of health literacy and the compliance with physical activity guidelines [62], on health literacy and poorer physical and mental health [14], on maternal health literacy and early parenting practices [15], and on numeracy and diabetes medication adherence [63].

3.2   Health Literacy and Coping Strategies Among Informal Caregivers

Researchers through the years have developed models to interpret people's coping behaviors. In Perlin's model, there are three types of coping strategies: problem-focused, emotion-focused, and meaning-focused. According to Pearlin [64], coping is defined as *"the things that people do to avoid being harmed by life-strains...any response to external life strains that serves to prevent, avoid, or control emotional distress."* The coping process is multidimensional; includes *"behaviors, cognitions, and perceptions;"* and has three functions *"management of the situation, management of the meaning and management of stress symptoms"* [64]. Perlin and Schooler discussed the coping efficacy meaning how effective the selection of a person's coping strategies is on the stress that derives from a situation. *"Effective coper"* is the person that feels no stress even in the most severe life situations. When a person has control over a role (e.g., family role), it is more effective to follow a problem-focused strategy. In the case where personal control over a role is lower (work, finances), the person may adopt emotion-focused or meaning-focused strategies, which reappraises the situation. In some cases, there are the so-called compensatory coping, when after reappraisal, the person may proceed to a problem-focused strategy to reinvest [65].

In the context of coping strategies in association with health literacy, in one study, the association between adjustment and caregiving experiences of informal caregivers of people with mental health disorders was reported [66]. Primary and secondary control engagement were the two dimensions of coping. Poorer adjustment was associated with disengagement. Life satisfaction was associated with secondary control engagement and caregiving confidence with primary control engagement [66]. In the case of informal caregivers of people with dementia, coping strategies were measured with brief-COPE, and lower levels of health literacy and eHealth literacy were associated with problematic coping and negative attitudes toward caring [25].

3.3   Health Literacy and Social Support Among Informal Caregivers

Human relationships play a crucial role in well-being and quality of life. Social support can be distinguished in tangible support, emotional support, or affirmation. The association of social support with health is well documented [67]. Depression, reduced immunological function, coronary heart disease, blood pressure, biological aging, and substance abuse have been documented to be related to lower levels of social support. Social support acts protectively to the life-threatening events during our lifetime, as it moderates the effects according to Cobb [68]. According to Thoits, the type of support affects the health outcomes: tangible support and emotional support (love, care, sympathy) seemed to be most effective for our health [69].

As part of the social networks' theory, Antonucci presented the Convoy model and discussed the importance of relationships through the lifetime of a person and personal and situational factors that influence these relationships [70]. The social networks are a protective net that promotes health (physical and mentally) and change as the person grows and changes, involving or excluding people based on the circumstances. As the person ages, the closest relationships of a person's social ties remain the same, even if the total number of relationships decreases. People with more extensive social networks have higher chances of receiving home care at a later age. The structure, access, and availability of the members in the network can be a predictor for potential informal caregivers and is differentiated from northern-western to southern-eastern European countries based on the familial model [71]. In Eastern countries, an extended family network can predict the informal care provision, but in the case of Northern countries, only the close partner is a predictor of informal care. Fernandez-Carro and Vlachantoni [72] identified the role of social networks taking into consideration the three models of care: Scandinavian, Continental, and Mediterranean. In another study from Spain representing the Mediterranean care model, by Serra et al., resilience and social support are protective factors of abuse to PwD and confirmed the mediating role of the burden for the association of social support and abuse [73]. In a cross-sectional study among Chinese informal caregivers of people with Alzheimer's disease, social support seemed to have a moderating effect on the way patient's cognitive impairment and depression associated with informal caregivers' burden. Informal caregivers with low social support express higher levels of burden because of disease progression and depression [74]. The social network received support and negative interactions were associated with self-rated health among informal caregivers, and informal caregivers' burden acts as a mediator in this relationship [75].

Health literacy and productive ageing were associated with social support in a sample of 992 older adults [76] and with positive impact on physical health of older adults [77]. Health literacy was associated to social support in a sample of informal caregivers of people with dementia [78]. Three profiles were identified in relation to the level of health and eHealth literacy of informal caregivers of people with dementia [79]: (1) informal caregivers with a high level of health and eHealth literacy and higher caregiving self-efficacy, (2) limited health and eHealth literacy and problematic coping, and (3) informal caregivers with a high level of health and eHealth literacy and strong social support and quality of support [18].

3.4   Interventions to Enhance Health and eHealth Literacy of Informal Caregivers and Health Care Professionals Working with Older People and Their Families

Interventions aiming at enhancing health literacy could be categorized as interventions focusing on enhancing health literacy, interventions tailored to the health literacy levels, and interventions aiming at promoting health outcomes [80].

Only recently do we find interventions directly targeting the informal caregivers' health literacy and eHealth literacy. In the last 4 years, European-funded projects are aimed in this direction. For example, the European-funded project eLILY aimed to provide a blended training program (face-to-face and eLearning course) for informal caregivers of frail older people and PwD based on Lily theory model developed by Norman and Skinner [26], integrating dimensions by Chan and Kaufman [27, 29] and Gilstad [29]. Five institutions from five countries participated (Poland, Cyprus, Greece, Italy, Bulgaria). The methodology followed included health and eHealth literacy survey on the existing policies in partners' countries, development of the step-by-step guide of the curriculum including six modules, a Delphi survey with informal caregivers, content development, and pilot testing.

The final contents included four core modules for informal caregivers of older people:

1. Module 1 Health literacy and communication skills. This module aimed to assist informal caregivers communicating effectively with physicians. It introduced health literacy concepts and provided the necessary information that health professionals required from the patients. The dimensions of burden and emergency needs were explained.
2. Module 2 Digital literacy. This module focused on the use of tablet and smartphones, providing the basic skills for their use. Informal caregivers in this module understand how to safely search online protecting their privacy.
3. Module 3 eHealth literacy, an introduction to selected sources. This module introduced the concept of eHealth literacy to informal caregivers, providing guidelines on the proper search of health information.
4. Module 4 Use of interactive services. The final module focused on the social media use. In this module, informal caregivers learned the different types of social media and understood how to use and assess health information available on social media.

Following this work, eLILY2 extended the work to nursing students and nurses working with older adults. The consortium this time included partners from Greece, Czech Republic, Lithuania, and Poland and was coordinated by partner from Cyprus. The blended course in this second European-funded project included four modules targeting nurses working with older adults and their families:

1. Module 1 Introduction to health literacy and eHealth literacy. This module introduced nurses and nursing students to the concepts of health and eHealth literacy and ways to assess online information.
2. Module 2 Patients with limited health literacy. In this models, nurses and nursing students focused on communication skills with older adults and their families, introducing concepts, for example, "Teach-Back" method and AskMe3.

3. Module 3 Feasibility and readability issues and eHealth challenges. This module focused on the assessment of written materials for older people and provided guidelines for clear communication in written language.
4. Module 4 Health literacy and patient safety. This module focused on medication adherence and ways to promote the use of new technologies, for example, apps.

Another study on informal caregivers of patients with multiple sclerosis used a randomized design to assess the impact of the family-centered empowerment program for health literacy and efficacy in a sample of 70 informal caregivers [81]. The model followed four phases: increasing knowledge on the disease, managing challenges and stress, increasing self-efficacy with the use of problem-solving strategies, providing information, and becoming a trainer for the patient and the final phase, evaluating the process.

4   Conclusion

Informal caregivers make health decisions for their own health and their relative's health. Health and eHealth literacy could act as an umbrella supporting these choices and facilitating caregiving. The informal caregivers' health literacy and eHealth literacy level is differentiated according to cultural, educational, and socioeconomical background and study designs, and more research is necessary to assess it. Future research could work in three pillars:

1. The development of disease-specific literacy scales. Disease-specific literacy scales could facilitate the work of healthcare professionals and healthcare services working with caregivers and patients with chronic diseases.
2. Healthcare services assisting caregivers need to adapt to a health and eHealth literacy-friendly policy, assisting informal caregivers by providing them all the necessary information and promoting caregivers' health and eHealth literacy skills when this is necessary.
3. The third step requires the development of sustainable interventions targeting caregivers with low level health and eHealth literacy.

References

1. Montoya S (2022) Defining literacy [Internet]. 2018. http://gaml.uis.unesco.org/wp-content/uploads/sites/2/2018/12/4.6.1_07_4.6-defining-literacy.pdf
2. Hillerich RL (1976) Toward an assessable definition of literacy. English J 65(2):50
3. OECD (2019) Skills matter: additional results from the survey of adult skills, OECD skills studies. OECD Publishing, Paris
4. Nes AAG, Steindal SA, Larsen MH, Heer HC, Lærum-Onsager E, Gjevjon ER (2021) Technological literacy in nursing education: a scoping review. J Profess Nurs WB Saunders 37:320–334

5. Jeong SH, Cho H, Hwang Y (2012) Media literacy interventions: a meta-analytic review. J Commun 62(3):454–472

6. Breivik PS (1991) Information literacy. Bull Med Libr Assoc 79(2):226–229

7. Liu C, Wang D, Liu C, Jiang J, Wang X, Chen H et al (2020) What is the meaning of health literacy? A systematic review and qualitative synthesis. Family Med Commun Health 8

8. Nutbeam D (2000) Health literacy as a public health goal: a challenge for contemporary health education and communication strategies into the 21st century. Health Promotion Int [Internet] 15(3):259–267. http://heapro.oxfordjournals.org/content/15/3/259

9. Sørensen K, van den Broucke S, Fullam J, Doyle G, Pelikan J, Slonska Z et al (2012) Health literacy and public health: a systematic review and integration of definitions and models. BMC public health [Internet] 12(8):80. http://www.pubmedcentral.nih.gov/articlerender.fcgi?artid=3292515&tool=pmcentrez&rendertype=abstract. http://ezproxy.deakin.edu.au/login?url=http://search.proquest.com/docview/1285089709?accountid=10445. http://library.deakin.edu.au/resserv?genre=arti

10. World Health Organization (2013) Health literacy the solid facts. Denmark: World Health Organisation Regional Office for Europe, 86 p. https://apps.who.int/iris/bitstream/handle/10665/128703/e96854.pdf

11. Healthy People 2030. Healthy People 2030 Objectives: Older people [Internet]. U.S. Department of Health and Human Services. [cited 2021 Feb 26]. https://health.gov/healthypeople/objectives-and-data/browse-objectives/older-adults

12. Brach C, Keller D, Hernandez LM, Baur C, Parker R, Dreyer B et al (2012) Ten attributes of health literate health care organizations

13. Xu XY, Yee A, Leung M, Chau PH (2018) Health literacy , self-efficacy, and associated factors among patients with Diabetes. 2(2):67–77

14. Kim SH, Yu X (2010) The mediating effect of self-efficacy on the relationship between health literacy and health status in Korean older adults: a short report. Aging Ment Health 14(7):870–873

15. Lee J-Y, Murry N, Ko JMTK (2018) Exploring the relationship between maternal health literacy, parenting self-efficacy, and early parenting practices among low-income mothers with infants. Ju-Young 29(4):1455–1471

16. Kim S, Song Y, Park J, Utz S (2019) Patients' experiences of diabetes self-management education according to health-literacy levels. Clin Nurs Res 105477381986587

17. Cajita MI, Cajita TR, Han HR (2016) Health literacy and heart failure a systematic review. J Cardiovasc Nurs 31(2):121–130

18. Davis T, Long S, Jackson R, Mayeaux E, George R, Murphy P et al (1993) Rapid estimate of adult literacy in medicine: a shortened screening instrument. Family Med 25:391–395. http://search.ebscohost.com/login.aspx?direct=true&db=mdc&AN=8349060&site=eds-live

19. Altin SV, Finke I, Kautz-Freimuth S, Stock S (2014) The evolution of health literacy assessment tools: a systematic review. BMC Public Health 14(1):1207. http://www.biomedcentral.com/1471-2458/14/1207

20. O'Neill B, Gonçalves D, Ricci-Cabello I, Ziebland S, Valderas J (2014) An overview of self-administered health literacy instruments. PLoS One 9(12):1–14

21. Efthymiou A (2020) The association of health literacy and eHealth literacy with caring concepts among carers of people with dementia. Limassol 31

22. Parker RM, Baker DW, Willia M, v., Nurss JR. (1995) The test of functional health literacy in adults: a new instrument for measuring patients' literacy skills. J Gen Intern Med 10(10):537–541

23. Weiss BD, Mays MZ, Martz W, Castro KM, DeWalt DA, Pignone MP et al (2005) Quick assessment of literacy in primary care: the newest vital sign 514–522

24. HLS-EU CONSORTIUM (2012) Comparative report on health literacy in EIght EU member states (Second Revised And Extended Version, Date July 22th, 2014). http://www.health-literacy.eu

25. Efthymiou A, Middleton N, Charalambous A, Papastavrou E (2021) Health literacy and eHealth literacy and their association with other caring concepts among carers of people with dementia: a descriptive correlational study. Health Soc Care Community 00:1–11
26. Norman CD, Skinner HA (2006) eHealth literacy: essential skills for consumer health in a networked world. J Med Internet Res e9
27. Chan C, v., Kaufman DR. (2011) A framework for characterizing ehealth literacy demands and barriers. J Med Internet Res 13(4):1–24
28. Norman C (2011) eHealth literacy 2.0: problems and opportunities with an evolving concept. J Med Internet Res 13(4):2–5
29. Gilstad H (2014) Toward a comprehensive model of eHealth literacy. CEUR Workshop Proceed 1251(Pahi):63–72
30. Koopman RJ, Petroski GF, Canfield SM, Stuppy JA Mehr DR (2014) Development of the PRE-HIT instrument: patient readiness to engage in health information technology. BMC Family Pract 15(1):18. http://www.biomedcentral.com/1471-2296/15/18
31. Cinelli M, Quattrociocchi W, Galeazzi A, Valensise CM, Brugnoli E, Schmidt AL et al (2020) The COVID-19 social media infodemic. Sci Rep 10:16598
32. Norman CD, Skinner HA (2006) eHEALS: the eHealth literacy scale. J Med Internet Res 8(4):1–7
33. van der Vaart R, van Deursen AJ, Drossaert CHC, Taal E, van Dijk JA, van de Laar MA (2011) Does the eHealth literacy scale (eHEALS) measure what it intends to measure? Validation of a Dutch version of the eHEALS in two adult populations. J Med Internet Res 13(4)
34. Lee J, Lee EH, Chae D (2021) eHealth literacy instruments: systematic review of measurement properties. J Med Internet Res 23
35. Efthymiou A, Middleton N, Charalambous A, Papastavrou E (2019) Adapting the eHealth literacy scale for carers of people with chronic diseases (eheaLS-cAREr) in a sample of Greek and Cypriot carers of people with dementia: reliability and validation study. J Med Internet Res 21(11):e12504
36. OECD (2011) The impact of caring on family carers. In: Help wanted? Providing and paying for long-term care, pp 85–120
37. World Health Organisation (2015) Supporting informal caregivers of people living with dementia supporting informal caregivers of people living
38. EUROCARERS. Carers in Europe [Internet]. 2009. http://www.eurocarers.org/userfiles/file/Factsheet2009_pages1to6.pdf
39. Perlesz A, Kinsella G, Crowe S (1999) Impact of traumatic brain injury on the family: a critical review. Rehabil Psychol 44(1):6–35
40. Salifu Y, Almack K, Caswell G (2021) 'My wife is my doctor at home': a qualitative study exploring the challenges of home-based palliative care in a resource-poor setting. Palliat Med 35(1):97–108
41. Efthymiou A, Papastavrou E, Middleton N, Markatou A, Sakka P (2020) How caregivers of people with dementia search for dementia-specific information on the internet: survey study, vol 3. JMIR Publications Inc., JMIR Aging
42. Meyer K. Carers' experiences accessing information on supports and services: learning the social care "dance." Qual Soc Work 2018;17(6):832–848
43. Yuen EYN, Knight T, Ricciardelli LA, Burney S (2018) Health literacy of caregivers of adult care recipients: a systematic scoping review. Health Social Care Community 26(2):e191–e206
44. Erickson SR, LeRoy B (2015) Health literacy and medication administration performance by caregivers of adults with developmental disabilities. J Am Pharm Assoc 55(2):169–177
45. Häikiö K, Cloutier D, Rugkåsa J (2020) Is health literacy of family carers associated with carer burden, quality of life, and time spent on informal care for older persons living with dementia? PLoS One 15
46. della Pelle C, Orsatti V, Cipollone F, Cicolini G (2018) Health literacy among caregivers of patients with heart failure: a multicentre cross-sectional survey. J Clin Nurs 27(3–4):859–865
47. Fagnano M, Halterman J, Conn K, Shone L (2012) Health literacy and sources of health information for caregivers of urban children with asthma. Clin Pediatr (Phila) 51(3):267–273

48. Garcia CH, Espinoza SE, Lichtenstein M, Hazuda HP (2013) Health literacy associations between hispanic elderly patients and their caregivers. J Health Commun 18(Suppl. 1):256–272
49. Jiang Y, Sereika S, Lingler J, Tamres K, Erien J (2018) Health literacy and its correlates in informal caregivers of adults with memory loss. Geriatr Nurs 39(3):285–291
50. Levin JB, Peterson PN, Dolansky MA, Boxer RS (2014) Health literacy and heart failure management in patient-caregiver dyads. J Cardiac Fail [Internet] 20(10):755–761. https://doi.org/10.1016/j.cardfail.2014.07.009
51. Metin S, Demirci H, Metin AT (2019) Effect of health literacy of caregivers on survival rates of patients under palliative care. Scand J Caring Sci 33(8):669
52. Moore C, Hassett D, Dunne S. Health literacy in cancer caregivers: a systematic review. https://doi.org/10.1007/s11764-020-00975-8
53. de Almeida KMV, Toye C, LVA S, Slatyer S, Hill K, Jacinto AF (2019) Assessment of functional health literacy in Brazilian carers of older people. Dementia Neuropsychol 13(2):180–186
54. Chen S, Wu Q, Qi C, Deng H, Wang X, He H et al (2017) Mental health literacy about schizophrenia and depression: a survey among Chinese caregivers of patients with mental disorder. BMC Psychiatry 17:89
55. Queiroz JPC, Machado ALG, Vieira NFC (2020) Health literacy for caregivers of elders with alzheimer's disease. Revista brasileira de enfermagem 73(Suppl 3):e20190608
56. Rohwer E, Mojtahedzadeh N, Neumann FA, Nienhaus A, Augustin M, Harth V et al (2021) The role of health literacy among outpatient caregivers during the covid-19 pandemic. Int J Environ Res Public Health 18(22)
57. Crellin NE, Orrell M, McDermott O, Charlesworth G (2014) Self-efficacy and health-related quality of life in family carers of people with dementia: a systematic review. Aging Mental Health [Internet] 18(8):954–969. https://doi.org/10.1080/13607863.2014.915921
58. Cheng ST, Lam LCW, Kwok T, Ng NSS, Fung AWT (2013) Self-efficacy is associated with less burden and more gains from behavioral problems of Alzheimer's disease in Hong Kong Chinese caregivers. Gerontologist 53(1):71–80
59. Gallagher D, Mhaolain AN, Crosby L, Ryan D, Lacey L, Coen RF et al (2011) Self-efficacy for managing dementia may protect against burden and depression in Alzheimer's caregivers. Aging Ment Health 15(6):663–670
60. Mausbach BT, Roepke SK, Chattillion EA, Harmell AL, Moore R, Romero-Moreno R et al (2012) Multiple mediators of the relations between caregiving stress and depressive symptoms. Aging Ment Health 16(1):27–38
61. Fong HF, Rothman EF, Garner A, Ghazarian SR, Morley DS, Singerman A et al (2018) Association between health literacy and parental self-efficacy among parents of newborn children. J Pediatrics 202:265–271.e3. https://doi.org/10.1016/j.jpeds.2018.06.021
62. Geboers B, de Winter AF, Luten KA, Jansen CJM, Reijneveld SA (2014) The association of health literacy with physical activity and nutritional behavior in older adults, and its social cognitive mediators. J Health Commun [Internet] 19 (Suppl 2):61–76. http://www.ncbi.nlm.nih.gov/pubmed/25315584
63. Huang YM, Shiyanbola OO, Chan HY (2018) A path model linking health literacy, medication self-efficacy, medication adherence, and glycemic control. Patient Educ Couns 101(11):1906–1913
64. Pearlin LI, Schooler C (1978) The structure of coping. J Health Soc Behav 19:2–21
65. Avison WR, Aneshensel CS, Schieman S, Wheaton B (2010) Advances in the conceptualization of the stress process, vol 1. Springer
66. Fraser E, Pakenham KI (2009) Resilience in children of parents with mental illness: relations between mental health literacy, social connectedness and coping, and both adjustment and caregiving. Psychol Health Med 14(5):573–584
67. Johnson RJ, Turner RJ, Link BG (2014) Sociology of mental health: selected topics from forty years 1970s–2010s [Internet], 172 p. https://www.google.com/books?id=3FhbBAAAQBAJ

68. Cobb S (1976) Social support as a moderator of life stress. Psychosomatic Medicine [Internet] 38(5):300–314. http://search.ebscohost.com/login.aspx?direct=true&db=edb&AN=11498321 8&site=eds-live
69. Thoits PA (2011) Mechanisms linking social ties and support to physical and mental health. J Health Soc Behav 52(2):145–161
70. Antonucci TC (2001) Social relations: an examination of social networks, social support, and sense of control. In: Handbook of psychology and aging, pp 427–53
71. Fernández-Carro C, Vlachantoni A (2019) The role of social networks in using home care by older people across continental Europe. Health Soc Care Community 1–17
72. Pommer E, Woittiez I, Stevens J (2007) Comparing care
73. Serra L, Contador I, Fernández-Calvo B, Ruisoto P, Jenaro C, Flores N et al (2018) Resilience and social support as protective factors against abuse of patients with dementia: a study on family caregivers. Int J Geriatr Psychiatry 33(8):1132–1138
74. Wang Z, Ma C, Han H, He R, Zhou L, Liang R et al (2018) Caregiver burden in Alzheimer's disease: moderation effects of social support and mediation effects of positive aspects of caregiving. Int J Geriatr Psychiatry 33(9):1198–1206
75. Xian M, Xu L (2019) Social support and self-rated health among caregivers of people with dementia: the mediating role of caregiving burden. Dementia
76. Yang Y, Zhang B, Meng H, Liu D, Sun M (2019) Mediating effect of social support on the associations between health literacy, productive aging, and self-rated health among elderly Chinese adults in a newly urbanized community. Medicine 98(16):e15162
77. Lee S-YD, Gazmararian JA, Arozullah AM (2006) Health literacy and social support among elderly medicare enrollees in a managed care plan. J Appl Gerontol 25(4):324–337
78. Li Y, Hu L, Mao X, Shen Y, Xue H, Hou P et al (2020) Health literacy, social support, and care ability for caregivers of dementia patients: structural equation modeling. Geriatr Nurs 41(5):600–607
79. Efthymiou A, Middleton N, Charalambous A, Papastavrou E (2021) Identifying the carer's profiles of health literacy, eHealth literacy and caregiving concepts. Eur J Pub Health [Internet]   31(Suppl   3):1.   https://academic.oup.com/eurpub/article/31/Supplement_3/ ckab164.275/6405684
80. Visscher BB, Steunenberg B, Heijmans M, Hofstede JM, Deville W, van der Heide I et al (2018) Evidence on the effectiveness of health literacy interventions in the EU: a systematic review. BMC Public Health 18(1)
81. Jafari Y, Tehrani H, Esmaily H, Shariati M, Vahedian-shahroodi M (2020) Family-centred empowerment program for health literacy and self-efficacy in family caregivers of patients with multiple sclerosis. Scand J Caring Sci 34(4):956–963

The Use of Information and Communication Technology Among Informal Caregivers

Evridiki Papastavrou ⓘ and Areti Efthymiou ⓘ

1   Introduction

The number and proportion of people over the age of 60 years is increasing dramatically and, according to the World Health Organization estimations, is expected to increase up to 2.1 billion by the year 2050 (https://www.who.int/health-topics/ageing#tab=tab_1). Aging is often associated with several health conditions, chronic diseases, comorbidities, and frequent limitations that affect the everyday life and reduce the ability of people to live an independent life. As regards patients with cognitive decline that greatly reduces their ability for independent living, an estimated 6.2 million Americans aged 65 and older are living with Alzheimer's dementia today, and this number could grow to 13.8 million by 2060 [1]. Support in managing conditions associated with old age and related diseases, for example, cognitive impairment, is usually provided by the family and people who identify themselves as "informal caregivers." In the United States, and only for patients suffering from Alzheimer's disease, caregivers report about 18 billion hours of unpaid care every year [2] meaning that this number is much higher if informal caregivers of all diseases are added in the equation. Although many informal caregivers find caregiving as rewarding and associated with positive feelings, still providing care to older adults and other patients with chronic disabilities is stressful, and there is evidence of adverse outcomes such as burden, depression, anxiety, family conflicts, and lower quality of life [3–5]. Additionally, most caregivers report that apart from support,

E. Papastavrou (✉)
Limassol, Cyprus
e-mail: e.papastavrou@cut.ac.cy

A. Efthymiou
Kaisariani, Greece
e-mail: al.efthymiou@edu.cut.ac.cy

© The Author(s), under exclusive license to Springer Nature   111
Switzerland AG 2023
A. Charalambous (ed.), *Informal Caregivers: From Hidden Heroes to Integral Part of Care*, https://doi.org/10.1007/978-3-031-16745-4_7

they need more information to manage the care they provide and to cope with the caring challenges and demands [6, 7]. Better caregiver preparation and training is also linked to lower rates of health care utilization and better communication of medical information. In a recent systematic review of the associated literature, it has been shown that caregivers who are more and better prepared for caregiving, demonstrate decrease in the related stress with a one-unit increase in caregiver preparedness connected to a 17% reduction in their stress [8]. The aim of this chapter is to investigate and report the importance and meaning of technological solutions for the informal caregivers of people living with chronic diseases in the community and especially for those caring of people with dementia. The discussion will follow with a scoping review conducted by the authors, aiming to explore e-health literacy of caregivers in relation to older persons and those suffering from dementia, the characteristics of those who are using the internet for the benefit of their patients, what they expect to find, and what they post in the social media.

2 Information and Communication Technology and Informal Caregivers

Information and communication technology (ICT) has emerged as a promising solution in the support of caregivers of chronically ill patients, and many researchers have demonstrated that technology-based interventions can improve outcomes among patients and can reduce burden and emotional strain among caregivers [9]. This type of solution consists of digital and related technologies, including hardware, software, networks, and media that facilitate collecting, capturing, storing, processing, transmitting, exchanging, and presenting information and/or communication [2]. Some examples for caregivers include interactive services, psychoeducational and stress management programs, informal caregivers' platforms, e-learning courses, telemedicine, and telehealth that all have the potential to support informal caregivers in the management of care. The importance of Information and Communication Technology is also recognized by the WHO [10] stating that:

> From technologies that allow people to manage their health more effectively, to better ways of diagnosing disease, to monitoring the impact of policies on population health, digital technologies for health, or digital health, are having a profound effect on how health services are delivered and how health systems are run.

The e-Health solutions targeted on informal caregivers that are most frequently described are mobile applications, web-based portals, and telehealth solutions delivering education, support, and stress management training, multimedia solutions for art viewing or music experiencing targeted at the caregiver–care receiver dyad to facilitate communication and enhance the relationship, or solutions targeting the psychological needs of caregivers [11]. The terms that are often used in the caring literature in recent years are electronic health (eHealth) and mobile health (mHealth), and according to the Global Observatory for eHealth, mHealth is defined as "a medical and public health practice supported by mobile devices, such as mobile phones, patient monitoring devices, personal digital assistants, and other wireless devices." Mobile devices can be of great advantage for informal caregivers as they are widely available and normally easier to use than PCs, they are user-friendly, and they also allow handy access to internet-based applications [10]. WHO defines eHealth as the cost-effective and secure use of information and communication technologies in support of health and health-related fields, including health care services, health surveillance, health literature, and health education, knowledge, and research [11].

2.1 Information and Communication Technology and Informal Caregivers in the Dementia Context

Language and communication problems are present early in almost all types of dementia; they involve speaking, expressing, and conversation, and it is a source of tension for the families and caregivers. The impaired communication skills and memory function may result in tension in the caregiving dyad and the quality of relationship increasing caregiver stress that influence the caregiver well-being, health, quality of life, and their ability to manage care. Communication is considered one of the most challenging caring issues, and the factors that can contribute and explain this problem are described in the conceptual model of Morris et al. [12]. These include difficulties in understanding the changing internal world that affects the memory capacity and the personality of the patient as well as the diminished linguistic resources that do not allow patients to express their needs clearly, leading to informal caregiver frustration [12]. The increased dependence of the patient and the associated role changes, the lack of appreciation to the caregiver's offer, grief due to the "loss" of the person used to be, tension related to the history of long attachment relationships, and practical pressures, fatigue, and isolation may explain the challenges for communication and interaction between the caregiver and the care receiver [12]. Research offers promising findings for the potential of technology to promote communication and relationships in a way that relieves caregiver strain, creates meaningful interactions, and minimizes social isolation [13]. Some systematic reviews are providing interesting results of studies related to ICT-based solutions that have the potential to support informal caregivers in home care settings. Bratches et al. [8], focusing on the impact of technological solutions on the caregiver and patient outcomes, found statistically significant improvements in key outcomes for caregivers receiving visit information, including caregiver happiness, caregiver activation, caregiver preparedness, and caregiver confidence in managing patient health. In their systematic review of ICT interventions for informal caregivers of patients with dementia, Lucero et al. [14] categorized the technology used in telephone, video, and computer interventions and found that a range of these interventions are successful in supporting caregivers and may prevent outcomes such as burden, depression, and anxiety. Other authors describe the emergence of new technologies that can empower and support caregivers, such as the robotics, connected sensors, virtual reality, voice, and interaction of multiple technologies [15]. Yet, several reservations have been expressed by some authors related to challenges such as the design and usability of technology, funding, and sustainability; ethical challenges associated with equity, inclusion, access, autonomy, and privacy of data; and political and regulatory factors [16, 17].

However, although seeking, assessing, evaluating, and understanding health care information is crucial both for caregivers to manage and provide better care and for patients to receive safe and quality care, research findings are not consistent [18–20]. The fact that some studies have found poor informal caregivers e-health literacy and others satisfactory literacy can partly be explained by differences in methodological approaches and the selection of samples, based on the difficulties in deciding who can be better described as a caregiver.

3   Informal Caregivers and Internet Use

Some systematic reviews provided much information on the type of internet use that informal caregivers of different chronic diseases make without any further recommendation regarding the level of eHealth literacy [21–23]. People usually search for information on their suggested treatment, questions that doctors have not replied to and information on healthy habits, and most users consider the information on the internet to be of good quality. Technology tools used by informal caregivers were mainly videoconferencing tools, followed by phone-based technology, and less web-based info or remote monitoring and telemetry. The technology-based interventions for informal caregivers were categorized as follows: (1) education using mainly telephone-based, web-based, and video interventions; (2) consultation using videoconferencing; (3) psychosocial/CBT intervention using the telephone and videoconferencing tools; (4) social support, using videoconferencing tools; (5) data collection/monitoring including response center, sensors, and fall detectors; and (6) clinical care delivery using videoconferences [23]. The interventions reported were befriending and peer support intervention, family support and social network interventions, and support group and remote interventions [27].

Results of the above systematic reviews provided positive outcomes of the use of the web-based interventions for informal caregivers as the improvement in psychological health, well-being (measured with depression measures), sense of competence, decision-making confidence, self-efficacy satisfaction, knowledge, quality of life (QoL), social support, problem-solving skills communication with providers, cost-saving, and physical health. On the other hand, results showed that internet interventions did not affect depression, anxiety, burden, QoL, or social isolation [21, 23, 24]. The outcomes had qualitative results on sharing, companionship, and improved relationships, but there were not any quantitative results supporting this [21]. In the case of randomized trials, mental health has improved [22]. Videoconferencing and online psychological support were promising, providing evidence of enhanced satisfaction, on self-efficacy, and reduced burden, distress and depression [21, 22]. There is a growing research field discussing the type, impact, quality, and implementation of web-based interventions of informal caregivers of PwD to understand the factors that may influence informal caregiver characteristics and needs that would facilitate the internet-based intervention use. On the other hand, there were very few reviews on the type of internet (health-related and dementia-specific) use made by informal caregivers, such as the one reported by Ottaviani et al. (2021) stating that informal caregivers of people living with dementia indicate that internet-based interventions are mostly effective, efficient, and satisfactory. Caregivers also considered these to be informative, relevant, and functional, highlighting the utility and intention of using the resource in the future.

The following scoping review aimed to identify the available literature of the health-related internet use made by informal caregivers of PwD and older people with disabilities or chronic diseases focusing on the type of use those informal caregivers make and the characteristics that may influence this use.

4   Scoping Review on the Dementia Informal Caregivers Internet Use

4.1   Review Methodology

The methodology followed the Preferred Reporting Items for Systematic Reviews and Metanalysis for scoping reviews [25] as well as the five stages of Arksey and O'Malley, [26] on scoping reviews. As part of the research questions, we searched for the characteristics of the informal caregivers that may predict the internet use and dementia-specific internet use, the way that informal caregivers use the internet, available theoretical frameworks for dementia-specific internet use, and the needs of informal caregivers with dementia when using the internet. In the second stage, we identified all relevant studies by searching all available resources: electronic databases, conference proceedings, and gray literature. We have included studies with informal caregivers in general and of older people and PwD, as in this way, we broaden our search, and it was possible to find related information on our topic that was important for us to understand the phenomenon. Based on this, we also included interventional studies, even if not related directly with internet use, as this type of research is an indicator of online service use, and we were also interested in mapping the existing research on online use and services. Additionally, usually in the interventional studies, there is always the usability issue and how ready and friendly the informal caregivers consider this type of technology, which was a question of interest in our research. Studies were excluded if the language was not English and if there was no full paper available. Systematic reviews of the relevant topic were also identified but not included. No type of study design was excluded as the area is new, and we were interested in identifying all possible aspects. The search resulted in 1223 papers, and after reading the titles, we included 208 papers. Through abstracts reading, we included 101 papers, and after full-text reading, we concluded 13 papers. Another six articles were included by the snowball effect. The final number of included papers for review raised to 19 full texts. The reviewers also included a quality appraisal section in the same sector for the selected papers used for qualitative studies (interviews and focus groups), the Consolidated Criteria for Reporting Qualitative research (COREQ), for the observational study Strengthening the Reporting of Observational Studies in Epidemiology Statement (STROBE), and for the online surveys, the Checklist for Reporting Results of Internet E-Surveys (Cherries). All the information regarding the scoping review is shown in Table 1.

Table 1 Results of the scoping review on the Dementia Informal Caregivers Internet Use

Authors, year	Country	Qualitative assessment	Participants	Design	Category	Main outcomes	Theory
(Chiu and Eysenbach, 2010)	CHINA	STROBE 17/22	46 family carers of PwD	Multiphase, longitudinal design, interventional quantitative	Understanding patterns of internet intervention use	Consideration stage (easy technology matters), initiation (acceptance of technology matters), utilisation (frequency of use matters)	Andersen's behavioral model of health service use and Venkatesh's unified theory of acceptance and use of technology
(Chiu and Eysenbach, 2011)	CHINA	COREQ: 12/32	14 family carers of PwD	Qualitative analysis (in depth interviews)	Conceptualization patterns of internet intervention use	Dimension of the web-based intervention use: (a) caregiver needs, influenced by personal capacity, social support, and caregiving belief; (b) information communication technology (ICT) factors (accessibility barriers and perceived efforts) and (c) style of using the technology	Anderson's model of health service utilization, Venkatesh's theory of technology acceptance, and Chatman's and Wilson's information behavior theories
(Kim, 2015)	USA	STROBE = 19/22	450 family carers of PwD	Descriptive correlational design	Internet use	59% identified as internet users. Health-related internet users were younger, more educated, higher income, fewer hours of caregiving. Sociodemographic characteristics and subjective response to stress indicators of health-related internet use, followed by the hours of caregiving	Stress process model

(Larner, 2003)	UK	STROBE = 5/22	Descriptive study	Use of internet and NHS help line of patients and carers	More than 50% of patients and families/ carers had internet access; 27% had accessed relevant information. 82% expressed interest in, or willingness to access, websites with relevant medical information if these were suggested by the clinic doctor. Although 61% had heard of the NHS Direct telephone helpline, only 10% of all patients had used this service	N/A
(Blackburn et al., 2005)	UK	STROBE = 16/22	Cross-sectional survey	Internet use	Half (50%) of all carers had previously used the Internet. Of this group, 61% had used it once a week or more frequently. Factors significantly associated with having previously used the Internet were carer's age, employment status, housing tenure and number of hours per week they spent caring. Frequency of Internet use was significantly associated with carer's age, sex, employment status and number of hours spent caring	N/A
(Alwan et al., 2011)	USA	REPORT	Quantitative online study	Usability and needs met by 12 technologies	Reported benefits of web-based use: saving time, facilitating caring, safety, self-efficacy and reduction of stress	N/A

(continued)

Table 1 (continued)

Authors, year	Country	Qualitative assessment	Participants	Design	Category	Main outcomes	Theory
(Kernisan et al., 2010)	USA	COREQ: 14/20 OR CHERRIES 30/30	2161 carers (50% caring for parents of elders	Five questions pop up survey	Internet use	People visiting a caregiving-related website search for general information on caring, specific assistance (custoial, medical, emotional and financial), training, disease progression and symptoms, caring support, peer support	N/A
(Lam and Lam, 2009)	AUST RALIA	STROBE: 16/20	784 carers of older adults over 60 with disability	National health survey	Internet use	Significant association between use of internet and better mental health status	N/A
(Fox and Brenner, 2012)	USA	REPORT	860 carers of adults	National telephone survey	Internet use	Caring is associated with being online and with online e-health behaviors. Carers are active health care consumers	N/A
(Kim, 2012)	USA	DISSERTATION	752 family carers of PwD	Telephone surveys	Internet use	Carers' stress may predict carers' perception of poor health status. Health-related Internet use did not mediate this relationship effectively	N/A
(Li, 2015)	USA	STROBE: 19/22	800 carers of older adults over 65		Internet use	Carers search for care receivers' conditions or treatments (77.2%), available services for care receivers (52.7%), and care facilities (35.3%). Only a small percentage search for support for themselves	Wilson's model of information-seeking behavior

(Anderson et al., 2017)	USA	COREQ 18/21	3245 carers' posts of PwD	Descriptive study/ qualitative research/ analysing samples of blogs	Internet use	Themes derived from carers' posting social support through communication and engagement, information gathering and seeking, reminiscing and legacy building, altruism	N/A
(Werner et al., 2017)	USA	COREQ 18/32	26 carers of PwD	Qualitative (4 focus groups)	Information needs assessment/internet use?	Authors find three critical information needs: (1) timely access to information, (2) access to information that is tailored to caregiver's needs and (3) usable information that can directly inform how caregivers' manage behaviors	System engineering initiative for patient safety
(Yoo et al., 2010)	USA	COREQ 9/21	798 carers' messages of PwD	Qualitative study/content analysis	Socio-affective regulation (SAR) and goods-and information acquisition (GIA)	The results indicated that Korean caregivers expressed more family burden than US caregivers. Also, the Korean caregivers expressed more negative emotions than the US caregivers	N/A
(Jeong et al., 2018)	USA / South Korea	STROBE = 16/22	104 dementia carers	Descriptive correlational design	Information seeking and forwarding- cybercoping	Information seeking is associated with the affective coping and physical coping than information forwarding. Information seeking is associated with problem focused coping	Chiu and Eysenbach, 2011 and Lazarus (emotion based and problem-based coping)

(continued)

Table 1 (continued)

Authors, year	Country	Qualitative assessment	Participants	Design	Category	Main outcomes	Theory
(Allen et al., 2018)	UK	CHERRIES 13/30	212 dementia carers	Online and postal survey (questions adapted from the US health and services 2014)	Dementia information seeking, access and understand	Source of information accessed: First source: Internet (almost all except 2 people)- 82% search dementia specific information, 57% accessed the web through mobile. Second source: health and social care professionals Factors related to frequency of use: Age in majority, they were searching info by dementia charities websites Relational information source: GP and friends and family Friends and family most popular information resource for emotional support Passive information resources: Newspapers, television and internet Health and social care professional as most inaccessible sources and internet as the most accessible source followed by the published material Most important characteristic of information source: trustworthiness, accessibility and answer questions	N/A

| (Lucero et al., 2018) | USA | COREQ21/32 | 20 carers and 11 caregiving counselors | Qualitative (6 focus groups of 4–6 people)/ exploratory study | Effectiveness of family-HIMS intervention | Three tasks and six skills were presented in the analysis: Tasks: medical management, role management and emotional management. Emotional management and resource utilization mentioned more often, by carers and counsellors, medical management more often by the caregivers. 6 self-management skills: (1) Problem-solving (2) Decision-making (3) Resource utilization (4) The formation of patient-provider partnership (5) Action planning (6) Self tailoring | *Chronic disease self-management program framework: Improvements in health status and outcome are result of an individual's knowledge ability and confidence in practicing self-management* |
| (Ruggiano et al., 2018) | USA | COREQ 14/32 | 36 dementia carers | Beta test interviews for care IT | Use of technology and an app | Current technology use: all had access to internet, spouses less active on the internet in comparison with children. They do not use the technology for caregiving activities. Only three people use apps for caregiving. Importance to the usefulness of the technology to generate interest to use: social networking, and personalized technology. Half of the participants support that IT would be helpful for medication management information | Technology acceptance model |

(continued)

Table 1 (continued)

Authors, year	Country	Qualitative assessment	Participants	Design	Category	Main outcomes	Theory
(Scharett et al., 2017)	USA	COREQ 11/19	250 posts and related responses (randomly selected) of dementia carers	Post qualitative analysis	Emotions of problems stated and given solutions	Categories from initial analysis of 500 posts: Problem categorization: Carers feelings/Symptoms/Doctors and nursing homes/physical safety/basic hygiene/ general info/medicines/conflicts/ solutions/ethics. Solution categories: informational resources for carers, contact professional assistance, assisted care facilities, doctor consultations, caregivers well-being, patients well-being, memory problems, safety, medication, bathing and sanitation, anxiety or depression, hallucinations, home care	Linguistic inquiry and word count system: provide an emotional rating 0 to 100 (0 negative emotion and 100 positive emotion)

4.2   Characteristics of the Studies Reviewed

Much of the internet use research among informal caregivers was based in the United States, with 11 out of 19 papers developed in the United States. Other countries of research were the United Kingdom ($n = 4$), China ($n = 2$), Australia ($n = 1$), and South Korea ($n = 1$). The total number of the study sample was 10,091, with five papers using a sample under 50 informal caregivers [1, 19, 34–36]. Furthermore, three research papers analyzed 3393 posts on social media and forums to understand how informal caregivers of PwD post online [20, 21, 37]. Most of the papers focused on informal caregivers of PwD ($n = 13$). In other cases, the research focused on informal caregivers of older people ($n = 3$), informal caregivers of adults ($n = 1$), informal caregivers without defining ($n = 1$), and informal caregivers of adults of mental and physical diseases ($n = 1$).

1. Quality of the studies

    In the analysis, nine qualitative studies and ten quantitative studies (including two reports and one dissertation) were included. In the case of the qualitative studies, three of them analyzed and discussed the findings from the text that was already uploaded on the internet by the informal caregivers of older people through related websites or open online support groups as ALZConnected.org and other blogs. In most of the qualitative studies, the authors did not provide information on the personal characteristics of the interviewers or moderators or the relationship that was established during and before the study. Information regarding methodology orientation, sampling, and data collection as well as the consistency of data and findings and presentation of major and minor themes were always included. On the other hand, authors usually did not provide information on data saturation, setting of data collection, involvement of the participants in the transcription and findings, and nonparticipation rates. The three papers that used online posted material and messages were the most difficult to be assessed as in COREQ most items were not related as in the case of the relationship with participants, nonparticipation, method of approach, presence of nonparticipants, setting, interview guide, duration, and transcription. In this case, we used items 1–5 regarding the characteristics of the coders, theoretical framework, participant (posts) selection, description of the sample, data collection, analysis, and findings items. Only in one case did the authors discuss this regarding the terminology of posts and if posts considered being handled as "participants" [27]. In six of the seven studies, the assessment of the observational studies was high with minimum score 16/22 and maximum 19/22. Only in one study did we find a low score of STROBE 5/22 including only items 3, 5, 13, 14, and 18. In this study, the topic discussed the use of the internet and NHS telephone line from people with cognitive disorders and was the first study that we included chronologically in the area, followed by Blackburn [28].

2. Theoretical underpinning of the studies reviewed

Most of the studies were not based on a certain theory, and only in nine out of the 19 papers, a theoretical framework supported the findings, although all studies used a different theoretical approach. In total, nine theories were presented:

The "Andersen's Behavioral Model of Health Service use: Model explaining service use including three main dimensions, predisposing, enabling and needs factors."

The Venkatesh's unified theory of acceptance and use of technology: intention to use information technology with four core dimensions—performance and effort expectancy, social influence, and facilitators.

The "Chatman's and Wilson's information behavior theories: dynamic relation among the user, information system and information resources."

The "Stress Process model" developed by Pearlin.

The "System Engineering Initiative for Patient Safety: sociotechnical system model."

"Lazarus coping strategies: primary and secondary appraisal, coping processes and coping styles: problem-focused and emotion-focused."

"Law of Attrition" by Eysenbach—stages of use: consideration, initiation of use, attrition or continuation of use, and outcomes."

"Chronic disease self-management program framework: improvements in health status and outcomes are a result of an individual's knowledge, ability and confidence in practicing self-management."

"Linguistic inquiry and word count system (to analyze the emotional level of posts online)."

5 Results of the Scoping Review

5.1 The Profile of the Caregivers Who Use the Internet for Caregiving

Caregivers' characteristics that affect the use of the internet for health-related or caregiving topics Internet access and use by informal caregivers seemed to be influenced by socioeconomic factors. The age of the informal caregivers and the age of the person cared for, gender, employment status, living conditions, and hours of care are factors associated with internet access and frequency of use. Being over 55 years old and with more hours of care was related to limited internet access and less frequent use. Being not in paid employment was also connected with not having use the internet. Being a female was the strongest predictor for using the internet less than once a week [28]. The health-related internet use was also related with sociodemographic characteristics of informal caregivers, such as age, education, income, hours of caregiving and relationship with the cared-for person, age of care recipient and instrumental of daily living (IADL) level of dependency, chronic condition, and having a recent crisis in health. More specifically, younger informal caregivers (children and grandchildren) more educated, with higher income, more financial hardships, and fewer hours of caregiving were most likely to be health-related internet users [29, 30]. Dementia-specific internet use was also associated with being informal caregivers or not [30]. Internet use was associated with better mental health after adjusting for confounders such as the age of the informal caregiver, being a primary informal caregiver and caring for a disabled person significant [31]. The frequency of internet searches for caregiving information was related to the informal caregivers' service needs, being or not a primary informal caregiver, informal caregivers' strain, and health status. The higher the service needs for informal caregivers, being a secondary informal caregiver, reporting better health status and higher caregiving strain, the more likely it was for informal caregivers to search the internet [32]. The percentages of internet use and access differed according to the study. Blackburn, Read, and Hughes [28] found that 61% were frequent users and almost half had internet access, and Kim [29] found that 59% of the informal caregivers used the internet for health-related reasons and caregiving information.

5.2   How Do Informal Caregivers Use the Internet?

Informal caregivers of older people visiting a caregiving website mostly looked for health information, practical issues, and legal and financial issues [33]. These preferences were directed from the type of caregiving. Informal caregivers also searched online to communicate and receive support by other informal caregivers, health professionals, and eHealth solutions. Kernisan et al.'s [33] group replies in four categories: (a) caring for a parent, (b) caring for themselves only, (c) other caregiving situations, and (d) unknown caregiving situations. In the case of the informal caregivers of older people, practical issues were the most frequently searched. According to Lam and Lam [31], the most common use of the internet among informal caregivers in Australia included chat sites and emails. This related to the informal caregivers needs to communicate. Furthermore, informal caregivers used the internet for information and for accessing government services, to pay bills. Informal caregivers who used the internet 12 months before the study had better mental health in comparison with the informal caregivers who had not used the internet during that period. In another study by Li [32], using secondary data of 812 informal caregivers from the US caregiver survey, informal caregivers searched for disease-specific information (77.2%) and services for the patients (52.7%), and only 11% searched for information for themselves. In the report by Pew Research Center "Family Caregivers Online" [30], 860 informal caregivers participated in the survey about internet use among informal caregivers in the United States. From most of the sample, 79% used the internet at home, 88% searched for health information online, and 55% had a laptop or another mobile device. Informal caregivers were more likely to search for health information for someone else, use social media for communication, and read clinicians, medical facilities, and drug reviews. They also considered the internet as useful when searching for health- related issues. In other research on information-seeking among the family of PwD, 171 out of 214 informal caregivers replied that they were searching for information mainly through dementia association websites (82%) and that 38% rated the information that they found on the internet about dementia as low quality [34]. The internet together with newspapers and television was considered as passive information sources, and the internet was considered the most accessible source (86%) and was the first source of the search for information followed by health professionals. Informal caregivers also considered access to online sources as important for the knowledge and skills of health self-management [2]. Informal caregivers considered technology use as important for networking and personalized care, being most useful for information management [35]. In the same study, spouses made less frequent use than children who cared for a parent with dementia, and only three informal caregivers used applications for caregiving.

5.3 What Do Informal Caregivers Post Online?

In the case of the research by Anderson et al. [27], 2345 posts were analyzed by nine websites and were categorized in four categories: (a) social support–communication and inclusion, (b) the search for information, (c) sharing of memories with the person with dementia, and (d) information to other informal caregivers and advocacy. In another study by Yoo et al. [36], 798 messages were analyzed by informal caregivers from South Korea, and they found that informal caregivers expressed mostly negative feelings in comparison with informal caregivers in the United States, and they looked for emotional support to online communities. More recently, 500 posts of the Alzheimer Association forum were categorized in ten categories: feelings, symptoms, doctors and services, physical safety, hygiene, general info, medicine, conflicts, solutions, and ethics. Another 250 posts randomly selected included their solutions and were included in the below categories. The problems were mostly negative, and solutions provided by other informal caregivers or moderators were neutral. The solutions were also categorized into six categories: information, communication with experts, assisted care facilities, memory problems, safety and care at home [37], and information search and coping, a model developed to associate information seeking and information forwarding among informal caregivers of PwD and coping strategies online. Information seeking was associated more with problem-solving techniques and information forwarding with emotion-based techniques [38]. Needs and benefit among informal caregivers of PwD informal caregivers considered as important elements for using the technology to have on-time access to related tailored information and be able to receive information online for direct behavioral management [39]. According to the American National Alliance for Caregiving [40], benefits for accessing online health-related information were: (a) time-saving, (b) support with caregiving, (c) safety of the person receiving care, and (d) a sense that the caregiver is effective.

6 Conclusions of the Internet Use Among Informal Caregivers Systematic Scoping Review

The scoping review searched all available published research of health-related or dementia-related internet use among informal caregivers of PwD, elderly, and adults with mental or physical chronic conditions. In the papers included, the importance of internet use was identified, and predictors of the use are reported such as age, relationship with the patient, education, socioeconomic position, and other characteristics. Informal caregivers searched online for dementia information and services, and they tried to communicate with other informal caregivers or health professionals. eHealth literacy was not reported in any of the above published papers of the search period (2000–2018) neither as a theory or as survey concept, even if in many cases, the related questions may have been part of the concept of eHealth literacy.

References

1. Alzheimer's Association (2021) Alzheimer's disease facts and figures. Alzheimer's and dementia, vol 17. Wiley
2. Lucero RJ, Jaime-Lara R, Cortes YI, Kearney J, Granja M, Suero-Tejeda N et al (2018) Hispanic dementia family caregiver's knowledge, experience, and awareness of self-management: foundations for health information technology interventions. Hispanic Health Care Int 154041531881922. https://doi.org/10.1177/1540415318819220
3. Chiao C, Wu H, Hsiao C, Hsiao C-Y (2015) Caregiver burden for informal caregivers of patients with dementia: a systematic review (110):340–350
4. Farina N, Page TE, Daley S, Brown A, Bowling A, Basset T et al (2017) Factors associated with the quality of life of family carers of people with dementia: a systematic review. Alzheimer's Dementia 13(5):572–581. http://search.ebscohost.com/login.aspx?direct=true&db=psyh&AN=2017-09842-001&site=eds-live
5. Huang S-S (2022) Depression among caregivers of patients with dementia: associative factors and management approaches. World J Psychiatry 12(1):59–76
6. Gilhooly KJ, Gilhooly MLM, Sullivan MP, McIntyre A, Wilson L, Harding E et al (2016) A meta-review of stress, coping and interventions in dementia and dementia caregiving. BMC Geriatr 16:106
7. Feast A, Orrell M, Charlesworth G, Melunsky N, Poland F, Moniz-Cook E (2016) Behavioural and psychological symptoms in dementia and the challenges for family carers: systematic review. Br J Psychiatry 208(5):429–434
8. Bratches RWR, Scudder PN, Barr PJ (2021) Supporting communication of visit information to informal caregivers: a systematic review. PLoS One 16
9. Sanders D, Scott P (2020) Literature review: technological interventions and their impact on quality of life for people living with dementia, vol 27. BMJ Health and Care Informatics. BMJ Publishing Group
10. World Health Organisation (2018) Digital technologies: shaping the future of primary health care. Geneva [cited 2022 Jan 16]. https://www.who.int/docs/default-source/primary-health-care-conference/digital-technologies.pdf?sfvrsn=3efc47e0_2
11. Dequanter S, Gagnon MP, Ndiaye MA, Gorus E, Fobelets M, Giguère A et al (2021) The effectiveness of e-Health solutions for aging with cognitive impairment: a systematic review. Gerontologist Gerontol Soc Am 61:E373–94

12. Morris L, Mansell W, Williamson T, Wray A, McEvoy P (2020) Communication empowerment framework: an integrative framework to support effective communication and interaction between carers and people living with dementia. Dementia 19(6):1739–1757

13. Hoel V, Feunou CM, Wolf-Ostermann K (2021) Technology-driven solutions to prompt conversation, aid communication and support interaction for people with dementia and their caregivers: a systematic literature review. BMC Geriatr 21(1):157

14. Lucero RJ, Fehlberg EA, Patel AGM, Bjarnardottir RI, Williams R, Lee K et al (2019) The effects of information and communication technologies on informal caregivers of persons living with dementia: a systematic review. Alzheimer's Dementia 5:1–12. https://doi.org/10.1016/j.trci.2018.11.003

15. Charalambous A (2019) Utilizing the advances in digital health solutions to manage care in cancer patients. In: Asia-Pac J Oncol Nurs, pp 234–237

16. Lindeman DA, Kim KK, Gladstone C, Apesoa-Varano EC, Hepburn K (2020) Technology and caregiving: emerging interventions and directions for research. Gerontologist Gerontol Soc Am 60:S41–S49

17. Hassan AYI (2020) Challenges and recommendations for the deployment of information and communication technology solutions for informal caregivers: scoping review, vol 3, JMIR Aging. JMIR Publications

18. Soleimaninejad A, Valizadeh-Haghi S, Rahmatizadeh S (2019) Assessing the eHealth literacy skills of family caregivers of medically ill elderly. J Pub Health Inf 11(2):e12

19. Verma R, Saldanha C, Ellis U, Sattar S, Haase KR (2021) eHealth literacy among older adults living with cancer and their caregivers: a scoping review. J Geriatric Oncol

20. Efthymiou A, Middleton N, Charalambous A, Papastavrou E (2021) Identifying the carer's profiles of health literacy, eHealth literacy and caregiving concepts. Eur J Public Health 31(Suppl 3):1. https://academic.oup.com/eurpub/article/31/Supplement_3/ckab164.275/6405684

21. Dam AEH, de Vugt ME, Klinkenberg IPM, Verhey FRJ, van Boxtel MPJ (2016) Review article: a systematic review of social support interventions for caregivers of people with dementia: are they doing what they promise? [Internet], vols. 85 OP-I, p 117. http://search.ebscohost.com/login.aspx?direct=true&site=eds-live&db=edselp&AN=S037851221530092X

22. Hopwood J, Walker N, McDonagh L, Rait G, Walters K, Iliffe S et al (2018) Internet-based interventions aimed at supporting family caregivers of people with dementia: systematic review. J Med Internet Res 20(6):e216

23. Chi N, Demiris G (2015) A systematic review of telehealth tool and interventions to support family caregivers. J Telemed Telecare 21(1):37–44

24. Boots LMM, Vugt ME, Knippenberg RJM, Kempen GIJM, Verhey FRJ (2014) A systematic review of Internet-based supportive interventions for caregivers of patients with dementia. [Internet], vol 29, p 331. http://search.ebscohost.com/login.aspx?direct=true&site=eds-live&db=pbh&AN=94777553

25. Tricco A, Lillie E, Zarin W, O'Brien K, Colquhoun H, Levac D et al (2018) PRISMA extension for scoping reviews (PRISMA-ScR): checklist and explanation. Ann Intern Med 169(7):467–473

26. Arksey H, O'Malley L (2005) Scoping studies: towards a methodological framework. Int J Soc Res Methodol: Theory Pract 8(1):19–32

27. Anderson JG, Hundt E, Dean M, Keim-Malpass J, Lopez RP (2017) "The Church of Online Support": examining the use of blogs among family caregivers of persons with dementia. J Fam Nurs 23(1):34–54

28. Blackburn C, Read J, Hughes N (2005) Carers and the digital divide: factors affecting internet use among carers in the UK. Health Soc Care Community 13(3):201–210. http://search.ebscohost.com/login.aspx?direct=true&site=eds-live&db=rzh&AN=106649859

29. Kim H (2015) Understanding internet use among dementia caregivers: results of secondary data analysis using the US caregiver survey data. Interact J Med Res 4(1). http://search.ebscohost.com/login.aspx?direct=true&db=mdc&AN=25707033&site=eds-live

30. Fox S, Brenner J (2012) Family caregivers online. Pew Internet Res

31. Lam L, Lam M (2009) The use of information technology and mental health among older care-givers in Australia. Aging Mental Health 13(4):557. http://search.ebscohost.com/login. aspx?direct=true&site=eds-live&db=rzh&AN=105395472
32. Li H (2015) Informal caregivers' use of the internet for caregiving information. Soc Work Health Care 54(6):532–546. http://www.ncbi.nlm.nih.gov/pubmed/26186424
33. Kernisan L, Sudore R, Knight S (2010) Information-seeking at a caregiving website: a qualitative analysis. J Med Internet Res 12(3). http://search.ebscohost.com/login.aspx?direct=true&d b=mdc&AN=20675292&site=eds-live
34. Allen F, Cain R, Meyer C (2018) Seeking relational information sources in the digital age: a study into information source preferences amongst family and friends of those with dementia. Dementia
35. Ruggiano N, Brown EL, Shaw S, Geldmacher D, Clarke P, Hristidis V et al (2018) The potential of information technology to navigate caregiving systems: perspectives from dementia caregivers. J Gerontol Soc Work 4372:1–19. https://doi.org/10.1080/01634372.2018.1546786
36. Yoo JH, Jang SA, Choi T (2010) Sociocultural determinants of negative emotions among dementia caregivers in the United States and in Korea: a content analysis of online support groups. Howard J Commun 21(1):1–19
37. Scharett E, Lopes S, Rogers H, Bhargava A, Ponathil A, Madathil KC et al (2017) An investigation of information sought by caregivers of Alzheimer's patients on online peer-support groups. Proc Hum Fact Ergonomics Soc 1773–1777
38. Jeong JS, Kim Y, Chon MG (2018) Who is caring for the caregiver? The role of cybercoping for dementia caregivers. Health Commun 33(1):5–13
39. Werner NE, Stanislawski B, Marx KA, Watkins DC, Kobayashi M, Kales H et al (2017) Getting what they need when they need it. Appl Clin Inf 8(1):191–205. https://doi.org/10.4338/ACI-2016-07-RA-0122
40. Alwan M, Orlov L, Schulz R, Vuckovic N (2011) E-connected family caregiver: bringing caregiving into 21st century

Family Caregivers in Palliative Care in the Hospital Setting

Elina Haavisto, Johanna Saarinen, and Anu Soikkeli-Jalonen

1 Introduction

Patients' palliative care situation affects their whole family, and with every patient comes a number of family caregivers requiring palliative care services both before and after the patient's death [1]. While family typically involves people with close affinity to the patient, the concept of family has varying definitions, both narrow and broad, in the literature. In the broadest sense, a family can be defined as a group of people who have continuous, personal relationships with the patient and are involved in the patient's life and care [2]. Apart from family [3], the following terms are also used: family caregiver [4], family member [5], relative [6], and next of kin [7]. Therefore, the terms family and family caregiver are used interchangeably in this chapter. Furthermore, the hospital context mentioned in this chapter refers to the ward environment and not the outpatient clinics.

Over 56.8 million people need palliative care each year, especially for long-term illnesses such as cardiovascular disease, cancer, chronic respiratory diseases, diabetes, and neurological conditions, and the need for palliative care increases as the

E. Haavisto (✉)
Department of Health Sciences, Nursing, Faculty of Social Sciences, Tampere University, Tampere, Finland

Department of Nursing Science, Faculty of Medicine, University of Turku, Turku, Finland
e-mail: elina.a.haavisto@tuni.fi

J. Saarinen
Department of Nursing Science, Faculty of Medicine, University of Turku, Turku, Finland
e-mail: johanna.ka.saarinen@utu.fi

A. Soikkeli-Jalonen
Department of Health Sciences, Nursing, Faculty of Social Sciences, Tampere University, Tampere, Finland
e-mail: anu.soikkeli-jalonen@tuni.fi

© The Author(s), under exclusive license to Springer Nature Switzerland AG 2023
A. Charalambous (ed.), *Informal Caregivers: From Hidden Heroes to Integral Part of Care*, https://doi.org/10.1007/978-3-031-16745-4_8

population ages [8]. Care systems and locations for palliative care vary by country, and there are differences in the palliative care systems across Europe [9]. Palliative care environments also vary, ranging from the patient's home to different clinical settings. Patients receive care in an inpatient setting for several reasons; for instance, they may not be able to manage the illness at home or may require treatments for the occurring symptoms [10]. When the patient care needs are complex, intense, and frequent, treatment is carried out in specialised palliative care units [11]. It has been shown that the majority of people in the developed world die in hospitals [12], although some patients also wish for the possibility of dying at home [13]. In meta-analysis concerning cancer patients' preferred place of death, about half of the patients hoped that they could die at home, while half of the patients preferred different health care settings [14]. In addition, while not just patients but also their families consider home to be the ideal place of death, their initial perspectives are not based on the actual emotional and practical requirements and strains associated with death. For this reason, when families face the actual demands of caring for a dying person, they often prefer hospital or other care facilities compared to home [15]. Furthermore, even patients' opinions change over time as the patient's disease progresses and the condition changes[16].

Palliative care treatment is demanding and requires special resources over time, which also induces economic challenges [17]. Although it is known that healthcare costs increase as people age, minimal research has been conducted on palliative care costs [18], and knowledge about the actual costs of palliative care is limited. Notably, palliative care encompasses aspects other than end-of-life care. The indirect costs, including informal caregiving, can account for half of the palliative care costs, thus emphasising the importance of the family's role and support in the care process [17]. In large data published in a systematic review, it has been observed that the service use and costs of care increase exponentially as death approaches, and the hospitalisation is the main cost driver [19]; furthermore, end-of-life care accounts for 25% of healthcare expenditure in the USA, 20% of hospital bed-days in the UK [20], and about 25% of healthcare expenditure in Finland [21].

The implementation of palliative care is regulated by national laws, norms, and guidelines [22] and ethical codes [23, 24] that regulate family status as part of patient care. The starting point for palliative care is to alleviate and support the suffering of patients and their families holistically. Family caregivers expect healthcare professionals to communicate information actively, understand their situation, and respond to their needs [25] because the palliative care situation causes emotional distress and the need for support in coping with the situation [26, 27]. Even though the family should be considered a unit of care, it is often seen as a distinct aspect of the patient's life [28], and its needs are not easily met [29]. Furthermore, there is a lack of feasible practices for guiding family involvement in palliative patient care.

The scarcity of research on family being part of patient care in the hospital context [27, 30, 31] and the factors with the greatest significance in relation to the patient, family, and quality of care are not evident [32]. Furthermore, what it means for the family to be part of care is that it has received little attention from researchers and theorists in the area of cancer nursing and palliative care [33]. Research concerning palliative care tends to focus on the healthcare perspective instead of the patient and family [34]. To the best of our knowledge, no comparative study in the hospital setting has been conducted between several countries. Furthermore, no known intervention studies have focused on family participation in palliative care in hospitals [31]. Overall, there is a lack of interventions aimed at the families of inpatient palliative care patients [30]. However, such interventions would be beneficial [35], making it necessary to gain more information about family involvement in palliative care and to define the problems and challenges therein [36].

2 Family-Centred Care in the Palliative Care Context

Family-centred care considers patients' families as integral for care provision and aims to promote their well-being and enable active participation [37]. It is also a core area of palliative care provision, as family caregivers form an integral part of the patient's life in the hospital setting [38]. Therefore, while the healthcare system is strongly organised around the patient, family-centred care is also a central and valued part of palliative care [33].

A recent concept analysis defined family-centred care as a philosophy of care provision that, despite originating in paediatrics, is relevant in diverse care contexts and age groups [39]. The Institute of Patient and Family Centred Care has defined the core concepts of patient- and family-centred care as a practice where healthcare professionals treat patients and families with dignity and respect, listening to and honouring their perspectives and choices. Additionally, their understanding, values, beliefs, and cultural background are considered in care planning and delivery. Healthcare professionals need to communicate clearly and honestly and share unbiased, complete, and accurate information with families. Furthermore, families' participation in decision-making and care processes must be encouraged and supported. Collaboration with families should also be promoted at all levels of care delivery, healthcare policy, and research [37]. However, while family caregivers are implicitly understood to be members of care units, articulated policies for the same are not always present [33].

A scoping review of the models and key components of family-centred care identified the common aspects of patient- and family-centred care in different illness populations and care contexts, thus confirming the core areas established in different care settings. The key components included (a) collaboration among healthcare professionals, patients, and families in care planning and care delivery, with better communication and information exchange to enable patient advocacy and participation in decision-making; (b) emotional support for families and educating family caregivers about the illness and care provision by different means, considering their needs and preferences; (c) consideration of the family context with the awareness that families are an essential part of patient care, providing emotional, physical, and practical support in line with the strengths and cultural values of the family; and (d) the need for policies and procedures, including those for resources and the opportunity to implement family-centred care and support [40]. McLeod et al. (2010) [33] identified two defining factors of high-quality family care practice: (a) getting to know the family and being known by the family; (b) addressing the family's concerns and anxiety. It is important to view each family as a unique unit with its own history and needs, requiring the skill of understanding non-verbal and para-verbal cues. Knowing patients' families involves understanding their relational and interactional responses to the patient's illness; this allows healthcare professionals to respond appropriately to the family's concerns and distress.

In this chapter, family involvement in palliative inpatient care in the hospital setting, or family-centred care, is understood in three parts (Fig. 1): (1) factors associated with family involvement in palliative inpatient care (see Sect. 3), (2) family involvement in palliative patient care based on two elements—family participation in patient care (see Sect. 4) and psychosocial support for family (see Sect. 5), and (3) consequences of family involvement (see Sect. 6).

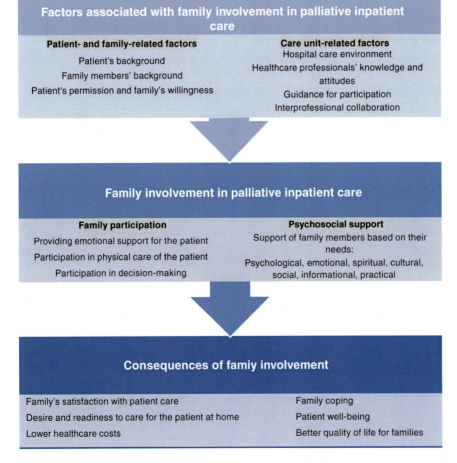

Fig. 1 Family involvement in palliative inpatient care—associated factors and consequences of involvement

3 Factors Associated with Family Involvement in Palliative Inpatient Care

Previous studies [41–44] have associated family involvement in palliative patient care with (a) patient- and family-related factors, such as patient and family caregivers' background and willingness to involve each other in the care process; and (b) care unit-related factors, such as the hospital care environment and climate, knowledge and attitudes of healthcare professionals, guidance that the family receives from healthcare professionals, and interprofessional collaboration (Fig. 1). Family involvement depends on the patient's consent and the family's desire to participate. Many patients want their families to be involved in the caregiving process. However, some patients do not want constant family involvement [45].

Patient background factors, such as status and diagnosis, are related to the family's desire to be involved in the care when the patient has different hospital admission times and care needs as well as the stage of the disease [44]. Patient condition is associated with family participation in concrete care with advanced cancer patients, and poor health conditions increase family involvement in the care [42]. The background and personal characteristics of family caregivers are associated with their past caregiver role, closeness to the patient, physical condition, age, gender, and education [41]. It has been shown that women give more importance to participation in care than men do, and they also participate more. Furthermore, younger family caregivers and those with higher primary education participate more than those with lower educational levels [42]. Family involvement may also be influenced by social and moral norms and the expectations of the family and community [46].

A positive and safe person-centred care environment [47] can significantly influence family involvement in palliative hospital care [43]. A physical environment that enables a family to be present [41] has been found to be important for participation. Furthermore, an environment that facilitates family attendance and participation and is considered welcoming has been identified to support families [3, 44, 48–50]. It is important that healthcare professionals do their best to acknowledge and strengthen the position of family caregivers in palliative care in the hospital setting [3]. However, family caregivers have also been found to experience uncertainty about their own position in the care setting, requiring them to negotiate and justify their position [51]. Families may find it difficult to get involved in patient care within the hospital context due to the new and unfamiliar environment [52].

Healthcare professionals' knowledge and attitudes are also essential factors for family involvement [43]. Palliative care requires comprehensive competence from healthcare professionals, which, in addition to good patient care, includes providing support and preparing the family for the end-of-life care of the patient, guiding the family caregivers, and supporting the family after the patient's death [53]. However, a lack of competence is one of the main obstacles to implementing high-quality palliative care [54]. Patient care staff should also support families in their role as intermediaries between patients and healthcare professionals [3]. Even if family involvement in palliative care is seen as important by healthcare professionals, the inclination to actively invite the involvement of families is rare [55]. Studies have also shown that nurses' attitudes towards the care of terminal patients are not always holistic [56].

The quality of the guidance and detailed, explicit information received from healthcare professionals about the patient's illness, condition, palliative care, prognosis, and different treatment opportunities are factors that enable family participation in the care and decision-making processes [41] as well as ensure that family caregivers understand the relevant information [43]. Family caregivers' ability to act as representatives of the patient increases when they are sufficiently informed and involved in decisions about treatment and care [6].

Interprofessional collaboration encourages active participation in care delivery and care planning; it involves sharing information with the family involved and knowledge and skills with different healthcare professionals [57]. For families, collaboration comprises mutual communication, team spirit, and teamwork. Involving family caregivers in interprofessional teamwork can convey the healthcare professionals' interest and enthusiasm. However, the deterioration of a patient's health changes the nature of an interprofessional team and the family caregiver's role. It has been shown that although families may not always recognise the need for teamwork and may have no opportunity to participate, they remain confident in healthcare professionals' interprofessional work [5]. Interprofessional collaboration has been identified as an essential aspect of building palliative care knowledge and skills [58], and it may improve health outcomes and care [59].

4 Family Participation in Palliative Inpatient Care

Family participation has been identified as a meaningful part of palliative patient care in the hospital setting [3, 31]. In this context, the focus is usually on the healthcare professionals who provide care for the patient; however, family caregivers are also important because they contribute to patient care and provide support [27, 31]. The benefits of familial support in patient care have also been acknowledged by healthcare professionals [60], since family presence can support the patient in different aspects of care and therefore it is also beneficial for healthcare professionals [61].

Every family caregiver has his or her own way of contributing to the patient's palliative care in a hospital setting [31]. The literature in this regard shows that family caregivers participate in different aspects of patient care in hospital settings: they provide emotional support for the patient, assist in the patient's physical care, and participate in making decisions related to patient care [27, 31] (Fig. 1); this includes being a part of care planning and advanced care planning (ACP) [62]. A literature review on family participation in hospital-based palliative care [31] conveys that studies on this topic have included patients, family caregivers, and healthcare professionals as study participants. Family participation has been studied in specialised palliative care settings as well as in medical, surgical, oncological, and acute settings using qualitative, quantitative, and mixed methods. Studies on family caregivers' participation in inpatient palliative care have been conducted since the 1980s, and the number of studies has increased over the last decade.

4.1 Providing Emotional Support for the Patient

A patient's family is an important resource of emotional as well as nursing support. Thus, family caregivers should be provided the opportunity to stay with the patient in the hospital, and their participation in patient care should be encouraged [63]. It is also important for the family to visit the patient in the hospital regularly [64]. Family caregivers can form a rotation-based visitation schedule; they also have the option of visiting for a short time, spending several hours a day with the patient, or even staying at night [65].

When in the hospital, patients can experience feelings of loneliness, especially when they don't have family caregivers visiting them or don't receive enough emotional support [64]. Family caregivers ensure that the patient does not feel alone [65, 66]. Their presence provides comfort [60, 66] and safety for the patient [61, 66] in unfamiliar environments. Spending time together also provides the opportunity to patients to share their emotional burden [64] and to family caregivers to show their support and love for the patient [6].

In addition, family caregivers can support the spiritual needs of the patient according to their culture and religion. In Abudari et al.'s study [67], nurses described how the families of Muslim patients supported the spiritual needs of the patients by praying with them. Apart from this, family caregivers also tend to be present at the moment of the patient's death [60, 63]; this requires healthcare professionals to communicate with the family and inform them about the patient's condition in a timely manner [68].

4.2 Participation in the Patient's Physical Care

In addition to emotional support, family caregivers can assist in the physical care of patients [61, 65, 66]. The patient's condition as well as family caregivers' abilities [61] and preference to participate [65] affect this aspect of care. A family caregiver's role in the hospital is similar to the assistance that he or she would provide for the patient at home. Common care tasks include assisting the patient with eating and drinking, personal hygiene, mobility, and position changes [65, 66]. Family caregivers help the patient get dressed, move around, go to the bathroom, and wash themselves as well as help ease the patient's pain, nausea, or vomiting. Furthermore, they increase stimulation and bring drinks and food to the patient [43].

Family caregivers can also participate in post-mortem care when the patient dies. This participation should be accommodated according to the wishes of the family caregivers, and they can participate to the extent that they feel comfortable. They may simply be present in the room during the final care, or they may participate in combing, grooming, anointing, washing, and dressing the body [68]. Family caregivers can be described as members of the patient care team in the hospital setting since they also assist the nursing staff with, for example, positioning the patient [61]; in turn, the nursing staff teaches them how to provide care [66].

4.3   Participation in the Decision-Making Process

Decisions concerning patient care can be made by healthcare professionals alone [69] or together with the patient and the patient's family [69, 70]. It has been noted that family caregivers' participation in making decisions about patient care and treatment is an important element of end-of-life care, even though these decisions can be difficult to make [44]. To participate, family caregivers need to be provided with information on different care and treatment options, and they need to understand the patient's condition and situation [44]. Healthcare professionals can also gather important information about a patient's condition from family caregivers, since they know the patient well and spend a lot of time with the patient. Family caregivers can provide details about the patient's food intake or complaints, for example, and might even identify changes in the patient's condition [61]. Family caregivers are not always offered the opportunity to participate in decision-making, but when they are, it is suitable to do so once the caregiver has been with the patient for a few entire days [6].

Family participation in the decision-making process involves the caregivers supporting and helping the patients express their wishes [70] or representing the patients when the patients are unable to express their own wishes [6, 70]. Family caregivers are satisfied with their role as the patient's representative in the decision-making process when they are fully aware of the various treatment options, feel like they have made the decisions together with the doctor [6], and that the decisions respect the patient's wishes [70].

When discussing treatment goals, it is important that family caregivers have a consistent understanding of the patient's situation and do not set unrealistic expectations. However, studies have revealed differences in goals between the patient and family, the patient and physician, and the family and physician [45]. The involvement of family caregivers is important because they can clarify the patient's description of the situation and act as an advocate for the patient, thus asking questions on behalf of the patient and participating in decision-making processes if the patient is unable to do so. Involving the family can also help the patients take an active role in their own care. For instance, a caregiver involved in the decision-making may want treatment to continue although the patient disagrees [45].

Advance care planning (ACP) in palliative care is a family-centred method that aims to ensure patients' right to self-determination [71]. The ACP procedure supports the consideration of patients' wishes and desires at the end of their lives [72]. ACP is employed to make decisions about patients' future care, especially to plan for situations wherein the patients are no longer able to express their wishes or capable of making decisions [73]. ACP is implemented in cooperation with the patient, healthcare professionals, and family caregivers [74]. Family participation in ACP has been observed to have several benefits, such as improvements in patient care and enhanced patient satisfaction. Furthermore, the direct benefits of a successful ACP on family caregivers include decreased anxiety, stress, and depressive symptoms, which supports their coping and survival [75, 76]. Additionally, patients also consider it important for families to be included in care planning [60].

However, the implementation of ACP in palliative care still has some limitations, such as often taking place too late in terms of the patient's condition [62]. This indicates why families do not fully understand the ACP policy or its meaning and realisation [77].

5 Psychosocial Support for Families in Palliative Hospital Care

5.1 Psychosocial Support

Family support is an essential aspect of palliative care, considering the family's important role in the care process; family needs should be noticed and taken care of, along with the patients' [38]. In hospital care, this broadly involves their physical, emotional, social, spiritual, and informational needs [78]. Therefore, psychosocial support is often implemented to comprehensively address families' needs. While the psychosocial approach to family support has various definitions, it typically considers the psychological and social aspects of life and may involve practical interventions such as providing financial support or aid in housing and daily living (Fig. 1) [79]. The US National Cancer Institute at the National Institutes of Health defines psychosocial support as *"support given to help meet patients' mental, emotional, social, and spiritual needs and families. Diseases such as cancer can affect a patient's thoughts, feelings, moods, beliefs, ways of coping, and relationships with family, friends, and co-workers. There are different kinds of psychosocial support that can help cancer patients. These include counselling, education, group support, and spiritual support"* [80].

It has been recommended that psychosocial support should be available to all families of a patient with advanced disease, since care requirements for severe illnesses are complex and result in special support needs for both the patient and family members [81]. Family caregivers with a patient in hospital care require support in their role due to the unfamiliar environment. Furthermore, in the hospital context, healthcare professionals need to inform family caregivers of the patient's treatment, condition, and prognosis; otherwise, they can end up as outsiders if only the patient is taken care of and informed [41], as it may be difficult for family caregivers to find their positions and places in such an unaccustomed and stressful situation [27, 52].

5.2 Psychosocial Support in Relation to Family Caregivers' Needs in Palliative Hospital Care

Family caregivers have several unmet needs that need to be considered by healthcare professionals in palliative hospital care [82]. Not only do they need support in coping with and adjusting to the palliative care situation in general but also in adapting to the hospital environment. Thus, there is a high need for family support in palliative care situations. [83]. When a patient receives palliative care, family caregivers are naturally concerned about losing their loved one; in addition, their role in a hospital setting is different from that at home, which complicates their adapting to the situation and increases the need for support [84–87]. The patient situation in palliative care is always serious and causes a severe fear of loss among families, a burden that is greater than that of the families in other care settings [88]. Despite this, families experience unsatisfactory support practices and information exchanges with healthcare professionals [82].

While family caregivers' support needs have been reported to be mainly informational, emotional, and social in nature, physical, financial, service-related, and spiritual needs are also common [82]. Psychosocial support encompasses those frequently occurring needs [79]. However, restrictions have been reported in meeting family caregivers' support needs in an inpatient environment, primarily with regard to sharing patient care information, such as symptom management and medication, limited interest in family caregivers' daily needs or emotional and psychological distress, or an absence of direct support [89]. Therefore, considering these constraints, the families of palliative care patients are often described as hidden patients, and they have been estimated to have even more unmet needs than the patients themselves [28]. This can be problematic since family caregivers may experience anxiety and depression when their needs are not fulfilled, leading to greater emotional burden and distress [90]. Furthermore, when family caregivers experience continuous anxiety during the patient's treatment, it affects all areas of their life over time and increases the risk of psychological [91] and physical morbidities that can impair the overall quality of life [92, 93].

5.3 Implementing Support During Palliative Inpatient Care

As previously stated, palliative care situations are stressful and complicated for family caregivers, due to which there is no single, easy approach to implementing systems of support [30, 94]. Healthcare professionals are in key positions for providing support in hospital environments [95], and family caregivers not only expect professional and safe care for the patient but also seek support for themselves [3]. However, studies indicate that healthcare professionals face challenges in providing support to families, and their competence in supporting family caregivers is not always optimal [47, 91, 92]. Healthcare professionals' education is commonly concentrated on patient care issues, especially physical care, but family care has received less attention. Therefore, the lack of training in practical care can hinder healthcare professionals from acknowledging and employing family support measures [97, 98].

Nevertheless, family caregivers are often supported by various interventions, usually implemented by healthcare professionals, to relieve their burdens and inhibit their morbidity [85, 99]. However, most of the interventions are designed for home and community care, and only a few aim to support families during the inpatient palliative care process [30]. Even though existing interventions were found to be beneficial in family support [29, 35, 100, 101], the studies implemented in home and community care have limited generalisability to hospital settings [89]. There are also mixed results concerning the effectiveness of different interventions for family support [96, 101–104]. It must be noted that the process of developing supportive interventions for palliative care family caregivers is not straightforward due to the increasing distress caused by the patient's worsening condition [30].

The interventions utilised in hospital settings largely involve three approaches: meetings, education, and therapy [30]. Meeting-based interventions are commonly used with families in palliative care settings; however, the effectiveness of the process remains uncertain, and more research is needed in this area [104]. Family meeting interventions are implemented with multidisciplinary groups, patients, and families [30], and they usually provide emotional [105, 106], communicational, and informational [107, 108] support for the families. In addition, several interventions involve educational methods that aim to develop family caregivers' preparedness and competence in patient care [109]. Educational interventions specifically address family caregivers' informational needs and help them adapt to their role in the hospital context [85]. Therapy-based interventions are also used in palliative care, involving, for example, behavioural and mindfulness-based approaches, and they need to be implemented by qualified therapists [30].

To be usable and feasible, interventions in the palliative care context should be easy to implement and not too strenuous for the families involved. However, it is important to note that the most effective interventions include multiple long, supportive sessions, and although they can be made more efficient, designing and implementing such interventions are complicated in the practical care environment of hospitals [30]. Studies indicate that decreasing family caregivers' anxiety and depressive symptoms is challenging, and frequent meetings are required to make progress [100]. The most effective, intensive, and therapy-based interventions can be burdensome for family caregivers and laborious to implement in the hospital setting, as they require lots of resources and time [30]. Behavioural interventions [110] and interventions based on psychoeducation [35] and mindfulness [111], as well as interventions combining various elements [112], have been found to be helpful. However, family caregivers' symptoms of anxiety and depression [100–102] and quality of life [103] tend to be difficult to improve through external support provided by the healthcare professionals.

6   Consequences of Family Involvement

Although family involvement is acknowledged as an important part of palliative care delivery, its consequences are poorly studied, and there is not much knowledge about the actual impact and influence of the same [31, 113]. However, there is some evidence that family involvement in palliative patient care can lead to many positive consequences (Fig. 1) and improve the overall quality of care [41, 103]. In general, involving both the patient and family in the care approach leads to better health outcomes [37, 114] and promotes care efficacy. Clinician and staff satisfaction may also improve, and resources may be better allocated to enable family care implementation in practice [37].

Family involvement also increases patient and family satisfaction with healthcare [37]. It is essential for family caregivers to be able to trust that the patient receives good-quality care [3, 47]. Families have their own expectations, and they assess whether and how these expectations were realised. Expectations are connected to the healthcare professionals' approach to care as much as their actions for themselves [115]. Furthermore, when these expectations are met and families experience good patient care, the positive experience increases their coping [115].

According to a systematic review regarding the most important elements of end-of-life care in hospital settings, family caregivers considered that the essential aspects relate almost entirely to patient's care. Families gave the most importance to symptom management and good physical care. Furthermore, they were found to expect effective communication and shared decision-making processes, respectful and compassionate care, adequate environmental and organisational characteristics, and recognition and support of the family's role in care, which includes valuing their expert knowledge of the patient and advocacy of the patient's needs, maintenance of patient safety and prevention of harm, preparation for death, extending care to the family after patient death, enabling patient choice at the end of life, and managing financial affairs [3].

Family caregivers are better able to cope with the palliative care situation when they desire to participate in [116], are seen as a part of, and can be present for the patient's care [117]. Family togetherness and time together are considered very important [118], and visiting the patient increases the family caregivers' adaptation [115]. Their coping levels also increase when healthcare professionals provide them with information and support [119]. Additionally, they feel important and are up to date on the patient's condition and decisions made when actively participating in patient's care [116].

Family-centred strategies have been shown to reduce the use of healthcare resources, number of referrals and diagnostic tests, and costs related to healthcare [40]. Family involvement can also economically benefit the healthcare system, such as when the family participates in concrete caring [28]. Involvement in patient care in the hospital setting can also lead to the ability to achieve home care and enhance the well-being of the patient [28]. Healthcare professionals have pointed out that family caregivers who contribute to patient care during hospitalisation learn the care tasks that they will handle at home after the patient's discharge [61].

7 Conclusion

Globally, there is a large population of patients needing inpatient palliative care. Since their families tend to be involved in the care experience, they become part of the patient's care in hospital settings. Although palliative care implementation is regulated by national laws, norms, and guidelines and ethical codes, as well as the preferences of the patient and family caregivers, family involvement is not optimally facilitated by healthcare professionals. It does not take place as per recommendations, and on some occasions, it may not even be possible. Family involvement in palliative patient care is associated with a variety of factors, some of which depend on the knowledge and attitude of healthcare professionals, hospital climate, and family guidance provided. More attention should be paid to these.

Family involvement in palliative care is seen in the patient- and family-centred approach, which considers families integral to the care delivery process. Dignified and respectful treatment, information exchange, participation, and collaboration are essential elements of family involvement in patient care. Family caregivers may participate in the emotional support and physical care of the patient and in decision-making processes during the hospitalisation period. However, they are also in need of psychosocial support during the palliative care situation, which tends to be burdensome. Despite the importance of psychosocial support, it is yet a difficult task for the healthcare professionals—family caregivers' needs are complex and not easily fulfilled in such a situation. Nevertheless, family caregivers' presence in the hospital and their participation in the care process support the well-being of the patient and also increase the caregivers' coping abilities and desire to care for the patient at home. Therefore, many positive consequences of family involvement in palliative patient care should be considered, and healthcare professionals should enable and support families' participation if desired and acknowledge their position in the unfamiliar hospital environment.

It is recommended that future research focuses on family involvement in the hospital setting, the factors most important to the patients, family caregivers, and healthcare professionals, and considers the family caregivers' point of view. Intervention studies and comparative research in several countries should also be conducted. Additionally, the consequences of family involvement, not only for the patients and families in palliative care but also for the whole healthcare system, require more attention in future research, as it is important to demonstrate the effects of family involvement at the individual, economic, and organisational levels through evidence-based methods.

References

1. World Health Organisation (WHO) (2022) WHO definition of palliative care. https://www.who.int/cancer/palliative/definition/en/
2. Mitchell ML, Chaboyer W (2010) Family Centred care—a way to connect patients, families and nurses in critical care: a qualitative study using telephone interviews. Intensive Crit Care Nurs 26:154–160

3. Virdun C, Luckett T, Lorenz K, Davidson PM, Phillips J (2017) Dying in the hospital setting: a meta-synthesis identifying the elements of end-of-life care that patients and their families describe as being important. Palliat Med 31:587–601

4. Hudson PL, Lobb EA, Thomas K, Zordan RD, Trauer T, Quinn K, Williams A, Summers M (2012) Psycho-educational group intervention for family caregivers of hospitalized palliative care patients: pilot study. J Palliat Med 15:277–281

5. Kesonen P, Salminen L, Haavisto E (2022) Patients and family members' perceptions of interprofessional teamwork in palliative care: a qualitative descriptive study. J Clin Nurs. https://doi.org/10.1111/jocn.16192

6. Witkamp E, Droger M, Janssens R, van Zuylen L, van der H (2016) How to deal with relatives of patients dying in the hospital? Qualitative content analysis of relatives' experiences. J Pain Symp Manage 52:235–242

7. Brobäck G, Berterö C (2003) How next of kin experience palliative care of relatives at home. Eur J Cancer Care 12:339–346

8. Connor SR (2020) Global atlas of palliative care, 2nd edn. Worldwide Hospice Palliative Care Alliance, London

9. Woitha K, Carrasco JM, Clark D, Lynch T, Garralda E, Martin-Moreno JM, Centeno C (2016) Policy on palliative care in the WHO European region: an overview of progress since the Council of Europe's (2003) recommendation 24. Eur J Public Health 26:230–235

10. Wallace EM, Cooney MC, Walsh J, Conroy M, Twomey F (2013) Why do palliative care patients present to the emergency department? Avoidable or unavoidable? Am J Hospice Palliat Med 30:253–256

11. Buss MK, Rock LK, McCarthy EP (2017) Understanding palliative care and hospice. Mayo Clin Proc 92:280–286

12. Broad J (2013) Where do people die? An international comparison of the percentage of deaths occurring in hospital and residential aged care settings in 45 populations, using published and available statistics. Int J Public Health 58:257–267

13. Haavisto E, Eriksson S, Cleland Silva T, Koivisto J-M, Kausamo K, Soikkeli-Jalonen A (2022) Palliative care cancer patients' experiences of encounters with healthcare professionals in palliative care inpatient units: a qualitative explorative study. Omega J Death Dying

14. Fereidouni A, Rassouli M, Salesi M, Ashrafizadeh H, Vahedian-Azimi A, Barasteh S (2021) Preferred place of death in adult cancer patients: a systematic review and meta-analysis. Front Psychol. https://doi.org/10.3389/fpsyg.2021.704590

15. Sathiananthan MK, Crawford GB, Eliott J (2021) Healthcare professionals' perspectives of patient and family preferences of patient place of death: a qualitative study. BMC Palliat Care 20:147

16. van Doorne I, van Rijn M, Dofferhoff SM, Willems DL, Buurman BM (2021) Patients' preferred place of death: patients are willing to consider their preferences, but someone has to ask them. Age Ageing 50:2004–2011

17. Haltia O, Färkkilä N, Roine RP, Sintonen H, Taari K, Hänninen J, Lehto JT, Saarto T (2018) The indirect costs of palliative care in end-stage cancer: a real-life longitudinal register- and questionnaire-based study. Palliat Med 32:493–499

18. Gardiner C, Ingleton C, Ryan T, Ward S, Gott M (2017) What cost components are relevant for economic evaluations of palliative care, and what approaches are used to measure these costs? A systematic review. Palliat Med 31:323–337

19. Langton JM, Blanch B, Drew AK, Haas M, Ingham JM, Pearson S-A (2014) Retrospective studies of end-of-life resource utilization and costs in cancer care using health administrative data: a systematic review. Palliat Med 28:1167–1196

20. Smith S, Brick A, O'Hara S, Normand C (2014) Evidence on the cost and cost-effectiveness of palliative care: a literature review. Palliat Med 28:130–150

21. Saarto F-S (2019) Recommendation on the provision and improvement of palliative care services in Finland. Final report of the expert working group. https://julkaisut.valtioneuvosto.fi/bitstream/handle/10024/161946/STM_2019_68_Rap.pdf?sequence=1&isAllowed=y

22. Radbruch L, Payne S (2010) White paper on standards and norms for hospice and palliative care in Europe: part 2. Eur J Palliat Care 17:22–33
23. International Council of Nurses (2012) The ICN codes of ethics for nursing. https://www.icn.ch/sites/default/files/inline-files/2012_ICN_Codeofethicsfornurses_%20eng.pdf
24. The World Medical Association (2018) WMA International Code of Medical Ethics. https://www.wma.net/policies-post/wma-international-code-of-medical-ethics/
25. Adams JA, Donald E, Bailey J, Anderson RA, Docherty SL (2011) Nursing roles and strategies in end-of-life decision making in acute care: a systematic review of the literature. Nurs Res Pract 2011:527815–527834
26. Lazarus PhD RS, Folkman PDS (1984) Stress, appraisal, and coping. Springer Publishing Company, New York
27. Partanen E, Lemetti T, Haavisto E (2018) Participation of relatives in the care of cancer patients in hospital—a scoping review. Eur J Cancer Care (Engl) 27:e12821-n/a
28. Hudson P, Payne S (2011) Family caregivers and palliative care: current status and agenda for the future. J Palliat Med 14:864–869
29. Harding R, List S, Epiphaniou E, Jones H (2012) How can informal caregivers in cancer and palliative care be supported? An updated systematic literature review of interventions and their effectiveness. Palliat Med 26:7–22
30. Soikkeli-Jalonen A, Mishina K, Virtanen H, Charalambous A, Haavisto E (2021) Supportive interventions for family members of very seriously ill patients in inpatient care: a systematic review. J Clin Nurs. https://doi.org/10.1111/jocn.15725
31. Saarinen J, Mishina K, Soikkeli-Jalonen A, Haavisto E (2021) Family members' participation in palliative inpatient care: an integrative review. Scand J Caring Sci. https://doi.org/10.1111/scs.13062
32. Sudore RL, Casarett D, Smith D, Richardson DM, Ersek M (2014) Family involvement at the end-of-life and receipt of quality care. J Pain Symptom Manag 48:1108–1116
33. McLeod DL, Tapp DM, Moules NJ, Campbell ME (2010) Knowing the family: interpretations of family nursing in oncology and palliative care. Eur J Oncol Nurs 14:93–100
34. Hasson F, Nicholson E, Muldrew D, Bamidele O, Payne S, McIlfatrick S (2020) International palliative care research priorities: a systematic review. BMC Palliat Care 19:16
35. Hudson PL, Remedios C, Thomas K (2010) A systematic review of psychosocial interventions for family carers of palliative care patients. BMC Palliat Care 9:17
36. Tarberg AS, Kvangarsnes M, Hole T, Thronæs M, Madssen TS, Landstad BJ (2019) Silent voices: family caregivers' narratives of involvement in palliative care. Nurs Open 6:1446–1454
37. IPFCC (2022) Patient- and family-centered care. In: Institute for Patient- and Family-Centered Care. https://www.ipfcc.org/about/pfcc.html
38. Steele R, Davies B (2015) Supporting families in palliative care. In: Social aspects of care. Oxford University Press, pp 51–72
39. Moradian ST (2018) Family-centered care: an evolutionary concept analysis. Int J Med Rev 5:82–86
40. Kokorelias KM, Gignac MAM, Naglie G, Cameron JI (2019) Towards a universal model of family centered care: a scoping review. BMC Health Serv Res 19:564
41. Bélanger L, Desmartis M, Coulombe M (2018) Barriers and facilitators to family participation in the care of their hospitalized loved ones. Patient Exp J 5:56–65
42. Eriksson E, Lauri S (2000) Participation of relatives in the care of cancer patients. Eur J Oncol Nurs 4:99–107
43. Mackie BR, Mitchell M, Marshall AP (2019) Patient and family members' perceptions of family participation in care on acute care wards. Scand J Caring Sci 33:359–370
44. Robinson J, Gott M, Ingleton C (2014) Patient and family experiences of palliative care in hospital: what do we know? An integrative review. Palliat Med 28:18–33
45. Lin JJ, Smith CB, Feder S, Bickell NA, Schulman-Green D (2018) Patients' and oncologists' views on family involvement in goals of care conversations. Psycho-Oncology 27:1035–1041
46. Papastavrou E, Charalambous A, Tsangari H (2009) Exploring the other side of cancer care: the informal caregiver. Eur J Oncol Nurs 13:128–136

47. Lindahl J, Elmqvist C, Thulesius H, Edvardsson D (2015) Psychometric evaluation of the Swedish language person-centred climate questionnaire - family version. Scand J Caring Sci 29:859–864
48. Bainbridge D, Giruparajah M, Zou H, Seow H (2018) The care experiences of patients who die in residential hospice: a qualitative analysis of the last three months of life from the views of bereaved caregivers. Palliat Support Care 16:421–431
49. Donnelly S, Prizeman G, Coimín DÓ, Korn B, Hynes G (2018) Voices that matter: end-of-life care in two acute hospitals from the perspective of bereaved relatives. BMC Palliat Care 17(117)
50. Røen I, Stifoss-Hanssen H, Grande G, Brenne A-T, Kaasa S, Sand K, Knudsen AK (2018) Resilience for family carers of advanced cancer patients—how can health care providers contribute? A qualitative interview study with carers. Palliat Med 32:1410–1418
51. Morris SM, Thomas C (2002) The need to know: informal carers and information [1]. Eur J Cancer Care 11:183–187
52. Lemetti T, Partanen E, Hupli M, Haavisto E (2020) Cancer patients' experiences of realization of relatives' participation in hospital care: a qualitative interview study. Scand J Caring Sci. https://doi.org/10.1111/scs.12918
53. Haavisto E, Soikkeli-Jalonen A, Tonteri M, Hupli M (2020) Nurses' required end-of-life care competence in health centres inpatient ward - a qualitative descriptive study. Scandinavian journal of caring sciences. Scand J Caring Sci. https://doi.org/10.1111/scs.12874
54. Abu-Saad Huijer H (2009) Palliative care in Lebanon: knowledge, attitudes and practices. Int J Palliat Nurs 15:346–353
55. Luttik M, Goossens E, Ågren S, Jaarsma T, Mårtensson J, Thompson D, Moons P, Strömberg A (2017) Attitudes of nurses towards family involvement in the care for patients with cardiovascular diseases. Eur J Cardiovasc Nurs 16:299–308
56. Iranmanesh S, Razban F, Tirgari B, Zahra G (2014) Nurses' knowledge about palliative care in Southeast Iran. Palliat Support Care 12:203–210
57. Way D, Jones L, Busing N (2000) In: Way D, Jones L, Busing N (eds) Implementation strategies: collaboration in primary care—family doctors & nurse practitioners delivering shared care, Toronto
58. Soikkeli-Jalonen A, Stolt M, Hupli M, Lemetti T, Kennedy C, Kydd A, Haavisto E (2020) Instruments for assessing nurses' palliative care knowledge and skills in specialised care setting: an integrative review. J Clin Nurs 29:736–757
59. Walters SJ, Stern C, Robertson-Malt S (2016) The measurement of collaboration within healthcare settings. JBI Database System Rev Implement Rep 14:138–197
60. Virdun C, Luckett T, Lorenz K, Davidson PM, Phillips J (2020) Hospital patients' perspectives on what is essential to enable optimal palliative care: a qualitative study. Palliat Med 34:1402–1415
61. da Silva MM, da Lima L (2014) Participation of the family in hospital-based palliative cancer care: perspective of nurses. Rev Gaucha Enferm 35:14–19
62. Kuusisto A, Santavirta J, Saranto K, Korhonen P, Haavisto E (2020) Advance care planning for patients with cancer in palliative care: a scoping review from a professional perspective. J Clin Nurs 29:2069–2082
63. Kuuppelomäki M (2003) Emotional support for dying patients–the nurses' perspective. Eur J Oncol Nurs 7:120–129
64. Çıracı Y, Nural N, Saltürk Z (2016) Loneliness of oncology patients at the end of life. Support Care Cancer 24:3525–3531
65. Andershed B, Ternestedt B-M (1998) Involvement of relatives in the care of the dying in different care cultures: involvement in the dark or in the light? Cancer Nurs 21:106–111
66. Miranda da S, Chagas Moreira M, Luzia Leite J, Lorenzini Erdmann A (2012) Analysis of nursing care and the participation of families in palliative care in cancer. Texto Contexto Enfermagem 21:658–666
67. Abudari G, Hazeim H, Ginete G (2016) Caring for terminally ill Muslim patients: lived experiences of non-Muslim nurses. Palliat Support Care 14:599–611

68. Hadders H, Paulsen B, Fougner V (2014) Relatives' participation at the time of death: standardisation in pre and post-mortem care in a palliative medical unit. Eur J Oncol Nurs 18:159–166
69. Kuuppelomaki M (1993) Ethical decision-making on starting terminal care in different health-care units. J Adv Nurs 18:276–280
70. Moon F, Mooney C, McDermott F, Miller A, Poon P (2021) Bereaved families' experiences of end-of-life decision-making for general medicine patients. BMJ Supportive & Palliative Care bmjspcare-2020-002743
71. Johnson S, Butow P, Kerridge I, Tattersall M (2016) Advance care planning for cancer patients: a systematic review of perceptions and experiences of patients, families, and health-care providers. Psycho-Oncology 25:362–386
72. Sudore RL, Lum HD, You JJ et al (2017) Defining advance care planning for adults: a consensus definition from a multidisciplinary Delphi panel. J Pain Symptom Manag 53:821–832.e1
73. Rietjens JAC, Sudore RL, Connolly M et al (2017) Definition and recommendations for advance care planning: an international consensus supported by the European Association for Palliative Care. Lancet Oncol 18:e543–e551
74. Rietjens J, Korfage I, Taubert M (2021) Advance care planning: the future. BMJ Support Palliat Care 11:89–91
75. Detering KM, Hancock AD, Reade MC, Silvester W (2010) The impact of advance care planning on end of life care in elderly patients: randomised controlled trial. BMJ 340:c1345
76. Kuusisto A, Santavirta J, Saranto K, Haavisto E (2021) Healthcare professionals' perceptions of advance care planning in palliative care unit: a qualitative descriptive study. J Clin Nurs 30:633–644
77. Kuusisto A, Saranto K, Korhonen P, Haavisto E (2022) Accessibility of information on patients' and family members' end-of-life wishes in advance care planning. Nurs Open 9:428–436
78. Hui D, Hoge G, Bruera E (2021) Models of supportive care in oncology. Curr Opin Oncol 33:259–266
79. Macleod R (2008) Setting the context: what do we mean by psychosocial care in palliative care? In: Lloyd-Williams M (ed) Psychosocial issues in palliative care. Oxford University Press, pp 1–20
80. NIH (2022) Psychosocial support. In: National Cancer Institute at the National Institutes of Health. https://www.cancer.gov/publications/dictionaries/cancer-terms/def/psychosocial-support
81. Rodin G, An E, Shnall J, Malfitano C (2020) Psychological interventions for patients with advanced disease: implications for oncology and palliative care. J Clin Oncol 38:885–904
82. Wang T, Molassiotis A, Chung BPM, Tan J-Y (2018) Unmet care needs of advanced cancer patients and their informal caregivers: a systematic review. BMC Palliat Care 17:29–96
83. Oechsle K, Ullrich A, Marx G et al (2019) Psychological burden in family caregivers of patients with advanced cancer at initiation of specialist inpatient palliative care. BMC Palliat Care 18:102
84. Ullrich A, Ascherfeld L, Marx G, Bokemeyer C, Bergelt C, Oechsle K (2017) Quality of life, psychological burden, needs, and satisfaction during specialized inpatient palliative care in family caregivers of advanced cancer patients. BMC Palliat Care 16:31
85. Li Q, Loke AY (2013) A spectrum of hidden morbidities among spousal caregivers for patients with cancer, and differences between the genders: a review of the literature. Eur J Oncol Nurs 17:578–587
86. Lee J, Cha C (2017) Unmet needs and caregiver burden among family caregivers of hospice patients in South Korea. J Hosp Palliat Nurs 19:323–331
87. Vermorgen M, de Vleminck A, Leemans K, van den Block L, van Audenhove C, Deliens L, Cohen J (2019) Family carer support in home and hospital: a cross-sectional survey of specialised palliative care. BMJ Support Palliat Care bmjspcare-001795

88. Papastavrou E, Charalambous A, Tsangari H, Karayiannis G (2012) The burdensome and depressive experience of caring: what cancer, schizophrenia, and Alzheimer's disease caregivers have in common. Cancer Nurs 35:187–194

89. Ullrich A, Marx G, Bergelt C et al (2021) Supportive care needs and service use during palliative care in family caregivers of patients with advanced cancer: a prospective longitudinal study. Support Care Cancer 29:1303–1315

90. Shaffer K, Jacobs J, Coleman J et al (2017) Anxiety and depressive symptoms among two seriously medically ill populations and their family caregivers: a comparison and clinical implications. Neurocrit Care 27:180–186

91. Grande G, Rowland C, van den Berg B, Hanratty B (2018) Psychological morbidity and general health among family caregivers during end-of-life cancer care: a retrospective census survey. Palliat Med 32:1605–1614

92. Choi S, Seo J (2019) Analysis of caregiver burden in palliative care: an integrated review. Nurs Forum (Auckl) 54:280–290

93. Areia NP, Fonseca G, Major S, Relvas AP (2019) Psychological morbidity in family caregivers of people living with terminal cancer: prevalence and predictors. Palliat Support Care 17:286–293

94. Areia NP, Góngora JN, Major S, Oliveira VD, Relvas AP (2020) Support interventions for families of people with terminal cancer in palliative care. Palliat Support Care 18:1–9

95. LaValley SA (2018) End-of-life caregiver social support activation: the roles of hospice clinicians and professionals. Qual Health Res 28:87–97

96. Candy B, Jones L, Drake R, Leurent B, King M (2011) Interventions for supporting informal caregivers of patients in the terminal phase of a disease. Cochrane Database Syst Rev 6:CD007617

97. Røen I, Stifoss-Hanssen H, Grande G, Kaasa S, Sand K, Knudsen AK (2019) Supporting carers: health care professionals in need of system improvements and education - a qualitative study. BMC Palliat Care. https://doi.org/10.1186/s12904-019-0444-3

98. Teixeira MJC, Alvarelhão J, Souza D, Teixeira HJC, Abreu W, Costa N, Machado FAB (2019) Healthcare professionals and volunteers education in palliative care to promote the best practice–an integrative review. Scandinavian journal of caring sciences. Scand J Caring Sci 33:311–328

99. Tang ST, Chang W-C, Chen J-S, Wang H-M, Shen WC, Li C-Y, Liao Y-C (2013) Course and predictors of depressive symptoms among family caregivers of terminally ill cancer patients until their death. Psychooncology 22:1312–1318

100. Northouse LL, Katapodi MC, Song L, Zhang L, Mood DW (2010) Interventions with family caregivers of cancer patients: meta-analysis of randomized trials. CA Cancer J Clin 60:317–339

101. Becqué YN, Rietjens JAC, van Driel AG, van der Heide A, Witkamp E (2019) Nursing interventions to support family caregivers in end-of-life care at home: a systematic narrative review. Int J Nurs Stud 97:28–39

102. Ahn S, Romo RD, Campbell CL (2020) A systematic review of interventions for family caregivers who care for patients with advanced cancer at home. Patient education and counseling. Patient Educ Couns. https://doi.org/10.1016/j.pec.2020.03.012

103. Alam S, Hannon B, Zimmermann C (2020) Palliative care for family caregivers. JCO 38:926–936

104. Cahill PJ, Lobb EA, Sanderson C, Phillips JL (2017) What is the evidence for conducting palliative care family meetings? A systematic review. Palliat Med 31:197–211

105. Carson SS, Cox CE, Wallenstein S, Hanson LC, Danis M, Tulsky JA, Chai E, Nelson JE (2016) Effect of palliative care-led meetings for families of patients with chronic critical illness: a randomized clinical trial. JAMA 316:51–62

106. White DB, Angus DC, Shields AM et al (2018) A randomized trial of a family-support intervention in intensive care units. N Engl J Med 378:2365–2375

107. Randall Curtis J, Treece PD, Nielsen EL, Gold J, Ciechanowski PS, Shannon SE, Khandelwal N, Young JP, Engelberg RA, Curtis JR (2016) Randomized trial of communication facilita-

tors to reduce family distress and intensity of end-of-life care. Am J Respirat Crit Care Med 193:154–162

108. Hannon B, O'Reilly V, Bennett K, Breen K, Lawlor PG (2012) Meeting the family: measuring effectiveness of family meetings in a specialist inpatient palliative care unit. Palliat Support Care 10:43–49

109. Preisler M, Rohrmoser A, Goerling U, Kendel F, Bär K, Riemer M, Heuse S, Letsch A (2019) Early palliative care for those who care: a qualitative exploration of cancer caregivers' information needs during hospital stays. Eur J Cancer Care 28:e12990-n/a

110. Chi NC, Demiris G, Lewis FM, Walker AJ, Langer SL (2016) Behavioral and educational interventions to support family caregivers in end-of-life care: a systematic review. Am J Hosp Palliat Care 33:894–908

111. Jaffray L, Bridgman H, Stephens M, Skinner T (2016) Evaluating the effects of mindfulness-based interventions for informal palliative caregivers: a systematic literature review. Palliat Med 30:117–131

112. Jadalla A, Ginex P, Coleman M, Vrabel M, Bevans M (2020) Family caregiver strain and burden: a systematic review of evidence-based interventions when caring for patients with cancer. Clin J Oncol Nurs 24:31–50

113. McCauley R, McQuillan R, Ryan K, Foley G (2021) Mutual support between patients and family caregivers in palliative care: a systematic review and narrative synthesis. Palliat Med 35:875–885

114. Bertakis KD, Azari R (2011) Patient-centered care is associated with decreased health care utilization. J Am Board Family Med 24:229–239

115. Eriksson E (2001) Caring for cancer patients: relatives' assessments of received care. Eur J Cancer Care 10:48–55

116. Benkel I, Wijk H, Molander U (2010) Using coping strategies is not denial: helping loved ones adjust to living with a patient with a palliative diagnosis. J Palliat Med 13:1119–1123

117. Saukkonen M, Viitala A, Lehto JT, Åstedt-Kurki P (2017) Syöpäpotilaan ja hänen läheisensä selviytymistä edistävät tekijät palliatiivisen hoidon aikana - systemaattinen kirjallisuuskatsaus. Hoitotiede 29:195–206

118. Ho AHY, Leung PPY, Tse DMW, Pang SMC, Chochinov HM, Neimeyer RA, Chan CLW (2013) Dignity amidst liminality: healing within suffering among Chinese terminal cancer patients. Death Stud 37:953–970

119. Juarez G, Branin JJ, Rosales M (2014) The cancer caregiving experience of caregivers of Mexican ancestry. Hispanic Health Care Int 12:120–129

Supporting Caregivers of Patients with Childhood Malignancies

Theologia Tsitsi and Koralia A. Michail

1 Introduction

1.1 Epidemiology of Cancer in Children

Childhood cancer remains a substantial global burden. Even though survival rates in high income countries reach 80%, only 10% of children reside in these countries [1, 2]. Additionally, there are no available screening programs for childhood cancers, as opposed to adults, resulting in delays in diagnosis and treatment [2].

Childhood cancer rates, as yielded from the Surveillance, Epidemiology and End Results Databases in 2015, reached 344,543 children [3]. Leukaemias were the most common cancer, accounting for 28.8%, followed by CNS tumours and Lymphomas, with an overall rate of 24% and 11.2%, respectively [3].

The use of a metric that factors in the mortality as well as the treatment-related morbidity of childhood and adolescent cancer, namely the disability-adjusted life years (DALYs), has been used from the Global Burden of Disease Study [2]. According to the aforementioned study, children aged 0 to 4 year old corresponded to the higher proportion of global childhood cancer DALYS, with leukaemias representing the highest DALY according to the cancer category, followed by brain and nervous system cancers. Rare adolescent cancers, namely testes, ovaries and thyroid, corresponded for the second highest DALY burden. The same study highlighted the role of a low sociodemographic index on the burden of the disease.

Adverse outcomes of cancer and cancer therapy can be detected even on long-term survivors [4]. The burden of both the disease as well as its consequences bears down not only the children but also their caregivers.

T. Tsitsi (✉) · K. A. Michail
School of Health Sciences, Department of Nursing, Cyprus University of Technology, Limassol, Cyprus
e-mail: theologia.tsitsi@cut.ac.cy; Koralia.michail@cut.ac.cy

A. Charalambous (ed.), *Informal Caregivers: From Hidden Heroes to Integral Part of Care*, https://doi.org/10.1007/978-3-031-16745-4_9

2   Childhood Cancer Burden for Caregivers

Parenting is rewarding but at the same time, it can also be challenging [5]. This is particularly true among parents of children with cancer. The threat of a possible death of their child (life-threatening nature of cancer), the often-intense treatment chemotherapy regimens, the accompanying short- and long-term consequences of the illness and treatment (e.g. cardiac toxicity, sterilisation, limb loss) [6] and the possibility that the child will not respond to treatment, pose severe challenges to parents with severe impact on their health and well-being [7, 8]. A study by Boman et al. [9] found that unlike paediatric diabetes, where levels of parental uncertainty decreased over time, paediatric cancer was associated with parents' constant fear of losing the child. This can be partly attributed to the fact that even in the cases where the treatment is followed by a remission period, paediatric oncologists cannot guarantee a full recovery [10].

In addition to these challenges generated by the childhood cancer and the treatment, parents often have to take on a number of new caregiving tasks [11]. Parents may have to continue taking household tasks and may have to adapt to a number of new roles, such as being a medical assistant, teacher or therapist [12], further complicating the balance of different life roles. Based on previous studies [6, 13, 14], it has been demonstrated that parents frequently take time off from work (sick leaves/unpaid leaves), or they quit their jobs, which can result in income variations and possibly financial difficulties. Adding to the financial toxicity that parents might face at the course of the cancer trajectory is the possibility of out-of-pocket expenses related to the management of the disease. Additionally, all these responsibilities may reduce the time that parents have to take care of themselves and their own health [6, 15] and they may give up leisure activities they had before the onset of the childhood cancer [10]. Consequently, the enormity of this responsibility for caregivers and its concomitant burden are associated with a wide range of health impairments for caregivers [16–18], such as sleep deprivation, eating disorders and psychological distress [7, 19]. In particular, parents of children with cancer are at far greater risk of psychological distress than caregivers of healthy children or caregivers of children with other forms of illness [20, 21]. These parents usually report more physical and psychological problems and visit physicians more frequently than others [22, 23]. Also, parents of children who have survived cancer are known to suffer long-term psychological effects, including post-traumatic stress disorder [24–27]. Previous studies show that the majority of parents experienced care burden, which was associated with the care of their child with chronic illness [28, 29].

As such, when parents face the diagnosis, a new and sudden role of caregiving is added to already existing roles. During this period of caregiving, studies showed that parents experience stress and burden resulting from the rigorous activity of caregiving [30–32], which can have a negative impact on their physical, personal, emotional, psychological health (depression, anxiety and post-traumatic stress) and social lives and may experience financial hardships, thereby decreasing their quality of life (QOL) [6, 33, 34].

2.1 Concept of Caregiving Burden (CB)

In the health literature, there is a lack of clarity around the concept of CB and the alternate usage of terms such as stress, distress, tension and burnout instead of burden [35, 36]. Stress is the most common synonym used by researchers to represent CB in the literature. Caregiver stress is considered both subjective and objective. Subjective stress refers to the emotional or cognitive responses of the caregiver, such as fatigue, inequality or the perception of the current state of caregiving. Objective stress mainly reflects the care responsibility [35] assumed by the caregiver, which is a measurement based on the need of care-recipients [37, 38]. Added to this, a child's cancer diagnosis is a primary source of stress that exerts its effects across various aspects of a parent's life, that is, physiologic, self-concept, role function and interdependence [39].

Also, there are various definitions available in the health literature. These have led to some confusion among professionals. According to Herdman [40] in nursing, caregiver role strain is an important nursing diagnosis that refers to difficulties in performing the family caregiver role. In medicine, primary caregiver syndrome, also known as stress in primary caregivers, is used to represent a combination of symptoms such as fatigue, loss of energy, exhaustion and tiredness that can occur from the care demands [41, 42]. Contributing to this confusion, burden and distress are often used synonymously in the health literature.

The concept of burden was first introduced by Hoenig [43] and believed that 'burden could be divided into subjective and objective burden'. 'Subjective burden primarily involves the personal feelings of carers generated while performing the caring function, while objective burden is defined as events or activities related to negative caring experiences' [43]. Afterwards, Zarit [44] defined CB 'as a state resulting from necessary caring tasks or restrictions that cause discomfort for the primary caregiver of an older adult and his or her health problems, psychological well-being, finances and social life'. In 1992, Given [45] revised the definition of caregiver burden and expanded the construct to include the caregiver's physical limitations (e.g. personal time and formal care resources) and role strain.

Meanwhile, Montgomery (1985) defined CB as 'the distress that caregivers feel as a result of providing care'. Measuring CB systematically, they identified three dimensions of CB: 'the objective demand burden', 'the subjective demand burden' and 'subjective stress' [46]. The objective demand burden is the perceived interruption of the daily lives of caregiver, and the subjective demand burden is the caregiver's perceived demand of responsibilities from caregiving. Finally, the subjective stress burden is the caregiver's emotional response to caregiving responsibilities [46, 47]. Although the approach of Montgomery [46] helps to measure the objective and subjective dimensions of CB, critics have argued that CB is too complex to be reduced into these contrasting categories [48].

Finally, two definitions of CB were suggested first by Choi et al. [48], after an integrated review, regarding the analysis of CB in palliative care with its attributes, antecedents, consequences and facilitators: 'CB, a multidimensional concept, is attributed to the perception of physical symptoms, psychological distress, impaired social relationships, spiritual distress and financial crisis that arise from caregiving tasks or care demands. Disruptive to a caregivers' daily life, CB involves role strain and increases the level of uncertainty during palliative care. The results of unresolved CB are the diagnosis of psychiatric illness, impaired physical health status, and poor quality of life'. The second definition came by Liu et al. [49], who after a concept analysis suggested that CB is 'the level of multifaceted strain perceived by the caregiver from caring for a family member and/or loved one over time (attributes)'.

However, CB is a complicated concept due to its multidimensional construction, and this is strongly supported by the literature [35, 50–52], thus this concept can be interpreted and evaluated differently according to caregivers' characteristics and their situations. This is because even if the number of caregiving tasks and the length of the caregiving period are likely to increase the level of caregiver burden, individual caregivers have different thresholds and there is variation in caregiver outcomes. Similarly, considering cancer as a multidimensional complex disease, parents take up the diagnosis of their child with cancer, trying to establish a balance between their personal needs and their children's needs, which seems to increase parents 'anxiety, depression, and the perceived burden' [53]. Also changes to the daily routines of all the family members confront them with new situations [54, 55]. It is worth noting that fathers and mothers face distinct demands and tend to deal differently with challenges. Mothers usually assume the role of primary caregiver and become emotionally involved while the fathers act as providers and tend to distance themselves emotionally from the situation [56]. Also, cultural gender roles may influence the manifestation of feelings, fears and expectations between parents [57]. Other important factors that may affect how parents perceived CB are their age, gender, economic status, the child's type of cancer and the parents' own health status [58–61]. Moreover, social support (SS) is another resource that can affect CB [62, 63]. According to the literature, feeling supported enhances caregivers' sense of self-efficacy in dealing with the patient and, in general, can reduce caregivers' emotional burden [64, 65].

In their study, Qadire et al. [53] found that parents children with cancer report high levels of burden. In particular, 75.4% of parents experienced mild-to-severe levels of burden. Raina et al. [66] emphasised CB as an important risk factor for poor parental adaptation outcomes and research has systematically found significant associations between parental distress and poor child adjustment [34, 67].

CB is related to the well-being of both the individual and caregiver; therefore, understanding the attributes associated with caregiver burden is important [49].

2.2   Attributes Associated with CB

Walker and Avant (2005) defined attributes as 'the features that appear repeatedly in the literature and are the critical attributes of the concept' [68]. The three key attributes of CB identified from the literature according to Liu (2020) [49] are: self-perception, multifaceted strain and over time.

2.2.1 Self-Perception (Perceived by an Individual)

Self-perception considers the caregiver reflecting on personal experience during the caregiving process [49], even though CB was found to be an individual's subjective evaluation of the present caregiving situation and measurement of the degree of difficulties. However, Liu et al. (2020) argued that 'CB includes both subjective and objective aspects and perception is seen as objective or subjective since it is the ability of an individual to observe or listen to things through their senses, or the way in which they regard, understand and interpret them'. According to Bhattacharjee [69], caregiver burden refers to 'the positive or negative feelings and perceptions of the caregiver associated with providing caregiving functions' (p. 114). Similarly, Kazak et al. (2009) argued that when parents are faced with childhood cancer, their perception about the illness and its treatment is an important predictor of parental adaptation [70]. In a study of parents of children undergoing treatment or children who have completed treatment for cancer, those who perceived their child's current medical condition in a more negative way reported poorer adjustment [71]. Furthermore, in Salvador et al. study [21], parents of children undergoing treatment reported more negative perceptions about the child's illness (severity and illness interference), higher levels of caregiving burden and poorer Quality of Life (QoL) than parents of children who were already off-treatment. It is obvious that among caregivers in the same context, the level of perceived burden varies [49]. For example, a longitudinal study among mothers of children with cancer reported a more beneficial finding [72]. Similarly, studies found that 90% of mothers and 80% of fathers of childhood cancer survivors mentioned at least one benefit (changed life perspective, emotional growth, family integration and healthier lifestyle) in having a child diagnosed with cancer or other chronic diseases [73, 74]. A study of de Korte-Verhoef [75] reported that more than half of caregivers experienced a high level of burden; however, only a quarter of the caregivers expressed that their burden negatively affected their daily life.

2.2.2 Multifaceted Strain

During the crisis of the child's cancer, parents struggle to balance stressors of the situation and their capabilities [76, 77] and pay limited attention to their own state of health. As a consequence, this leads to physical and psychological symptoms such as fatigue [78], insomnia or a lack of sleep due to anxiety or interruptions at night from caregiving demands [79], depression and an increased risk of developing mental illness [78]. Moreover, caregiving stress has been shown to impair parents' immune response to anti-inflammatory signals [80]. In a study conducted by Ghufran [81], 78% of the mothers (as the primary caregiver) were diagnosed with depression during the processes of their children's cancer treatments. Mothers were in psychological distress when they had to watch their children suffer through treatments and their side effects and felt strong negative emotions such as shock, anger and fear regarding the conditions and prognoses [82]. It has been documented that some parents of children who have survived cancer, suffer long-term psychological effects, including post-traumatic stress disorder [8, 24, 25] and as a result may experience negative health effects [17, 18]. Mothers, especially, are at risk for posttraumatic stress symptoms (PTSS) [7, 83], with an incidence as high as 40% [84, 85]. Consequently, family caregivers (either mothers or fathers) of children with cancer have a heavy caregiving burden, which negatively affects their Quality of Life (QoL) [86]. One of the factors explaining the poorer QoL reported by parents of children with cancer is CB [79].

Parents have also been shown to experience substantial socioeconomic impact as a result of the child's illness-related care, including direct expenses, lost income, work disruptions and increased out-of-pocket expenses [87, 88]. Studies have shown reductions in employment and work absenteeism, along with difficulties with unsupportive employers and finding flexible jobs [89]. A more recent research conducted by Borrescio-Higa et al. [90] in Chile found that economic fragility increases following a diagnosis of childhood cancer, as many caregivers report job loss and absenteeism. A previous study conducted in UK estimated the economic burden of caregiving in families of 917 children, showed that the economic burden on parents was high and especially so for caregivers of younger children with leukaemia [91]. The literature shows a strong association between the level of financial difficulties reported by caregivers and the degree to which they experienced psychological distress and social isolation in the general population [92] including depressive symptoms in parents of children with cancer [93, 94]. However, medical costs are not the only burden on patients and their families. Psychosocial costs are intangible, not precisely defined and are less documented than economic costs, even though they represent a large and significant part of the total burden of illness [95].

2.2.3 Over Time Attributes of CB

Caregiver burden is a rather dynamic concept [55, 96]. The needs and demands of the patient vary at different points in the disease trajectory and so does the caregiver's burden [97]. A growing body of literature suggests that the longevity of caregiving, social/family support and the trajectory of disease are all factors that significantly affect the level of burden on caregivers [55, 96]. A study by Klassen (2008) indicated that a timeline of parental health-related quality of life (HRQL) is seen, with most psychological distress at the point of diagnosis [15]. In addition, Katz (2018) found in his research study that parental anxiety can be elevated in the first 2 months after the child's diagnosis and they may have high levels of depression during the first 10 months [98]. Significant distress remains during treatment [56, 99] and significantly correlated positively with the intensity of treatment (especially chemotherapy) [71, 100]. Variations in the duration and persistence of psychological disturbances have been reported in the literature and such levels are higher among mothers [72, 101]. Compas [102] found that 29% of mothers and 13% of fathers of children with newly diagnosed cancer experienced moderate-to-severe depressive symptoms. A systematic review by Wakefield et al. [103] noted that completion of treatment can provoke intensified parental anxiety and additional stress as parents lose the security of the treatment regime and fear recurrence or relapse. Fear of recurrence was also linked to persistent fatigue in parents. Another study identified that significantly increased psychological distress may be experienced for as long as 5 years after the completion of the treatment [7]. In Salvador's study [21], parents of children undergoing treatment reported more negative perceptions about the child's illness (severity and illness interference), higher levels of caregiving burden and poorer QoL than parents of children who were already off-treatment.

On the contrary, in a descriptive qualitative study conducted by Kaushal [104], most mothers expressed coming to a stage of acceptance and shifting their focus to positive thoughts. This is consistent with Lazarus and Folkman's definition of coping as a purposeful cognitive or behavioural change to deal with the appraised external or internal demands [105]. Some mothers in the same research focused on 'blessings in disguise', such as closer family relationships and relatively good prognoses, and such positive reframing enabled them to endure through the treatment processes with their children [104]. Similarly, the perception of better-quality family relationships contributed prospectively to benefit finding among caregivers of children with cancer or Type 1 diabetes [85].

3 Support Needs of Caregivers of Patients of Childhood Malignancies Across the Cancer Continuum

When a child is diagnosed with cancer, the whole family is diagnosed. The caregiving role is multiplied and shifts towards a new role that demands new skills while trying to preserve the family equilibrium [106–108]. This new role is accompanied with unique needs that are differentiated according to the diagnosis and treatment phase, the family structure and the cultural and spiritual background of caregivers [107].

3.1 Diagnosis: Initial Phase of Treatment

The treatment initiation phase provokes the highest level of uncertainty and stress to parents, leading to the need for information and verification of the diagnosis [109]. The timely provision of necessary information has been highlighted in order to resolve uncertainty to these caregivers [109]. The uncertainty and difficulty of accepting the child's diagnosis highlight the need for professional assistance for emotional concerns like fear, worry and sadness [110, 111].

The need to accept the reality of what is happening, so that they can then begin to take control and deal with the situation has been described by parents [112]. Acceptance may serve as an important mediating role in the relationship between childhood cancer and parent's later distress [112]. On the contrary, avoidance around the time of diagnosis is predictive of higher distress in due course of child's treatment [113]. Caregivers of children with cancer should have early and ongoing assessment of their mental health needs [110].

3.2 During Treatment

During treatment, attention of caregivers of children undergoing cancer therapy shifts towards the support of their children. Parents have expressed the need for continuing their child's education during the hospital stay as well as the need for social programs including opportunities for play and art [5, 111].

The need for communication between departments has emerged, with caregivers feeling distressed when having to repeat their child's clinical history due to the lack of appropriate sharing of information between in-hospital services, including emergency departments [5, 114].

The need for emergency care during a child's treatment phase is a major stressor since caregivers find themselves unable to decide whether the child should be transferred to the hospital, for symptoms that would be otherwise be treated at home. The decision of taking an immunocompromised child to the ER comes with anxiety and stress that the child won't be isolated as ordered or even fear that the healthcare workers will not be able to manage the port catheters [114, 115]. The need for the existence of protocols involving the fast and safe management of these children in the ER is apparent.

Caregivers can find comfort during hospital stays by being with other parents and feeling their support and company [116]. Parents and caregivers of childhood malignancies often express their wish to meet other parents or be part of support groups, since having a group in similar situations can relieve distress [5]. The need for support groups can often be met with the use of social media platforms. With the use of such platforms, caregivers provide and receive information from other cancer families and obtain tools or knowledge that will help with their child's cancer treatment [117, 118].

Caregivers during the treatment of their child have concerns regarding information about the illness as well as the physical changes the child might be subjected to [111]. The need for information regarding their child's diagnosis and therapy can lead parents to the use of online sources [5]. Even though utility of social media as a cancer-related resource could be helpful for caregivers within specific communities, cancer information shared on Facebook was found to be inaccurate by 19%, stressing the need for recommending reliable, evidence-based sources to patients and caregivers [119].

The role of spirituality and religion on coping with the stress of caregiving has been described in the past [120], whereas religious and spiritual interventions have been found to play a significant role in reduction of stress and depression [121]. In a study performed by Abdoljabbari (2018), caregivers of children with cancer believed that conducting religious activities gave them a means to achieve composure, have hope in future and tolerate hardships and critical conditions related to the disease [122]. Spiritual needs of parents have been described independently of religious belief orientation during the treatment of their children in the form of the need of a prayer room, and availability of a spiritual/religious person in the hospital [111], even though these needs are often overlooked [123].

The family structure can influence parental well-being. Single parents are at an adverse position compared to two-parent families, since they have to balance the emotional, physical and financial strains of caring for their families while taking care of the child with cancer. The synergy of these cumulative stresses with the added strain of caregiving for a child with cancer can lead to long-term health and financial implications for parents [11]. Rosenberg-Yunger (2013) found that social-emotional, practical and financial support were crucial for single parents' abilities to cope with their role as the primary caregiver. Additionally, these parents needed encouragement to seek help for practical support, including the full range of resources available to them [124].

In a study by Wiener (2016), lone parents could be demographically single or with a partner who was absent, making them feel alone during the child's active therapy. Lone parents were found to experience significant worsening of relationships with their friends and their other children compared with non-lone parents [125]. This finding implies that healthcare workers should not rely only on demographic characteristics of caregivers but rather try exploring their need for support.

Immigrant caregivers of children with cancer account for a population with discrete needs, mainly due to language barriers [126–128]. Living in a country with different languages and culture constitutes a burden on its own for parents. The admission of the child to the hospital due to a malignancy is usually the first point of contact of these parents with the health services [128], whereas lack of necessary immigration documents might cause a delay in the diagnosis of these children since parents deem entering into the healthcare system as a threat [126]. Language poses a significant barrier for informed decision-making, access of available financial and other resources and advocating for the child's needs [126–128]. Language barriers can complicate paediatric cancer care for parents, regardless of the language [129]. Moreover, cultural differences and beliefs concerning health and sickness can affect parent's response to child's treatment as wells as towards healthcare providers [130]. Therefore, the need for a permanent interpreter and culturally available information is imperative. Moreover, HCPs should be educated to develop cultural awareness, knowledge, attitudes and communication skills towards immigrant caregivers, which is imperative [127, 128, 131].

The COVID-19 pandemic generated additional concerns for caregivers of children with malignancies. Unemployment rate skyrocketed, whereas the continuity of therapy was disturbed [132–134]. The hospital was longer perceived as a safe place for children, whereas the insecurity of caregivers intensifies the need for proper information [132]. Interventions that would secure the continuation of care, including logistics, guidance for government aid applications, food provision and the use of technology for connectivity support, were found to be substantial [135]. Depressive and anxiety symptoms of primary caregivers of children with cancer were similar in incidence with those reported from frontline healthcare workers during the pandemic, underlying the need for mental health support services [133, 134].

3.3 Post Therapy Needs: Remission Phase

The period that follows the completion of treatment, mainly the first two years after which children are considered long-term survivors, is of high importance [136].

During this period, caregivers begin to worry about the inefficacy of treatments, the possibility of relapse and death, as well as the effects of treatments in the future [137]. Parents with lower educational and socioeconomic status were found to be more prone to stress after the completion of therapy, whereas parents with higher education were more able to communicate with healthcare professionals and make informed decisions, indicating the importance of health literacy [137]. Caregivers share the need for education and information concerning worrisome symptoms and were to turn if those symptoms emerge. Moreover, they need reassurance that in the case of relapse, they will stay connected with their primary oncology caregiver [138, 139]. Additionally, caregivers need information regarding risk factors and late site effects of treatment. This information should not be provided immediately after the completion of treatment, since parents and children need time to adapt to their new normality [139].

4 Interventions Described in the Literature for Supporting Caregiver's Needs

Supporting caregivers of children with malignancies can be challenging. As mentioned above, support needs may vary according to treatment phase and family structure. Methods of support described in the literature and their focus vary in order to adjust to caregiver's needs.

4.1 Education and Information

Education concerning the child's disease and information regarding what to expect have been the main desideratum for caregivers of children with cancer during its whole trajectory. Provision of timely education and information to caregivers can significantly lower stress levels and resolve uncertainty [109]. Educational support should include diet education, environmental infection control and provision of information about the current patient's status and prognosis [109].

The use of video-assisted education prior to medical procedures has shown to enhance caregiver's knowledge and lower anxiety related to the procedure. Knowledge enhancement can provide a basis for informed decision-making. The information content and themes included must be balanced and medical terminology should be avoided [140].

Providing information in simple language or with the use of visuals including videos, pictures or theatre while considering cultural differences for the use of translated material is of high importance for immigrant caregivers [128]. Translation should be achieved by trained interpreters rather than ad-hoc or family members. Ad-hoc interpretation has been linked to diminished trust in doctors, breach of confidentiality, inaccurate communication, inadequate treatment and greater errors in translation [128].

In order to provide information and cover educational needs of caregivers after the completion of therapy, Hobbie et al. (2010) developed a booklet that focused on the informational needs of parents in the immediate post-treatment phase [139]. Furthermore, the review of late effects, scheduling of follow-up appointments and communication with school staff were considered helpful in the long run for caregivers [138].

De la Maza (2020) described a structured educational program which included topics related to cancer pathophysiology, diagnosis and treatment of cancer, medication side effects, infection prevention, Central Venous Catheter—CVC care, awareness of febrile neutropenia (FN) and understanding when an ER visit is necessary [141]. Education was provided in individual sessions by a nurse specialised in paediatric cancer, whereas a hardcopy of the educational content was also available for caregivers. The results showed enhanced knowledge for caregivers receiving the educational intervention, as well as improved clinical outcomes for the paediatric patients, especially concerning CVC infections and unnecessary ER visits [141].

A discharge-planning program to meet the physical needs of children with cancer was described by Yilmaz (2010) [142]. The program included an ongoing discharge teaching, home visits and telephonic consultation. Determination of care needs, namely infection management, bowel control, nutrition, fatigue and pain was made during home visit interviews, whereas education and counselling were initiated according to emerged needs. Telephonic consultation was available to caregivers 12 h daily. Results of the study showed that the intervention decreased infection-related problems, including unplanned visits and readmissions and nutritional problems, including nausea and vomiting [142]. The Children's Oncology Group has developed a standardised education checklist that can be used by nurses to guide the initial education provided to parents of children newly diagnosed with cancer before the initial hospital discharge [143]. As paediatric cancer patient care shifts towards a more home-based care, it is of paramount importance that caregivers are educated and feel competent to provide adequate care to their child. Moreover, communication of the healthcare agency, family and hospital should be enhanced [144].

Parents of a dying child will need support in order to recognise what is happening when and to make the best decisions to enhance the child's quality of life. Healthcare providers should be able to clarify ambiguities and provide information in a form that will secure the feeling of confidence to caregivers [145].

4.2 Emotional Support

Caregiving of a child with cancer is a distressful experience that can lead to reduction of quality of life and depression [146]. The need for emotional support should be assessed and provided as soon as diagnosis is made.

Interventions that aim on stress relief should begin prior to child's therapy and should be going on until child's discharge from the hospital. Liu et al. provided a three-stage intervention in caregivers of children with stem cell transplantation focused on four areas: (a) sharing past experiences, (b) promoting support for the caregiver, (c) providing medical information relevant to each caregiver's child and (d) reducing caregiver distress. The support intervention was provided 5 days pre-transplant, 14 days after and a week prior to discharge. Results showed a decrease of distress and an increase in quality of life for caregivers of children during the process of hematopoietic stem cell transplantation (HSCT) and hospitalisation, underlining the importance of early initiation of such interventions [147].

Support groups are defined as groups of people with common experiences and concerns who provide emotional and moral support to one another, while they can be combined with comprehensive education, thus simultaneously meeting parent's information needs [111]. Moreover, according to experienced healthcare professionals, in-hospital group therapy can benefit more caregivers, facilitate the interaction among group members, reduce the feeling of being alone, improve social support and offer better clarification of concepts, compared to individual psychotherapy sessions [104].

Berry-Carter (2021) described a mentoring program with parents having the role of mentor after training, which provides support and understanding to caregivers of children with cancer. Mentors and parents are trained to validate feelings, fears, concerns, regrets, grief, encourage parental self-care and assess for referral needs [148]. Parents reported that the mentor's support, the sharing of stories and the mutual communication and feedback were beneficiary [148]. Parents of children on terminal stage need insight and support on how to communicate with their dying child concerning death. Being able to talk with other parents was found especially important for parents and caregivers of these children [149].

The use of alternative relaxation intervention has also been described for reducing anxiety levels of parents of children with malignancies. Tsitsi et al. used progressive muscle relaxation and guided imagery techniques that significantly reduced anxiety symptoms and improved mood states [150].

4.3   Spiritual and Religious Support

Parents and caregivers often find support in spirituality. Spiritual practices were reported as a form of support and coping strategy that some mothers relied on, whereas their religious beliefs enabled them to go through the treatment processes [5]. Moreover, spiritual interventions based on the Richards and Bergin pattern [151], namely activities such as prayer, contemplation, reading sacred writings, forgiveness, repentance, worship, fellowship, spiritual direction and moral instruction, were found to reduce depression, anxiety and stress scores of caregivers of children with leukaemia [152]. It is therefore of high importance for caregivers to have a place during the child's treatment where they can pray and practice their religion, regardless of what it is [111]. Additionally, the availability of a priest or spiritual person in the hospital could facilitate spiritual and belief practices.

4.4   Social and Financial Support

Caring for a child with cancer more than often means that one parent should be able to stay with the child during hospitalisation. This can lead to loss of income which added to the cost of treatment and can be a source of considerable stress and financial hardship for families [6, 153]. Moreover, the absence of income and social support networks has been correlated with increase in therapy abandonment [154, 155].

Rosenberg-Yunger recommends the provision of educational sessions for both parents and their support networks with a scope to ensure that they know the full range of resources available to them, and for the latter to ensure that they know the kinds of assistance parents of children with cancer will need. Additionally, having a financially supportive work environment was important for single parents caring for a child with cancer, especially retaining access to extended benefits to ensure that the child's medications were covered [124].

Support networks can relief parents from direct caregiving and other responsibilities, so that they can focus on their child with cancer [107]. Timely education about their child's health status from healthcare providers and emotional support from family members, friends and others have been recognised as the most helpful forms of assistance to relieve caregiver burden [19].

All families should be assessed, offered support and informed of existing resources on an ongoing basis beginning at diagnosis [153].

4.5 Support with the Use of Technology

The use of technology, especially smartphone apps can facilitate meeting the support needs of caregivers [156]. mHealth tools could enable caregivers to become more efficient, effective, safer and less stressed while managing their children's care—oncology advice incorporated [114, 157]. Mueller et al. have developed an mHealth tool, namely COPE, to support parents in planning and manage emergencies for their children with cancer [157]. The tool provides components that include child's medical history inputted by the caregivers, documentation of common symptoms and provision of advice based on the inputted information. The tool also features contacting with the child's medical team, finding a nearby emergency department, as well as access resources such as sanitation and port access videos [157].

Developing social media-based interventions could help provide caregivers with accurate cancer information to reduce misinformation found online and create a space in which caregivers can have positive interactions with other families who have a child with cancer [118]. Facebook groups have been successfully used for peer support by sharing preventive health behaviour education and behavioural prompts while serving as a platform for parents to interact with each other [158].

5 Conclusions

Caregivers of children with malignancies carry an unbearable burden which may be due to the change of their role, fatigue, social isolation, loss of work and income or/ and to the financial burden. The needs of these individuals differ according to family status, the child's diagnosis, the stage of therapy and other contributing factors.

These needs should be recognised by health professionals in a timely manner in order to provide them with the necessary intervention. There are several ways to support parents of children with cancer and these are constantly evolving. It is the duty of health professionals working in the field to know both the ways and the bodies to support these caregivers, as the support will have an impact on the treatment outcomes of the child with cancer.

References

1. Bhakta N, Force LM, Allemani C et al (2019) Childhood cancer burden: a review of global estimates. Lancet Oncol 20:e42–e53. https://doi.org/10.1016/S1470-2045(18)30761-7
2. Force LM, Abdollahpour I, Advani SM et al (2019) The global burden of childhood and adolescent cancer in 2017: an analysis of the Global Burden of Disease Study 2017. Lancet Oncol 20:1211–1225. https://doi.org/10.1016/S1470-2045(19)30339-0
3. Johnston WT, Erdmann F, Newton R et al (2021) Childhood cancer: estimating regional and global incidence. Cancer Epidemiol 71:101662. https://doi.org/10.1016/J.CANEP.2019.101662
4. Robison LL, Hudson MM (2013) Survivors of childhood and adolescent cancer: life-long risks and responsibilities. Nat Rev Cancer 14:1 14:61–70. https://doi.org/10.1038/nrc3634
5. Tan R, Koh S, Wong ME et al (2020) Caregiver stress, coping strategies, and support needs of mothers caring for their children who are undergoing active cancer treatments. Clin Nurs Res 29:460–468. https://doi.org/10.1177/1054773819888099
6. Fletcher PC (2010) My child has cancer: the costs of mothers' experiences of having a child with pediatric cancer. Issues Comprehensive Pediatric Nurs 33:164–184. https://doi.org/1 0.3109/01460862.2010.498698
7. Jantien Vrijmoet-Wiersma CM, van Klink JMM, Kolk AM et al (2008) Assessment of parental psychological stress in pediatric cancer: a review. J Pediatric Psychol 33:694–706. https://doi.org/10.1093/JPEPSY/JSN007
8. Kazak AE, Baxt C (2007) Families of infants and young children with cancer: a post-traumatic stress framework. Pediatr Blood Cancer 49:1109–1113. https://doi.org/10.1002/pbc.21345
9. Boman KK, Viksten J, Kogner P, Samuelsson U (2004) Serious illness in childhood: the different threats of cancer and diabetes from a parent perspective. J Pediatrics 145:373–379. https://doi.org/10.1016/j.jpeds.2004.05.043
10. McCaffrey CN (2006) Major stressors and their effects on the well-being of children with cancer. J Pediatric Nurs 21:59–66. https://doi.org/10.1016/J.PEDN.2005.07.003
11. Granek L, Rosenberg-Yunger ZRS, Dix D et al (2014) Caregiving, single parents and cumulative stresses when caring for a child with cancer. Child: Care Health Dev 40:184–194. https://doi.org/10.1111/CCH.12008
12. Lindahl Norberg A, Mellgren K, Winiarski J, Forinder U (2014) Relationship between problems related to child late effects and parent burnout after pediatric hematopoietic stem cell transplantation. Pediatric Transplant 18:302–309. https://doi.org/10.1111/petr.12228
13. Patterson JM, Holm KE, Gurney JG (2004) The impact of childhood cancer on the family: a qualitative analysis of strains, resources, and coping behaviors. Psycho-Oncology 13:390–407. https://doi.org/10.1002/pon.761
14. McGrath P, Paton MA, Huff N (2005) Beginning treatment for pediatric acute myeloid leukemia: the family connection. Issues Comprehensive Pediatric Nurs 28:97–114. https://doi.org/10.1080/01460860590950881
15. Klassen AF, Klaassen R, Dix D et al (2008) Impact of caring for a child with cancer on parents' health-related quality of life. J Clin Oncol 26:5884–5889. https://doi.org/10.1200/JCO.2007.15.2835

16. Shaffer KM, Chow PI, Cohn WF et al (2018) Informal caregivers' use of internet-based health resources: an analysis of the health information national trends survey. JMIR Aging 1:e11051. https://doi.org/10.2196/11051
17. Spitzer C, Barnow S, Völzke H et al (2009) Trauma, posttraumatic stress disorder, and physical illness: findings from the general population. Psychosomatic Med 71:1012–1017. https://doi.org/10.1097/PSY.0B013E3181BC76B5
18. Breslau N (2002) Epidemiologic studies of trauma, posttraumatic stress disorder, and other psychiatric disorders. Can J Psychiatry 47:923–929. https://doi.org/10.1177/070674370204701003
19. James K, Keegan-Wells D, Hinds PS et al (2002) The care of my child with cancer: parents' perceptions of caregiving demands. J Pediatric Oncol Nurs 19:218–228. https://doi.org/10.1177/104345420201900606
20. Pinquart M (2018) Parenting stress in caregivers of children with chronic physical condition—a meta-analysis. Stress Health 34:197–207. https://doi.org/10.1002/SMI.2780
21. Salvador Á, Crespo C, Martins AR et al (2015) Parents' perceptions about their child's illness in pediatric cancer: links with caregiving burden and quality of life. J Child Family Stud 24:1129–1140. https://doi.org/10.1007/s10826-014-9921-8
22. Rafii F, Oskouie F, Shoghi M (2014) Caring for a child with cancer: impact on mother's health. Asian Pac J Cancer Prev 15:1731–1738. https://doi.org/10.7314/APJCP.2014.15.4.1731
23. Young B, Dixon-Woods M, Heney D (2002) Identity and role in parenting a child with cancer. Pediatric Rehabilitation 5:209–214. https://doi.org/10.1080/1363849021000046184
24. Norberg AL, Boman KK (2009) Parent distress in childhood cancer: a comparative evaluation of posttraumatic stress symptoms, depression and anxiety. 47:267–274. https://doi.org/10.1080/02841860701558773
25. Pöder U, Ljungman G, von Essen L (2008) Posttraumatic stress disorder among parents of children on cancer treatment: a longitudinal study. Psycho-Oncology 17:430–437. https://doi.org/10.1002/PON.1263
26. Stuber ML, Kazak AE, Meeske K, Barakat L (1998) Is posttraumatic stress a viable model for understanding responses to childhood cancer? Child Adolescent Psychiatric Clin North Am 7:169–182. https://doi.org/10.1016/S1056-4993(18)30266-9
27. Barakat LP, Kazak AE, Meadows AT et al (1997) Families surviving childhood cancer: a comparison of posttraumatic stress symptoms with families of healthy children. J Pediatric Psychol 22:843–859. https://doi.org/10.1093/JPEPSY/22.6.843
28. Adelman RD, Tmanova LL, Delgado D et al (2014) Caregiver burden: a clinical review. JAMA 311:1052–1059. https://doi.org/10.1001/JAMA.2014.304
29. Rubira EA, Santo E, Aparecida Munhoz Gaíva M, et al (2011) Taking care of children with cancer: evaluation of the caregivers' burden and quality of life Elizete Aparecida Rubira do Espírito Santo 1
30. Hansen T, Slagsvold B (2015) Feeling the squeeze? The effects of combining work and informal caregiving on psychological well-being. Eur J Ageing 12:51–60. https://doi.org/10.1007/S10433-014-0315-Y/FIGURES/1
31. Vitaliano PP, Strachan E, Dansie E et al (2014) Does caregiving cause psychological distress? The case for familial and genetic vulnerabilities in female twins. Ann Behav Med 47:198–207. https://doi.org/10.1007/S12160-013-9538-Y
32. Prince M, Brodaty H, Uwakwe R et al (2012) Strain and its correlates among carers of people with dementia in low-income and middle-income countries. A 10/66 Dementia Research Group population-based survey. Int J Geriatr Psychiatry 27:670–682. https://doi.org/10.1002/gps.2727
33. Caputo J, Pavalko EK, Hardy MA (2016) The long-term effects of caregiving on women's health and mortality. J Marriage Family 78:1382–1398. https://doi.org/10.1111/JOMF.12332
34. Wolfe-Christensen C, Mullins LL, Fedele DA et al (2010) The relation of caregiver demand to adjustment outcomes in children with cancer: the moderating role of parenting. Stress. 39:108–124. https://doi.org/10.1080/02739611003679881

35. Grandón P, Jenaro C, Lemos S (2008) Primary caregivers of schizophrenia outpatients: burden and predictor variables. Psychiatry Res 158:335–343. https://doi.org/10.1016/J. PSYCHRES.2006.12.013
36. Joyce J. Fitzpatrick and Geraldine McCarthy (2016) Nursing concept analysis: applications to research and practice, 1st edn. Springer, New York
37. Llanque S, Savage L, Rosenburg N, Caserta M (2014) Concept analysis: Alzheimer's caregiver stress an independent voice for nursing
38. Sisk RJ (2000) Caregiver burden and health promotion. Int J Nurs Stud 37:37–43. https://doi.org/10.1016/S0020-7489(99)00053-X
39. Roy C (2011) Research based on the Roy adaptation model: Last 25 years. Nurs Sci Q 24:312–320. https://doi.org/10.1177/0894318411419218
40. Herdman TH, Kamitsuru S, North American Nursing Diagnosis Association NANDA International, Inc. Nursing diagnoses: definitions & classification 2018-2020. 473
41. Peñarrieta De Córdova MI, Canales R, Krederdt S et al (2016) The relationship of the quality of life and burden of informal caregivers of patients with cancer in Lima, Peru. J Nurs Educ Pract 6. https://doi.org/10.5430/jnep.v6n8p36
42. Veloso VI, Tripodoro VA (2016) Caregivers burden in palliative care patients: a problem to tackle. Curr Opin Support Palliat Care 10:330–335. https://doi.org/10.1097/SPC.0000000000000239
43. Hoenig J, Hamilton MW (1966) The schizophrenic patient in the community and his effect on the household. Int J Soc Psychiatry 12:165–176. https://doi.org/10.1177/002076406601200301
44. Zarit SH, Reever KE, Bach-Peterson J (1980) Relatives of the impaired elderly: correlates of feelings of burden. Gerontologist 20:649–655. https://doi.org/10.1093/GERONT/20.6.649
45. Given CW, Given B, Stommel M et al (1992) The caregiver reaction assessment (CRA) for caregivers to persons with chronic physical and mental impairments. Res Nurs Health 15:271–283. https://doi.org/10.1002/NUR.4770150406
46. Montgomery RJ, Gonyea JG, Hooyman NR (1985) Caregiving and the experience of subjective and objective burden
47. Ferrell BR, Mazanec P (2009) Family caregivers. Geriatric Oncol 135–155. https://doi.org/10.1007/978-0-387-89070-8_7
48. Choi S, Seo JY (2019) Analysis of caregiver burden in palliative care: an integrated review. Nurs Forum 54:280–290. https://doi.org/10.1111/nuf.12328
49. Liu Z, Heffernan C, Tan J (2020) Caregiver burden: a concept analysis. Int J Nurs Sci 7:438–445. https://doi.org/10.1016/j.ijnss.2020.07.012
50. Bastawrous M (2013) Caregiver burden—a critical discussion. Int J Nurs Stud 50:431–441. https://doi.org/10.1016/J.IJNURSTU.2012.10.005
51. Costa-Requena G, Espinosa Val M, Cristòfol R (2015) Caregiver burden in end-of-life care: advanced cancer and final stage of dementia. Palliat Support Care 13:583–589. https://doi.org/10.1017/S1478951513001259
52. Chou KR (2000) Caregiver burden: a concept analysis. J Pediatric Nurs 15:398–407. https://doi.org/10.1053/JPDN.2000.16709
53. al Qadire M, Aloush S, Alkhalaileh M et al (2020) Burden among parents of children with cancer in jordan: prevalence and predictors. Cancer Nurs 43:396–401. https://doi.org/10.1097/NCC.0000000000000724
54. Given B, Wyatt G, Given C et al (2004) Burden and depression among caregivers of patients with cancer at the end-of-life. Oncol Nurs Forum 31:1105. https://doi.org/10.1188/04.ONF.1105-1117
55. Oechsle K, Ullrich A, Marx G et al (2020) Prevalence and predictors of distress, anxiety, depression, and quality of life in bereaved family caregivers of patients with advanced cancer. Am J Hospice Palliat Med 37:201–213. https://doi.org/10.1177/1049909119872755
56. Kohlsdorf M, Luiz Á, Junior C (2012) Psychosocial impact of pediatric cancer on parents: a literature review 1

57. Brody AC, Simmons LA (2007) Family resiliency during childhood cancer: the father's perspective. J Pediatric Oncol Nurs 24:152–165. https://doi.org/10.1177/1043454206298844

58. Rezende G, Gomes CA, Rugno FC et al (2017) Burden on family caregivers of the elderly in oncologic palliative care. Eur Geriatric Med 8:337–341. https://doi.org/10.1016/J.EURGER.2017.06.001

59. Williams PD, Williams KA, Williams AR (2014) Parental caregiving of children with cancer and family impact, economic burden: nursing perspectives. Comprehens Child Adolescent Nurs 37:39–60. https://doi.org/10.3109/01460862.2013.855843

60. Harding R, Gao W, Jackson D et al (2015) Comparative analysis of informal caregiver burden in advanced cancer, dementia, and acquired brain injury. J Pain Symp Manage 50:445–452. https://doi.org/10.1016/J.JPAINSYMMAN.2015.04.005

61. Shahi V, Lapid MI, Kung S et al (2014) Do age and quality of life of patients with cancer influence quality of life of the caregiver? J Geriatric Oncol 5:331–336. https://doi.org/10.1016/J.JGO.2014.03.003

62. Burnette D, Duci V, Dhembo E (2017) Psychological distress, social support, and quality of life among cancer caregivers in Albania. Psycho-Oncology 26:779–786. https://doi.org/10.1002/PON.4081

63. Chiou CJ, Chang HY, Chen IP, Wang HH (2009) Social support and caregiving circumstances as predictors of caregiver burden in Taiwan. Arch Gerontol Geriatrics 48:419–424. https://doi.org/10.1016/j.archger.2008.04.001

64. Shiba K, Kondo N, Kondo K (2016) Informal and formal social support and caregiver burden: the AGES caregiver survey. J Epidemiol 26:622–628. https://doi.org/10.2188/JEA.JE20150263

65. Erker C, Yan K, Zhang L et al (2018) Impact of pediatric cancer on family relationships. Cancer Med 7:1680–1688. https://doi.org/10.1002/cam4.1393

66. Raina P, O'donnell M, Schwellnus H, et al (2004) Caregiving process and caregiver burden: conceptual models to guide research and practice

67. Robinson KE, Gerhardt CA, Vannatta K, Noll RB (2007) Parent and family factors associated with child adjustment to pediatric cancer. J Pediatric Psychol 32:400–410. https://doi.org/10.1093/JPEPSY/JSL038

68. Walker LOAKC (2005) Strategies for theory construction in nursing, 4th edn. Pearson Prentice Hall, Upper Saddle River

69. Bhattacharjee M, Vairale J, Gawali K, Dalal PM (2012) Factors affecting burden on caregivers of stroke survivors: population-based study in Mumbai (India). Ann Indian Acad Neurol 15:113. https://doi.org/10.4103/0972-2327.94994

70. Kazak AE, RMT, NN (2009) Families and other systems in pediatric psychology. In: Handbook of pediatric psychology. Guilford, New York

71. Hussin Z, Othman A, Mohamad N, et al (2011) Factors related to parental well-being in children with cancer. In: International conference on social science and humanity

72. Kolbrun E, Svavarsdottir EK (2005) Caring for a child with cancer: a longitudinal perspective. J Adv Nurs 50:153–161. https://doi.org/10.1111/J.1365-2648.2005.03374.X

73. Barakat LP, Alderfer MA, Kazak AE (2006) Posttraumatic growth in adolescent survivors of cancer and their mothers and fathers. J Pediatric Psychol 31:413–419. https://doi.org/10.1093/JPEPSY/JSJ058

74. Affleck G, Allen DA, Tennen H et al (2011) Causal and control cognitions in parents' coping with chronically ill. Children 3:367–377. https://doi.org/10.1521/JSCP.1985.3.3.367

75. de Korte-Verhoef MC, Pasman HRW, Schweitzer BP et al (2014) Burden for family carers at the end of life; a mixed-method study of the perspectives of family carers and GPs. BMC Palliat Care 13:1–9. https://doi.org/10.1186/1472-684X-13-16/TABLES/5

76. Bigalke K (2015) Coping, hardiness, and parental stress in parents of children diagnosed with cancer. Dissertations

77. Joa J, Patterson JM (2002) Integrating family resilience and family stress theory. J Marriage Fam 64:349–360. https://doi.org/10.1111/J.1741-3737.2002.00349.X

78. Fernanda D, Alves S, de Brito GE, Kurashima AY (2013) Stress related to care: the impact of childhood cancer on the lives of parents 1. Rev Latino-Am Enfermagem 21:356–362
79. Klassen AF, Raina P, McIntosh C et al (2011) Parents of children with cancer: which factors explain differences in health-related quality of life. Int J Cancer 129:1190–1198. https://doi.org/10.1002/ijc.25737
80. Miller GE, Cohen S, Ritchey AK (2002) Chronic psychological stress and the regulation of pro-inflammatory cytokines: a glucocorticoid-resistance model. Health Psychol 21:531–541. https://doi.org/10.1037/0278-6133.21.6.531
81. Ghufran M, Andrades M, Nanji K (2014) Frequency and severity of depression among mothers of children with cancer: results from a teaching hospital in Karachi, Pakistan. Br J Med Pract 7:701
82. Ljungman L, Boger M, Ander M, et al (2016) Impressions that last: particularly negative and positive experiences reported by parents five years after the end of a child's successful cancer treatment or death. https://doi.org/10.1371/journal.pone.0157076
83. Schepers SA, Sint Nicolaas SM, Maurice-Stam H et al (2018) Parental distress 6 months after a pediatric cancer diagnosis in relation to family psychosocial risk at diagnosis. Cancer 124:381–390. https://doi.org/10.1002/CNCR.31023
84. Kazak AE, Boeving CA, Alderfer MA et al (2005) Posttraumatic stress symptoms during treatment in parents of children with cancer. J Clin Oncol 23:7405–7410. https://doi.org/10.1200/JCO.2005.09.110
85. Kazak AE, Alderfer M, Rourke MT et al (2004) Posttraumatic stress disorder (PTSD) and posttraumatic stress symptoms (PTSS) in families of adolescent childhood cancer survivors. J Pediatric Psychol 29:211–219. https://doi.org/10.1093/JPEPSY/JSH022
86. Mohammadi F, Rakhshan M, Houshangian M, Kyle H (2020) Evaluation of psychometric properties of the caregiver burden inventory in parents of Iranian children suffering from cancer. Nurs Midwifery Stud 9:102–109. https://doi.org/10.4103/nms.nms_22_19
87. Roser K, Erdmann F, Michel G et al (2019) The impact of childhood cancer on parents' socio-economic situation-a systematic review. Psycho-oncology 28:1207–1226. https://doi.org/10.1002/PON.5088
88. Santacroce SJ, Tan KR, Killela MK (2018) A systematic scoping review of the recent literature (~2011-2017) about the costs of illness to parents of children diagnosed with cancer. Eur J Oncol Nurs 35:22–32. https://doi.org/10.1016/J.EJON.2018.04.004
89. Kish AM, Newcombe PA, Haslam DM (2018) Working and caring for a child with chronic illness: a review of current literature. Child: Care Health Dev 44:343–354. https://doi.org/10.1111/CCH.12546
90. Borrescio-Higa F, Valdés N (2022) The psychosocial burden of families with childhood blood cancer. Int J Environ Res Public Health 19. https://doi.org/10.3390/IJERPH19010599
91. Pagano E, Baldi I, Mosso ML et al (2014) The economic burden of caregiving on families of children and adolescents with cancer: a population-based assessment. Pediatric Blood Cancer 61:1088–1093. https://doi.org/10.1002/PBC.24904
92. Frankham C, Richardson T, Maguire N (2020) Psychological factors associated with financial hardship and mental health: a systematic review. Clin Psychol Rev 77. https://doi.org/10.1016/J.CPR.2020.101832
93. Creswell PD, Wisk LE, Litzelman K et al (2014) Parental depressive symptoms and childhood cancer: the importance of financial difficulties. Support Care Cancer 22:503–511. https://doi.org/10.1007/S00520-013-2003-4
94. Keegan Wells D, Kelly James C, Janet Stewart RL, et al (2002) The care of my child with cancer: a new instrument to measure caregiving demand in parents of children with cancer. https://doi.org/10.1053/jpdn.2002.124114
95. Essue BM, Iragorri N, Fitzgerald N, de Oliveira C (2020) The psychosocial cost burden of cancer: a systematic literature review. Psycho-Oncology 29:1746–1760
96. Abrams HR, Leeds HS, Russell H, Hellsten MB (2019) Factors influencing family burden in pediatric hematology/oncology encounters. J Patient-Centered Res Rev 6:243–251. https://doi.org/10.17294/2330-0698.1710

97. Lukhmana S, Bhasin SK, Chhabra P, Bhatia MS (2015) Family caregivers' burden: a hospital based study in 2010 among cancer patients from Delhi. Indian J Cancer 52:146. https://doi. org/10.4103/0019-509X.175584

98. Katz LF, Fladeboe K, Lavi I et al (2018) Trajectories of marital, parent-child, and sibling conflict during pediatric cancer treatment. Health Psychol 37:736–745. https://doi.org/10.1037/ HEA0000620

99. Firoozi M, Besharat MA, Rahimian Boogar E (2013) Emotional regulation and adjustment to childhood cancer: role of the biological, psychological and social regulators on pediatric oncology adjustment 6

100. Jurbergs N, Long A, Ticona L, Phipps S (2009) Symptoms of posttraumatic stress in parents of children with cancer: are they elevated relative to parents of healthy children? J Pediatric Psychol 34:4–13. https://doi.org/10.1093/jpepsy/jsm119

101. Sahler OJZ, Dolgin MJ, Phipps S et al (2013) Specificity of problem-solving skills training in mothers of children newly diagnosed with cancer: results of a multisite randomized clinical trial. J Clin Oncol 31:1329–1335. https://doi.org/10.1200/JCO.2011.39.1870

102. Compas BE, Bemis H, Gerhardt CA et al (2015) Mothers and fathers coping with their children's cancer: individual and interpersonal processes. Health Psychol 34:783–793. https:// doi.org/10.1037/HEA0000202

103. Wakefield CE, McLoone J, Goodenough B et al (2010) The psychosocial impact of completing childhood cancer treatment: a systematic review of the literature. J Pediatric Psychol 35:262–274. https://doi.org/10.1093/JPEPSY/JSP056

104. Kaushal T, Satapathy S, Chadda RK et al (2019) Hospital based psychosocial support program for children with ALL and their families: a comprehensive triad's perspective. Indian J Pediatrics 86:118–125. https://doi.org/10.1007/s12098-018-2679-z

105. Biggs A, Brough P, Drummond S (2017) Lazarus and Folkman's psychological stress and coping theory. Handb Stress Health 349–364. https://doi. org/10.1002/9781118993811.CH21

106. Young B, Dixon-Woods M, Findlay M, Heney D (2002) Parenting in a crisis: conceptualising mothers of children with cancer. Soc Sci Med 55:1835–1847. https://doi.org/10.1016/ S0277-9536(01)00318-5

107. Jones BL (2012) The challenge of quality care for family caregivers in pediatric cancer care. Semin Oncol Nurs 28:213–220. https://doi.org/10.1016/j.soncn.2012.09.003

108. Lewandowska A (2021) Influence of a child's cancer on the functioning of their family. Children 8. https://doi.org/10.3390/children8070592

109. Park M, Suh EE, Yu SY (2021) Uncertainty and nursing needs of parents with pediatric cancer patients in different treatment phases: a cross-sectional study. Int J Environ Res Public Health 18. https://doi.org/10.3390/ijerph18084253

110. Kearney JA, Salley CG, Muriel AC (2015) Standards of psychosocial care for parents of children with cancer. Pediatric Blood Cancer 62:632–683. https://doi.org/10.1002/pbc

111. Rao VN, Anantharaman Rajeshwari R, Rajagopal R et al (2021) Inception of a pediatric cancer caregiver support group guided by parental needs. Cancer Rep 1–6. https://doi. org/10.1002/cnr2.1469

112. López J, Velasco C, Noriega C (2021) The role of acceptance in parents whose child suffers from cancer. Eur J Cancer Care 30. https://doi.org/10.1111/ecc.13406

113. Sultan S, Leclair T, Rondeau et al (2016) A systematic review on factors and consequences of parental distress as related to childhood cancer. Eur J Cancer Care 25:616–637. https://doi. org/10.1111/ECC.12361

114. Mueller EL, Cochrane AR, Moore CM et al (2020) Assessing needs and experiences of preparing for medical emergencies among children with cancer and their caregivers. J Pediatric Hematol/Oncol 42:e723–e729. https://doi.org/10.1097/MPH.0000000000001826

115. Mueller EL, Cochrane AR, Lynch DO et al (2019) Identifying patient-centered outcomes for children with cancer and their caregivers when they seek care in the emergency department. Pediatric Blood Cancer 66:e27903. https://doi.org/10.1002/pbc.27903

116. Ångström-Brännström C, Norberg A, Strandberg G et al (2010) Parents' experiences of what comforts them when their child is suffering from cancer. J Pediatric Oncol Nurs 27:266–275. https://doi.org/10.1177/1043454210364623
117. Gage-Bouchard EA, Devine KA, Heckler CE (2013) The relationship between socio-demographic characteristics, family environment, and caregiver coping in families of children with cancer. J Clin Psychol Med Settings 20:478–487. https://doi.org/10.1007/s10880-013-9362-3
118. Nagelhout ES, Linder LA, Austin T et al (2018) Social media use among parents and caregivers of children with cancer. J Pediatric Oncol Nurs 35:399–405. https://doi.org/10.1177/1043454218795091
119. Gage-Bouchard EA, LaValley S, Warunek M et al (2018) Is cancer information exchanged on social media scientifically accurate? J Cancer Educ 33:1328–1332. https://doi.org/10.1007/S13187-017-1254-Z/TABLES/3
120. Weaver AJ, Flannelly KJ (2004) The role of religion/spirituality for cancer patients and their caregivers. South Med J 97:1210–1214
121. Gonçalves JPB, Lucchetti G, Menezes PR, Vallada H (2015) Religious and spiritual interventions in mental health care: a systematic review and meta-analysis of randomized controlled clinical trials. Psychol Med 45:2937–2949. https://doi.org/10.1017/S0033291715001166
122. Abdoljabbari M, Sheikhzakaryaee N, Atashzadeh-Shoorideh F (2018) Taking refuge in spirituality, a main strategy of parents of children with cancer: a qualitative study. Asian Pac J Cancer Prev 19:2575–2580. https://doi.org/10.22034/APJCP.2018.19.9.2575
123. Kelly JA, May CS, Maurer SH (2016) Assessment of the spiritual needs of primary caregivers of children with life-limiting illnesses is valuable yet inconsistently performed in the hospital. 19:763–766. https://home.liebertpub.com/jpm. https://doi.org/10.1089/JPM.2015.0509
124. Rosenberg-Yunger ZRS, Granek L, Sung L et al (2013) Single-parent caregivers of children with cancer: factors assisting with caregiving strains. J Pediatric Oncol Nurs 30:45–55. https://doi.org/10.1177/1043454212471727
125. Wiener L, Viola A, Kearney J et al (2016) Impact of caregiving for a child with cancer on parental health behaviors, relationship quality, and spiritual faith: do lone parents fare worse? J Pediatric Oncol Nurs 33:378–386. https://doi.org/10.1177/1043454215616610
126. Zamora ER, Kaul S, Kirchhoff AC et al (2016) The impact of language barriers and immigration status on the care experience for Spanish-speaking caregivers of patients with pediatric cancer. Pediatric Blood Cancer 63:2173–2180. https://doi.org/10.1002/PBC.26150
127. Klassen AF, Gulati S, Watt L et al (2012) Immigrant to Canada, newcomer to childhood cancer: a qualitative study of challenges faced by immigrant parents. Psycho-Oncology 21:558–562. https://doi.org/10.1002/pon.1963
128. Gulati S, Watt L, Shaw N et al (2012) Communication and language challenges experienced by Chinese and South Asian immigrant parents of children with cancer in Canada: implications for health services delivery. Pediatric Blood Cancer 58:572–578. https://doi.org/10.1002/pbc.23054
129. Chino K, Sasaki Y, Miyagawa N et al (2019) Pediatric cancer care can be complicated by language barriers: a case involving parents with limited Japanese proficiency. Pediatric Blood Cancer 66. https://doi.org/10.1002/PBC.27563
130. Banerjee AT, Watt L, Gulati S et al (2011) Cultural beliefs and coping strategies related to childhood cancer: the perceptions of South Asian immigrant parents in Canada. J Pediatric Oncol Nurs 28:169–178. https://doi.org/10.1177/1043454211408106
131. Liang HF (2002) Understanding culture care practices of caregivers of children with cancer in Taiwan. J Pediatric Oncol Nurs 19:205–217. https://doi.org/10.1177/104345420201900605
132. Darlington ASE, Morgan JE, Wagland R et al (2021) COVID-19 and children with cancer: parents' experiences, anxieties and support needs. Pediatric Blood Cancer 68. https://doi.org/10.1002/pbc.28790
133. Wimberly CE, Towry L, Caudill C et al (2021) Impacts of COVID-19 on caregivers of childhood cancer survivors. Pediatric Blood Cancer 68. https://doi.org/10.1002/pbc.28943

134. Parambil BC, Goswami S, Moulik NR, et al (2021) Psychological distress in primary caregivers of children with cancer during COVID-19 pandemic-A single tertiary care center experience. Psycho-oncology pon.5793. https://doi.org/10.1002/pon.5793

135. Zuleta V, Berliner J, Rossell N, Zubieta M (2021) Securing continuation of treatment for children with cancer in times of social unrest and pandemic. Cancer Rep 1–6. https://doi.org/10.1002/cnr2.1430

136. Quast LF, Williamson Lewis R, Lee JL et al (2021) Psychosocial functioning among caregivers of childhood cancer survivors following treatment completion. J Pediatric Psychol 46:1238–1248. https://doi.org/10.1093/jpepsy/jsab061

137. Lemos MS, Lima L, Silva C, Fontoura S (2020) Disease-related parenting stress in the post-treatment phase of pediatric cancer. Comprehens Child Adolescent Nurs 43:65–79. https://doi.org/10.1080/24694193.2019.1570393

138. Karst JS, Hoag JA, Chan SF et al (2018) Assessment of end-of-treatment transition needs for pediatric cancer and hematopoietic stem cell transplant patients and their families. Pediatric Blood Cancer 65:e27109. https://doi.org/10.1002/PBC.27109

139. Hobbie WL, Ogle SK, Reilly M et al (2010) Identifying the educational needs of parents at the completion of their child's cancer therapy. J Pediatric Oncol Nurs 27:190–195. https://doi.org/10.1177/1043454209360778

140. Bany Hamdan A, Ballourah W, Elghazaly A et al (2020) The effect of video-assisted education prior intrathecal chemotherapy on anxiety and knowledge enhancement. J Cancer Educ 1–6. https://doi.org/10.1007/s13187-020-01787-1

141. de la Maza V, Manriquez M, Castro M et al (2020) Impact of a structured educational programme for caregivers of children with cancer on parental knowledge of the disease and paediatric clinical outcomes during the first year of treatment. Eur J Cancer Care 29:e13294. https://doi.org/10.1111/ECC.13294

142. Yilmaz MC, Ozsoy SA (2010) Effectiveness of a discharge-planning program and home visits for meeting the physical care needs of children with cancer. Support Care Cancer 18:243–253. https://doi.org/10.1007/S00520-009-0650-2

143. Rodgers C, Bertini V, Conway MA et al (2018) A standardized education checklist for parents of children newly diagnosed with cancer: a report from the children's oncology group. J Pediatric Oncol Nurs 35:235. https://doi.org/10.1177/1043454218764889

144. Jibb LA, Chartrand J, Masama T, Johnston DL (2021) Home-based pediatric cancer care: perspectives and improvement suggestions from children, family caregivers, and clinicians. JCO Oncol Pract 17:e827–e839. https://doi.org/10.1200/op.20.00958

145. Markward MJ, Benner K, Freese R (2013) Perspectives of parents on making decisions about the care and treatment of a child with cancer: a review of literature. Families Syst Health 31:406–413. https://doi.org/10.1037/a0034440

146. Pierce L, Hocking MC, Schwartz LA et al (2017) Caregiver distress and patient health-related quality of life: psychosocial screening during pediatric cancer treatment. Psycho-Oncology 26:1555–1561. https://doi.org/10.1002/pon.4171

147. Liu YM, Wen YC, Weng PY et al (2020) Effectiveness of a three-stage intervention in reducing caregiver distress during pediatric hematopoietic stem cell transplantation: a randomized controlled trial. J Pediatric Oncol Nurs 37:377–389. https://doi.org/10.1177/1043454220911358

148. Berry-Carter K, Barnett B, Canavera K et al (2021) Development of a structured peer mentoring program for support of parents and caregivers of children with cancer. J Pediatric Nurs 59:131–136. https://doi.org/10.1016/j.pedn.2021.03.031

149. Kenney AE, Bedoya SZ, Gerhardt CA et al (2021) End of life communication among caregivers of children with cancer: a qualitative approach to understanding support desired by families. Palliat Support Care 19:715–722. https://doi.org/10.1017/S1478951521000067

150. Tsitsi T, Charalambous A, Papastavrou E, Raftopoulos V (2017) Effectiveness of a relaxation intervention (progressive muscle relaxation and guided imagery techniques) to reduce anxiety and improve mood of parents of hospitalized children with malignancies: a random-

ized controlled trial in Republic of Cyprus and Gree. Eur J Oncol Nurs 26:9–18. https://doi.org/10.1016/j.ejon.2016.10.007

151. Richards PS, Bergin AE (2006) Religious and spiritual practices as therapeutic interventions. A spiritual strategy for counseling and psychotherapy, 2nd edn, pp 251–279. https://doi.org/10.1037/11214-009

152. Zafarian Moghaddam E, Behnam Vashani HR, Reihani T, Namazi Zadegan S (2016) The effect of Spiritual education on depression, anxiety and stress of caregivers of children with leukemia. J Torbat Heydariyeh Univ Med Sci 4:1–7

153. Tsimicalis A, Stevens B, Ungar WJ et al (2011) The cost of childhood cancer from the family's perspective: a critical review. Pediatric Blood Cancer 56:707–717

154. Ospina-Romero M, Portilla CA, Bravo LE et al (2016) Caregivers' self-reported absence of social support networks is related to treatment abandonment in children with cancer. Pediatric Blood Cancer 63:825–831. https://doi.org/10.1002/pbc.25919

155. Atwiine B, Busingye I, Kyarisiima R et al (2021) 'Money was the problem': caregivers' self-reported reasons for abandoning their children's cancer treatment in southwest Uganda. Pediatric Blood Cancer 68:e29311. https://doi.org/10.1002/pbc.29311

156. Mehdizadeh H, Asadi F, Mehrvar A et al (2019) Smartphone apps to help children and adolescents with cancer and their families: a scoping review. Acta Oncol (Stockholm, Sweden) 58:1003–1014. https://doi.org/10.1080/0284186X.2019.1588474

157. Mueller EL, Cochrane AR, Moore CM, et al (2020) The children's oncology planning for emergencies (COPE) tool: prototyping with caregivers of children with cancer. AMIA. Annual Symposium proceedings AMIA Symposium 2020, pp 896–905

158. Wilford JG, McCarty R, Torno L et al (2020) A multi-modal family peer support-based program to improve quality of life among pediatric brain tumor patients: a mixed-methods pilot study. Children 7:35. https://doi.org/10.3390/children7040035

Informal Caregivers: The Advocacy and Policy Perspective

Elizabeth Hanson and Claire Champeix

1 Introduction

The crucial role played by informal carers in caring for a relative/significant other with a health and/or care need is increasingly being recognised by policy makers and governments globally, mainly as a result of ageing demographic trends and finite economic resources concerning publicly funded health and long-term care services [1]. In addition, health policies advocating more people centred, integrated health and care systems [2] have led to a stronger focus on community care and care provided at home, making the role of the informal carer more prominent [3]. More recently, the COVID-19 pandemic has helped to shed a spotlight on informal carers and their situation given the governmental restrictions operating in many countries which led to many carers providing more care to frail older, disabled and/or chronically ill relatives living at home [4].

Thus, the adage that you are either currently a carer, or have been a carer, alternatively that you will be a carer at some point later in your life is increasingly the case within our societies today as informal carers represent the backbone of long-term care systems around the world [5]. It is estimated that between 12 and 18% of the EU population aged 18–75 provide informal long-term care at least once a week [6] and that nearly 16% of adults in the USA provide unpaid care to people with care needs [7]. In countries where community and residential long-term care services are less prevalent, nearly all long-term care is provided by informal carers [8].

E. Hanson (✉)
Department of Health and Caring Sciences, Linnaeus University, Swedish Family Care Competence Centre, Kalmar, Sweden

Eurocarers, Brussels, Belgium
e-mail: elizabeth.hanson@lnu.se

C. Champeix
Eurocarers, Brussels, Belgium
e-mail: cc@eurocarers.org

© The Author(s), under exclusive license to Springer Nature Switzerland AG 2023
A. Charalambous (ed.), *Informal Caregivers: From Hidden Heroes to Integral Part of Care*, https://doi.org/10.1007/978-3-031-16745-4_10

A life course perspective is highly relevant when it comes to informal care as people of all ages engage in caring activities. Indeed, it is estimated that at least 3–8% of all children and youth provide care to parents, siblings or friends, so called "young carers" [9]. Many carers are of working age, some of whom combine paid work with providing care to aged parents and/or to a child with a long-standing illness or disability, so-called "working carers". Informal caring is also common in old age where care is usually provided to a spouse/partner. Further, a gender perspective is important to highlight with regard to informal care as the majority of informal carers are women—at least 75% in the USA and approximately 55–60% in Europe [10, 11]. However, in their later years (70+), a higher proportion of male spouses are informal carers. Nevertheless, overall women are often the main carers and tend to carry out more personal caring activities. Further, their subjective mental and physical health is more adversely affected compared to men.

Having provided an overview for understanding the context and prevalence of informal caring, we will now turn our attention to outlining carers movements and their key advocacy role.

2   The Carers Movement(s) and Their Advocacy Role

Carers movements are largely grassroots movements that have been growing in recent years to include more countries internationally. Informal carers' collective voices are often formalised in local, regional and national carers associations who play an important role in both supporting carers in their individual caring situation and also collectively by lobbying and advocating for informal carers as a whole to improve their situation. In particular, to work for changes and improvements in practices, policies, legislation and research. Some of these associations also offer a range of information, education/training and support services to informal carers depending on their size and source(s) of funding. Many associations depend entirely on membership fees, private donations and sponsorships, external development and/ or research funding, whilst some associations receive some level of direct or indirect government funding. A number of well-established carers organisations were set up in the 1990s such as Carers Australia, the National Alliance of Caregiving, USA, the Taiwan Association of Family Caregivers and Carers Sweden and also around 2000 such as the French Association of Caregivers and Carers Canada. The earliest known carers organisation is Carers UK that began as a grassroots movement initiated by the Reverend Mary Webster who wrote a letter to the newspapers about the difficulties of working and caring for ageing parents. In 1965 Mary formed the National Council for the Single Woman and Her Dependents which later became Carers UK (https://www.carersuk.org).

It is important to note however that the establishment of carers' organisations remains uneven across countries. For example, currently, to the best of our knowledge. There are no carers organisations operating in the eastern European countries. We would argue that the growth of the carers' movement and the establishment of carers associations in countries where previously there were none is partly related to a couple of factors. Firstly, that in some countries the recognition of carers with some allowance(s) being granted, provides the basis for carers to gather. Second, progress in research shedding light on the weaknesses of the existing situation also acts as a catalyst as explained further below in the reference to Baroness Jill Pitkeathley.

As well as national associations there are also umbrella carers organisations at EU and international level. Eurocarers was established in 2006 and acts as the European voice for informal carers. The overall goal being to advance the situation of informal carers across Europe. It is a European network consisting of a total of over 75 members comprising of carers organisations together with relevant research institutes and universities. It has had a secretariat in Brussels since 2014 and its core funding is secured via European Union social funding programmes. The rather unique combination of membership—both carers members and researcher members—helps to bring about evidence-based advocacy at both national and EU levels. It does this primarily by firstly documenting and raising awareness about the significant contribution made by carers to health and social care systems and the economy as a whole, and of the need to safeguard this contribution. Secondly, by ensuring that both EU and national policies take account of carers. In other words, policies that: (1) promote carers' social inclusion and combat poverty, (2) the development of responsive support services, (3) enable carers to remain active in paid employment and maintain a social life and (4) to have the same rights and life chances as other citizens with regard to their health and well-being, education and employment (https://eurocarers.org).

Importantly, Eurocarers advocate for choice when it comes to caregiving: informal carers should have the possibility to make choices as to the type and the intensity of the care they provide, and the duration. Also, the preferences of those in need of care should be met. Eurocarers call for long-term care systems which not only take into account the essential role of informal carers and support them, but also offer formal qualitative care alternatives, be it in a residential setting or at home. The premise being that only by ensuring all people in need of care can access quality and affordable formal care, can we ensure that informal care arrangements reflect the personal preferences of the people concerned. It is also recognised that a combination of formal and informal care should be an option, supported by an adequate assessment and coordination of care needs. Therefore, informal and formal care should be considered as complementary, rather than two distinct and opposite care pathways (https://eurocarers.org).

Eurocarers provide the secretariat to the European Parliament Interest Group on Carers which was officially launched in 2007 and which brings together Members of the European Parliament from different countries and political parties who are willing to support the development of carer-friendly policies (https://eurocarers.org/ep-interest-group-on-carers/) (for further details of the work of the Interest Group, see below).

At an international level, IACO—the International Association of Carer Organisations—was established in 2012 and is an umbrella network organisation that brings together national non-governmental carers organisations from across the globe who work together to advocate for carers at an international level and in individual countries. It currently consists of 15 members and 4 associate members from 16 countries worldwide. The network relies on donations from members and sponsors and secures foundation and project grants for specific initiatives. The rationale for setting up IACO was the recognition by the founding members that once seen as a personal and private matter in family life, unpaid caring has become one of the most important social and economic policy issues worldwide. Thus, the overall aim of the international association is to foster international action for carers and to increase the awareness of the situation of caregivers and influence policy, programmes and services in individual countries. IACO members work collaboratively and independently to raise awareness of carers, identify and disseminate best practices and enhance carer well-being. IACO provides research, awareness and education regarding family carers on a global scale. It also encourages and provides assistance to countries interested in developing carer organisations (https://internationalcarers.org). [Please note that the terms carer, caregiver, and family caregiver are used interchangeably by IACO members.] In 2021 it produced an online resource—the Global State of Caring which profiles carer policies and practices in 18 countries [12].

An advocacy perspective is seen to be crucial to the growth of the carers movement(s) as it helps to ensure that the voices of carers and those of the people they care for are heard, so that the issues that matter most to them are actively addressed by the carers organisations and umbrella European and international networks. Taken together with evidence from rigorous research results, it helps to provide the impetus for more carer-friendly policies. In this way, advocacy, research and policy go "hand in hand" as the "mother" of the carers movement in the UK, Baroness Jill Pitkeathley has previously explained, the stories of carers are important as together with reliable data on the numbers of carers and their situation they are the essential ingredients for "selling the message" to the media, decision makers, policy makers and governments and providing the necessary evidence for change/improvements in policies [13].

In more recent years, there has been a growing momentum for a more rights-based perspective with regard to carers and their situation, similarly to the earlier disability rights movement. Luke Clements (2013) in a paper called "Does your carer take sugar" [14] highlighted the similarities in the struggles waged earlier by disabled people in the 1970s—which led to concrete international legal provisions some 30 years later—with those of carers, in challenging their social exclusion. He argued that we are witnessing a similar global trend in domestic legislation recognising the rights of carers, largely as the result of an ageing population and governments reducing the public provision of social welfare support, causing carers, especially working carers, to be "stretched to breaking point", hence necessitating some level of recognition and support for carers. At the same time, it is recognised that no matter how generous a welfare state is for people with health and care needs, this does not negate the necessity for carers to exist—which was traditionally a common argument in the Nordic countries with a prior history of a generous state funded welfare state "from the cradle to the grave". Clements argued that carers often have an innate sense of duty to care that can be taken to mean a human right to care that relates to the civil and political right "privacy/private life" and that being a carer should and will become a protected status for the purposes of non-discrimination legislation, on the same basis as other protected statuses (such as disability). Indeed, non-discrimination legislation for working carers was recently reflected in the EU Work Life Balance directive that was ratified by Member States at the end of December 2021 (see EU policy section for more details).

3 A Shift in the Policy Environment Concerning Carers

Carers organisations working with advocacy recognise that it is important to lobby for carer-friendly policies that both support and empower carers. Namely, to enable family members and friends to, as far as feasibly possible, make a choice as to whether to take on board a carer role and, if so, the type and extent of their caring activities. As well, for those carers who wish to care to receive support in their role so that they are able to live their life as they choose similarly to other citizens in society. Further, it is increasingly recognised that carer-friendly policies need to be widespread and cross-cutting across different government departments so that they not only solely focus on health and social care, but also on all spheres of life affecting carers. For example, education given the impact of caring by children and youths on their ability to complete their basic education and also the opportunity for them to continue with further and higher education [15]. Also, on employment and pensions due to the negative impact of caring—especially high intensity caring—on working carers' ability to continue in paid work, leading to a substantial number having to reduce their working hours or leave the workforce altogether with an immediate effect on their financial situation and, in the long term, on their future pensions [16]. Thus, there is a need to work proactively and as widely as possible with a range of government departments. Currently, relatively few countries have managed to work so broadly, with the notable exception of several countries such as England [17], Scotland [18] and Australia [19]. In this regard, a cross-government plan as part of a proactive and comprehensive carers strategy that covers all dimensions of a carer's experience has seen to be instrumental to their long-term, strategic goals.

Currently, to the best of our knowledge, and at the time of writing this chapter, there are six countries within Europe that have a comprehensive national carers strategy in place (that is, a holistic and coordinated set of measures in place): England [17], Scotland [18], Ireland [20], Norway [21], France [22] and Sweden [23].

Eurocarers' [24] EU strategy to support and empower informal carers across Europe entitled "Enabling Carers to Care" is currently being used by a number of members of the network as part of their lobbying efforts with governments and policy makers for a carers strategy in their own respective country (for example, in Finland and Portugal). The Strategy defines 10 core steps identified by Eurocarers network to implement a carer-friendly policy environment that seeks to recognise, support and empower carers across Europe in a comprehensive and coherent manner. The aim of the strategy is to help policy makers (as well as all other stakeholders who can improve the lives of carers, in partnership with them, and who can influence the support provided to carers) acting at EU, national and regional level to consolidate existing but sometimes tokenistic approaches and to highlight new evidence-informed initiatives in favour of carers' rights. The Steps are closely interconnected and are designed to be approached as part of a whole. The Strategy is premised on the assumption that people should have the right to choose freely whether they want to be a carer and to what extent they want to be involved in caring. As well, that people in need of care should have the right to choose who they wish to be their carers. Each of the 10 Steps with key arguments/rationales and action points are summarised below. An Explanatory Note was also produced to accompany the Strategy which provides a more detailed rationale for and explanation of the Strategy.

3.1   Step 1 Define and Acknowledge Carers

Step 1 emphasises the central role that carers play in the care of people with long-term conditions and disabilities living in the community and as a result, to the economy of EU countries. It also highlights that decision makers often fail to meet carers' needs and preferences because they use narrowly-focused definitions of informal care or definitions are entirely missing in relevant legislation.

A major point of action is for public authorities at international/EU, national and regional level to seek agreement on a clear and wide-ranging definition of informal care, such as the definition used by Eurocarers as follows:

> A carer is a person who provides usually unpaid care to someone with a long-term illness, disability or other long-lasting health or care need, outside a professional or formal framework.

It is proposed that such a broad definition should serve to drive the implementation of more systematic and proactive approaches to consolidate carers' existing legal rights and to set out principles for carer support.

3.2   Step 2 Identify Your Carers

In Step 2 it is argued that despite a growing momentum around care and caring, carers still form a largely invisible and undervalued workforce in many European countries. It is acknowledged that when carers are identified early and fully supported, they are better able to continue in their caring roles and maintain a healthy lifestyle.

Actions points are that public authorities should seek to raise awareness about informal care and collect data about the number, typology, needs and preferences of carers through national census, surveys and self-identification tools.

Further, as care professionals are in the forefront of carers' support, measures should be put in place to inform them about informal care and to train them to identify, support and work in partnership with carers.

3.3 Step 3 Assess the Needs of Your Carers

Step 3 emphasises that carers should have access to an assessment of the measures that could help make their life easier. In turn, it is argued that this will facilitate the development of a personalised set of support measures which, in turn, can help to improve their situation. It is acknowledged that carers organisations have a key role to play in this process by engaging carers in co-designing these assessment tools and by supporting the dissemination and uptake process.

Key action points include public authorities taking steps to develop and—when already in existence—improve the uptake and quality of carers assessment tools in order to personalise support plans to the actual needs of carers.

Second, public authorities should seek to identify, support and involve organisations representing carers in the design of carers assessment tools.

3.4 Step 4 Support Multisectoral Partnerships for Integrated and Community-Based Care Services

Step 4 proposes that carers should be central to the planning, shaping and delivery of services both for people with care needs and with regard to support for themselves. It recommends that carers are approached as partners in care.

A key action point is that partnerships of relevant actors, including informal carers, should be set up in order to ensure that care services respond to the needs of the community effectively and in a personalised and holistic manner.

3.5 Step 5 Facilitate Carers' Access to Information and Advice About Care, Caring and Care-Life Balance

In Step 5 it is recognised that carers often need to take on caregiving responsibilities without prior warning or planning. Many of them do not realise that they are carers and, when they do, they often struggle to access basic information about what it means to be a carer, benefits and entitlements, support services, employment, carers' breaks, training opportunities or the potential consequences for them and the person they care for.

Key action points for service provides include the development of one-stop shops for carers to access information about care, caring and the support measures available to provide quality care while maintaining a productive and healthy life. It is argued that Information and Communication Technology (ICT) based solutions and peer support initiatives offer significant potential in this respect and should therefore be encouraged and supported.

3.6   Step 6 Pay Attention to Carers' Health and Prevent Negative Health Outcomes

Step 6 notes that carers frequently suffer poor physical and mental health outcomes as a result of their caregiving activities when not adequately supported. Therefore, early identification and support along with specific preventive measures are deemed essential to maintain carers' health and well-being, prevent negative health outcomes and avoid creating a vicious circle where carers themselves become unwell and require care themselves.

Key action points are firstly that care professionals should be informed about the health risks of informal care on carers themselves and health checks should be organised more systematically to assess carers' health and well-being.

Second, it is acknowledged that health promotion, counselling and training offer great potential to prevent negative health outcomes among informal Carers. It is proposed that tailor-made resources on issues relating to physical/mental health and caring should be produced and actively promoted.

Third, access to emotional support through carers' centres, condition-specific organisations or via primary care physicians or other primary care professionals should be supported.

3.7   Step 7 Give Carers a Break

Step 7 highlights that respite care is often perceived as the most important and common form of support to alleviate caregiving burden and stress. Respite care can provide carers a break from usual caring duties for a short period or a longer time. It is acknowledged that without respite, carers may develop serious health and social risks due to the stress associated with continuous caregiving, and may also lack the time for essential personal and social needs or feel isolated.

Key action points include the development and enactment of policies that ensure ease of access to respite, for example via financial support to pay for such breaks, geographical proximity and sufficient availability and quality of respite services should be developed.

Also, local authorities/municipalities should actively provide and support access to short breaks which can be delivered in partnership with the voluntary sector and include respite within the home and elsewhere.

3.8   Step 8 Provide Carers with Access to Training and Recognise Their Skills

In Step 8 it is acknowledged that carer training promotes carer confidence and enables carers to provide better quality care for longer and in better conditions for themselves and the person they care for. It notes that the preventive aspects of well-trained and well-supported informal carers in avoiding or delaying hospital admission and long-term institutional care are well documented. Further, by recognising, developing and validating the numerous—sometimes highly technical—skills gained by informal carers while performing their caregiving tasks also offers significant potential to improve the quality of life of carers and the care recipient, but also to contribute to the sustainability of our care systems and to the EU (female) employment objectives.

Key action points include investments in carer training in order to strengthen carers' skills, improve the quality of the care they provide, maximise their opportunities to maintain an active professional life and exercise their acquired talents beyond their caregiving situation. It is argued that the expertise developed by carer organisations in the topic as well as the potential offered by ICT-based solutions are significant and should be further explored.

Second, the possibility and added value of a certification process to apply to the competences developed by carers in the framework of their caregiving activities should be explored in order to value their skills and facilitate their adherence, (re-) entry in the labour market.

3.9 Step 9 Prevent Carers' Poverty and Allow Them to Maintain an Active Professional/Educational Life

In Step 9 it is argued that taking on a caring role should not mean that people have to face financial hardship and social exclusion or give up work or education to care. Also, that carers who want and are able to study or work should be enabled to do so, and should not be discriminated against—they should be supported at school/university and in the workplace to maintain their employment status. Further, carers should also have access to lifelong learning opportunities, further and higher education and skills development in ways which take account of their caring responsibilities. It is recognised that this is essential to avoid poverty and social exclusion and is also important in the light of the gender pay and pension gap in Europe and the EU objectives in the fields of education, employment and growth.

In addition to action point 8 above, further key action points for Step 9 include the further development and regulation of financial support to carers—through care allowances or cash benefits that can be passed on to them. The level of financial support should be adequate enough to prevent carers from falling into poverty.

Third, carer-friendly employment practices (e.g. flexible working hours, part-time work, care leave, care brokerage, mental health in the workplace, etc.) should be actively encouraged and promoted. All relevant stakeholders (workers, employers, social partners and public authorities) should be involved in shaping and implementing these legislative and practical measures.

Fourth, young carers should be identified as early as possible (via improved vigilance and screening tools of professionals), their needs should be addressed and the needs of the whole family should be assessed. This requires good joint working between adult and children's services. The educational sector should also be made aware of the impact of informal care on (young) carers' ability to achieve educational attainment.

3.10 Step 10 Adopt the Carers' Perspective in All Relevant Policies

In Step 10 it is recognised that the success of initiatives aiming to address the needs and preference of carers largely depends on the interplay between a broad set of health and social policies. It highlights the need for better strategic planning and collaborative working between a wide range of services to ensure the effective delivery of coordinated support measures that meet the multidimensional needs of carers.

Key action points include public authorities and stakeholders helping to ensure that this happens by supporting the implementation and achievement of the objectives defined in this document and by considering the carers' perspective in all policy developments that could potentially impact their daily life.

Second, civil society organisations are invited to use the Strategy document to emphasise the consequences of public policies on the daily lives of carers and to improve the accountability of policy makers for the impacts of their decision at all levels of policy making.

Having explained the Eurocarers strategy, we will now highlight the key policy hooks that the carers' movement can use to help ensure that care is on the policy agenda. We begin at an international level before focusing on relevant policy hooks at European level.

Globally, the UN Sustainability Goals [25] act as the main policy instrument with regard to informal carers, care and caring. The 2030 Agenda for Sustainable Development, including 17 Sustainable Development Goals (SDGs) was adopted by all Member States of the United Nations, providing a roadmap towards sustainable prosperity, social inclusion and equality, while at the same time "preserving our planet and leaving no one behind". The European Union contributed to the development of the 2030 Agenda, and also committed to implement the SDGs in all its policies, whilst encouraging EU countries to do the same.

The EU Pillar of Social Rights [26] appears as a key step forward in this regard and acts as the major policy at EU level to have clear entry points for informal carers and caring. Proclaimed by EU institutions on the 17 November 2017 at the Social Summit for Fair Jobs and Growth in Gothenburg, Sweden, it is widely seen by civil society as a laudable attempt by the Commission to bring the social dimension of the union back on the EU policy agenda. It comprises a set of 20 principles under three headings: "equal opportunities and access to the labour market", "fair working conditions", and "social protection and inclusion", supporting the EU's efforts in delivering on the SDGs.

It was followed by a series of initiatives aimed at ensuring a concrete implementation of these principles, having an impact on the situation of carers. Importantly, a Directive on Work Life Balance was adopted in 2019 [27], establishing a right to a minimum of 5 days of leave per year per worker for caring purposes, and a right for carers to request flexible working arrangements. This Directive was welcomed as the first EU legislative instrument recognising informal carers. However, these new rights for parents and informal carers remain limited, and Member States retain significant room for manoeuvre in implementing these rights by August 2022 [28, 29].

The European Pillar of Social Rights Action Plan, adopted by the European Commission in the beginning of 2021 [30], sets out a number of EU actions that the Commission is committed to take during the current mandate, including an initiative on long-term care. Eurocarers has been advocating for social rights of informal carers to be enhanced, in particular in the areas of pensions, adequate income and access to social protection, presenting positive initiatives already taken in some countries [31].

In view of the importance of the issues at stake and the difficulties encountered across EU countries in providing lifelong care, which have been exacerbated since the outburst of the Covid 19 pandemic, [4], Ursula Van der Leyen, President of the European Commission, in her state of the union address (September 2021) [32] announced an even broader policy initiative, covering not only long-term care provision, but also early childhood care and education. In order to support care professionals and informal carers, but also parents, the policy initiative will take the form of a "Care package" to be unveiled in the third quarter of 2022, comprising a Commission Communication on a European Care Strategy, a proposal for a Council Recommendation on Long-term care and a proposal for a Council Recommendation on the revision of the Barcelona targets on early childhood education and care.

In support of its approach, the European Commission states that our response to care needs is key to social cohesion, labour market participation and economic growth. The Commission recognises that "the scale of the current problems demands a focused and comprehensive approach at EU level"—"one which provides a response to and recognition of the societal and economic importance of care while proposing concrete supportive actions". They also note the "increasing relevance of long-term care to the single market, as care providers and recipients take advantage of the freedom to move and to establish and provide services, including digitally enabled ones" [33]. Consultations are ongoing in preparation of the initiatives, but it is already expected that it will focus on accessibility, affordability and quality of long-term care, and address the issues of the care workforce, considering both care workers and informal carers under this heading. It is hoped that Member States will manage to agree on a common set of indicators in the area of long-term care, though the availability and comparability of data remain an issue [34].

Importantly, the announced care strategy appears also as a first action taken to address the ongoing demographic transition, following the publication in January 2021 of a Green Paper on Ageing by the Commission [35], setting out the speed and scale of the demographic changes in our society, as well as the impact this has across EU policies, ranging from health promotion, and lifelong learning to strengthening health and care systems to cater for an older population, looking at the impact of ageing on citizens' careers, well-being, pensions, social protection and productivity.

We recognise that the combination of a common vision and common objectives enshrined in a European Care Strategy, monitoring and mutual learning activities, has the potential to contribute to a better awareness of the issues at stake, broader debate, and policy commitment for better care across the life-cycle. Importantly, it can also help target EU financial support towards long-term care. The European

Recovery and Resilience Facility tool adopted in 2021 [36] puts a budget of up to 672 billion euros at the disposal of Member States to support reforms and investments by the end of 2026. The implementation of this financial effort across Member States will be monitored through the annual "European Semester process". This process serves as an important mechanism enabling the EU member countries to coordinate their fiscal, economic and social policies throughout the year and address the common challenges facing the EU. Every year, member states share information about the reforms they undertake or plan in order to contribute to European common fiscal, economic and social objectives. Building on a detailed analysis of each country's situation by the European Commission's services, Country Specific Recommendations are issued to guide member states' efforts, and importantly how they use the European funding instruments at their disposal. In more recent years, the EU Semester has increasingly addressed issues related to health and long-term care.

To date, long-term care has remained the "poor relation" in planned investments. However, it is expected that the adoption of the European Care Strategy will help member states seize the opportunity of the Recovery and Resilience Facility tool to initiate much needed reforms and investment in long-term care [37].

In addition to the initiative on long-term care within the Social Pillar Action plan, in March 2021, the Commission adopted the first comprehensive EU Strategy on the Rights of the Child [38], as well as a proposal for a Council Recommendation establishing a European Child Guarantee [39]. The Child Guarantee serves to provide guidance and tools to all member states in their efforts to support children in need. It acknowledges that reinforced and targeted support has to be put in place to ensure that all children have equal opportunities in enjoying their social rights.

As a result of the dissemination and exploitation work of a Eurocarers consortium EU Horizon 2020 adolescent young carers research project, "ME-WE" (https://me-we.eu), both the Child Guarantee itself and the Council Recommendation establishing the Guarantee explicitly recognise young carers as a group at risk of poverty and social exclusion that requires specific attention. The ME-WE project helped to raise awareness of adolescent young carers and the risks to their mental health and well-being arising from their caring responsibilities (https://me-we.eu). Previously, policy makers at EU level and at national level in many countries globally have largely been unaware of the situation of young carers and their needs for support to ensure that they thrive and enjoy the same rights regarding their health, education and opportunities in life as other children and young people.

It is worth noting that alongside the above-mentioned developments in the areas of social rights and long-term care, the situation of informal carers of people with cancer has gained visibility in the course of the development of European initiatives against cancer. The Europe's Beating Cancer Plan adopted by the European Commission in 2021 [40] specifically recognises the essential role of informal carers, "to support and provide care to cancer patients", as well as the often-negative impact of caring on the lives of carers in terms of their work-life balance, income, but also their physical and mental health and well-being, including the perpetuation of gender-related inequalities when it comes to care responsibilities.

The European Parliament has been usefully highlighting the role of informal cancer carers, and more particularly the European Parliament's Special Committee on Beating Cancer (BECA), which was created in June 2020 and ended its mandate on 23 December 2021. This committee organised an unprecedented consultation process through a series of public hearings. The European Parliament Resolution on "Strengthening Europe in the fight against cancer" adopted in January 2022 [41], calls for the recognition of informal cancer carers, including through their integration into health and care teams, their empowerment and the formalisation of informal care, which is argued in the Resolution to help ensure the recognition of a certain minimum standard of rights, especially for those carers who are providing long-term care.

Such a statement in favour of the recognition and support of informal carers is in line with the continuous work of the European Parliament Informal Carers Interest Group (previously outlined above), that brings together MEPs from different countries and political parties who are willing to support the development of carer-friendly societies. The Group aims to critically monitor and analyse EU policy development for its impact on carers and to propose and advocate concrete actions in order to improve the day-to-day situation for Europe's many carers, working in close partnership with relevant stakeholders.

Finally, last but by no means least, we highlight the importance of funding geared to research and life-long learning with the aim of strengthening the evidence base on informal carers, care and caring which in turn can contribute to evidence-based policy making and advocacy work in the area. In this regard, we recognise the importance of finding possible entry points with regard to operating grants, for example, at EU level within the current Horizon Europe funding in the area of Health and Culture, Creativity and Inclusive Societies (HE, 2021–22 Work programme) [42]. As well, the Erasmus+ funding with a focus on education, training, youth and sport [43]. In the context of informal carers, relevant entry points include lifelong learning and validation of skills among informal carers, youth initiatives that may relate to the topic of young carers and exchange of and development of best practices for teaching and learning in the area of informal carers, care and caring among European member states. Within the framework of European Cohesion Policy, specific funds target all regions and cities in the European Union in order to support job creation, business competitiveness, economic growth, sustainable development, and improve citizens' quality of life. Two of these financial instruments in particular, can also be instrumental in supporting informal carers. These comprise the European Regional Development Fund (ERDF), to invest in social and economic development and the European Social Fund Plus (ESF+) to support jobs and create a fair and socially inclusive society (https://ec.europa.eu/regional_policy/en/2021_2027/).

4 Conclusions

Our chapter has attempted to explain how an advocacy and policy perspective based on solid evidence is central to the support and empowerment of informal carers across the life course in countries across the world. We conclude with the following three take home messages:

(i) the importance of a strong carers movement globally to advocate for and with informal carers to ensure their voices are heard and that they remain, together with the people they care for, at the centre of polices, practices and research that concern them.

(ii) the importance of widespread policies embedded in a comprehensive carers strategy that places carer recognition and rights at the centre and advocates for: (i) services for users and carers that are reliable, flexible, affordable and technology enabled, (ii) work-care reconciliation—workplace and life course flexibility for employees, employers, labour force and (iii) adequate financial support measures to prevent financial hardship for carers.

(iii) the importance of getting the right balance: formalisation should not go with instrumentalization. While carers welcome the steps taken towards better recognition and support, including through the possibility of a formalisation of their role, ensuring they have access to social rights, they should always have the opportunity to make an informed choice as to the care responsibility they are willing and able to take on board. Recognition of informal care should go together with further investment in formal care services, against the backdrop of comprehensive strategies centred around the value of care and ensuring access for all to quality long-term care.

References

1. UNECE (2019) The challenging role of informal carers, policy brief. Policy Brief on Ageing 22
2. WHO (2016) Framework on integrated, people centred health services: WHO
3. Eurocarers (2016) Towards community-based people-centred integrated care: the role of informal care, Factsheet. Eurocarers, Brussels
4. Eurocarers/IRCCS-INRCA (2021) Impact of the Covid-19 outbreak on informal carers across Europe - final report. Eurocarers/IRCCS-INRCA, Brussels
5. Lorenz-Dant K, Comas-Herrera A (2021) The impacts of COVID-19 on unpaid carers of adults with long-term care needs and measures to address these impacts: a rapid review of evidence up to November 2020. J Long-Term Care 124–53
6. European Commission (2021) Long-term care report. Trends, challenges and opportunities in an ageing society vol 1. Joint report prepared by the social protection committee (SPC) and the European Commission (DG EMPL). Publications Office of the European Union, Luxembourg
7. US Bureau of Labour Statistics (2019) Unpaid Eldercare in the United States-2017-2018 Summary, USDL-19-2051 U.S: USDL
8. Wimo A, Gauthier S, Prince M (2018) Alzheimer's disease international. Global estimates of informal care, Alzheimer's international. ADI, Karolinska Institutet, London

9. Joseph S, Sempik J, Leu A, Becker S (2020) Young carers research, practice and policy: an overview and critical perspective on possible future directions. Adoles Res Rev 5:77–89
10. European Institute for Gender Equality (EIGE) (2019) Gender Equality Index 2019. Work-life balance. EIGE, Vilnius
11. Verbakel E, Tamlagsronning S, Winstone L, Fjaer EL, Eikemo TA (2017) Informal care in Europe: findings from the European social survey (2014) special module on the social determinants of health. Eur J Pub Health 27(1):90–95
12. International Alliance of Carer Organizations (IACO) (2021) The Global State of Caring IACO
13. Pitkeathley JB (2014) The carers' movement, opening plenary address at the 6th International Carers Conference, Gothenburg
14. Clements L (2013) Does your carer take sugar? Carers and human rights: the parallel struggles of disabled people and carers for equal treatment. Carers NSW, Sydney
15. Becker S, Sempik J (2018) Young adult carers; the impact of caring on health and education. Child Soc 33(4):377–386
16. Fast J (2015) Caregiving for older adults with disabilities. Present costs, future challenges, IRPP Study, 58. IRPP
17. England Carers Strategy (2008) Carers at the heart of 21st-century families and communities "A caring system on your side. A life of your own" London: HM Government
18. Scottish Carers Strategy (2019) The Scottish Government Carers strategic policy statement: consultation
19. Australian Carers Strategy (2011) National Carers Strategy Action plan 2011–2014. Australian Government, Canberra
20. Ireland Carers Strategy (2012) The National Carers' Strategy recognised, supported, Empowered: Department of Social Protection
21. Norway Carers Strategy (2020) The Norwegian Government's carers strategy and action plan
22. France Carers Strategy (2019). Available from: https://handicap.gouv.fr/agir-pour-les-aidants
23. Sweden Carers Strategy (2022) The National Carer Strategy within health care and social care: Department of Health and Social Affairs
24. Eurocarers (2018) Enabling carers to care - an EU strategy to support and empower informal carers. Eurocarers, Brussels
25. United Nations (2015) Transforming our world: the 2030 agenda for sustainable development A/RES/70/1: UN
26. European Parliament Council and Commission (2017) European pillar of social rights proclaimed by the European Parliament, the council and the Commission: European Parliament, Council and Commission
27. European Commission (2019) Directive (EU) 2019/1158 of the European parliament and of the council of 20 June 2019 on work-life balance for parents and carers and repealing council directive 2010/18/EU: Official Journal of the European Union
28. Eurocarers (2019) The work life balance directive: what's in it for carers? Eurocarers, Brussels
29. Eurocarers. (2020) Implementation of work-life balance directive and new carers' rights – where do we stand? Eurocarers, Brussels
30. European Commission (2021) The European pillar of social rights action plan. European Commission, Brussels
31. Eurocarers (2020) Enhancing the rights of informal Carers – Eurocarers' response to the consultation on the social pillar action plan. Eurocarers, Brussels
32. European Commission (2021) State of the union address by president von der Leyen. European Commission, Brussels
33. European Commission (2022) Call for evidence for an Initiative – European Care Strategy _ Ares(2022)1514879. European Commission, Brussels
34. Eurocarers (2021) The EU strategy on care: a new paradigm for Carers across Europe? Eurocarers, Brussels
35. European Commission (2021) Green paper on ageing: Fostering solidarity and responsibility between generations. COM (2021) 50 final. European Commission, Brussels

36. European Parliament and Council (2021) Regulation (EU) 2021/241 of the European Parliament and of the Council of 12 February 2021 establishing the Recovery and Resilience Facility: Official Journal of the European Union
37. Eurocarers (2021) Without greater investment in care, the European Union will fail to rebuild resilient societies at the service of people. Eurocarers, Brussels
38. European Commission (2021) EU strategy on the rights of the child. COM(2021) 142 final. Brussels, European Commission
39. European Commission D-GfE, Social Affairs and Inclusion (2021) Proposal for a Council recommendation establishing the European child guarantee. Publications Office of the European Union: European Commission
40. European Commission (2021) Europe's beating cancer plan: a new EU approach to prevention, treatment and care. European Commission, Brussels
41. European Parliament (2022) Resolution of 16 February 2022 on strengthening Europe in the fight against cancer – towards a comprehensive and coordinated strategy (2020/2267(INI)): European Parliament
42. European Commission (2021) Horizon Europe work programme 2021–2022. General Annexes. European Commission, Brussels
43. European Commission (2022) Erasmus+ Programme Guide, Version 2, 2022. European Commission, Brussels

Health Behavioral Change Interventions in Caregivers: The Prolepsis Project

Andri Christou and Maria Christodoulou Fella

1   Introduction

Many of the leading causes of death in developing and developed countries seem to be corelated with the human behaviors [1–3]. Behavior change communication is vital for increasing the enactment of behaviors known to promote health and growth [4]. Behaviors such as dietary physical activity tobacco and alcohol play a key role and can have substantial effects on population health outcomes [1, 5].

Health behavior encompasses many facets, and so behavioral interventions are broad as well. Such interventions have been targeted at behavioral risk factors (e.g., smoking, drug addiction [6] encouraging protective behaviors (e.g., health screening; [7, 8] e.g., adoption skin cancer protective behaviors, [9], enhancing adaptation to chronic and acute illness (e.g., following medical advice) [10] and improving the quality and efficiency of services by changing health professional behavior (e.g., hand hygiene compliance); [5, 11].

Historically, infectious diseases have been responsible for the greatest human death tolls in human history. For example, the bubonic plague killed approximately 25% of the European population. Even in such conditions the human behavior played a vital role in the outcomes of the pandemic. Therefore, it is important how people like to perceive and respond to threats and risk during a pandemic by adjusting their behavior accordingly [12].

Behavioral interventions are targeted to other factors, that are not classified as medical and genetic factors [13]. A simplistic form of intervention would be encouraging people to stop smoking (simple in the goals at least; smoking cessation is

A. Christou (✉) · M. Christodoulou Fella
School of Health Sciences, Department of Nursing, Cyprus University of Technology, Limassol, Cyprus
e-mail: andri.christou@cut.ac.cy

A. Charalambous (ed.), *Informal Caregivers: From Hidden Heroes to Integral Part of Care*, https://doi.org/10.1007/978-3-031-16745-4_11

189

quite complex to achieve). A more comprehensive intervention would make sure to target individuals with a variety of risk factors and encourage them to make several lifestyle changes, such as quitting smoking, eating fewer fatty foods, exercising more frequently, visiting physicians for hypertension screenings, and adhering to medication recommendations. As a matter of fact, behavioral changes are necessary for effective medical care and sustainable results over time. Rather than acting passively on individuals, the aim is to change the behavior of each individual toward more healthy practices.

The physical and emotional burden of caring for a functionally impaired person may adversely affect the preventive health behavior of the caregiver [6]. A caregiver's lifestyle, health behaviors, and use of preventive services are affected by the caregiving. Caregivers are significantly more likely than non-caregivers to not get enough rest, not exercise enough, forget about taking prescription medications, and not have time to recuperate from illness. Additionally, caregivers of ovarian cancer patients frequently fail to meet health guidelines and about half describe negative changes they have experienced as a result of caring for them [14]. Family members with chronic medical conditions, such as dementia, are primarily cared for by women [15]. Gender differences among caregivers have shown a considerable distinction with respect to physical and psychosocial health status [16]. Specifically, female caregivers report higher levels of depressive symptoms than their male counterparts, and are at greater risk for clinical depression [17]. Moreover, compared to their male counterparts, female caregivers report worse physical health and more emotional distress as a result of caregiving [18, 19]. Family caregivers continue to face significant stress and burden when caring for someone they love [20–23]. Caregivers' burden has been defined as a multidimensional aspect of physical, psychological, emotional, social, financial, and social stressors associated with the caregiving experience. It has been hypothesized as an acute reaction to the addition of new demands on caregivers and the intensifying of existing ones [24].

2   The Nature of Behavioral Interventions

Having a theoretical understanding of behavior change is necessary to maximize the potential efficacy of interventions. It includes the a priori assumptions about what human behavior is and what influences it, as well as the mechanisms of action (mediators) and moderators of change. As part of intervention design, evaluation, and evidence synthesis, theories are advocated as integral components [4, 25, 26]. The advantage is that theory-based interventions can be used to test theories. As a result, more useful theories are developed, which assists in optimizing interventions [27–29].

There is a predictable pattern in behavior and in the way that behavior changes over the past century based on basic psychological research. The accumulated science must therefore inform and guide interventions accordingly. It was found that there are a variety of theories covering a wide range of behaviors that can be applied to the design and evaluation of interventions that enhance public health and address issues including environmental sustainability and public safety [30].

In the areas of health education, health promotion, patient education, and psychotherapy, health behavior change interventions are considered complex interventions. Behavioral interventions are interventions designed to change the way people behave regarding their health and well-being [31]. It is important to change patient behavior with behavioral interventions. There is a tendency to emphasize individual abilities and motivations as well as social factors with regard to public health interventions.

Women who take on the job of the informal caregiver, encounter additional hurdles when it comes to participating in health promotion activities like breast cancer screening. In contrast to non-carers, studies on carers' health behaviors explicitly highlight the occurrence of worsened health behaviors such as missing healthcare appointments, eating a poor-quality diet, having restricted exercise time, and forgetting to take prescribed medications. Prolepsis (https://prolepsis.eu/) is an EU funded project which aimed the health promotion of breast cancer screening for informal care givers. In order to achieve this, a mobile phone application was developed, with tailored individual messages for informal caregivers, covering broad content areas, as a means to enhance preventive healthcare behavior of these carers. The Prolepsis Mobile Application is available to women who are informal caregivers, supporting the process of breast cancer awareness and healthy living. The success of the mobile application relies on its best utilization by the user.

3   Health Belief Model

There is a plethora of divergent and overlapping theories in this context [27, 32]. The Prolepsis project has a very specific aim and target population and therefore it was necessary to identifying which theories were more likely to be relevant and useful for the project.

According to Glanz and Bishop [26], a general trend in public health and behavior change interventions is to put more emphasis on individual and interpersonal factors than broader social and environmental factors. Most often, the focus is on abilities and motivation (individual factors), but context (social and environmental factors) is much less common.

Health-related behavior change interventions that are based on adequate theories are typically more effective [4]. The Prolepsis project was based on the health belief model to mobilize the caregivers for their own health. Most theories applied to public health interventions tend to emphasize individual capabilities and motivation, with limited reference to context and social factors [4, 33]. The Prolepsis project has created a digital application for mobile phones that, taking into account the special characteristics and data of the user, aims to mobilize for the adoption of preventive health behavior.

The behavior change approach promotes health through individual changes in lifestyle that are appropriate to people's settings [33]. The assumption of the Prolepsis project is that, changing a person's lifestyle can be achieved if they have a basic knowledge of health issues, adopt key attitudes, learn a set of skills and are provided with appropriate resources and support. The simple logic which described by Bernier et al. [34] was adopted during the whole design of the prolepsis project, that some behaviors leads to ill-health, and so persuading people directly to change their behaviors must be the most efficient and effective way to reduce illness.

People do not resist change, but they do resist being changed [35, 36]. Knowing when and how to apply science to produce an outcome is the art of health promotion [35]. The interventions of the Prolepsis project are addressed to a specific target population. Specifically, to women who have the responsibility of caring for an individual in their family environment. In order to meet the special needs of this specific population, three focus groups were done by the three participating countries: Cyprus, Italy, and Portugal.

The following elements can be included to make behavior change and health promotion more effective and sustainable: a strong policy framework that creates a supportive environment [35], an enablement of people to empower themselves to make healthy lifestyle decisions. Along the breast cancer prevention policies implemented in the participating countries, the creation of the digital mobile application by the Prolepsis project aims to empower women caregivers to manage stressful situations. A way that this was achieved was through text messages reminders for the adoption of simple habits that have a significant contribution to maintaining health.

4   Behavior Change and Health Promotion

It is known that diseases are driven by a complex interaction of factors, specifically those that are affected by political, social, and economic factors [37]. Despite decades of recognition on the direct effects of poverty, unemployment, and housing on people's health, these policy problems are often defined as behavioral risks such as physical inactivity. Work in health promotion that goes beyond the individual behavior model recognizes the importance of a broader determinants approach. The understanding of health policy agendas must, however, take into account the structural features of societies and the political nature of societies themselves [38].

Interventions to promote health that directly target behavioral risks can be effective at best but at worst can worsen societal inequalities. Due to their limited impact on broader conditions causing poor health, behavior change approaches do not have much bearing for vulnerable groups like migrants and low socioeconomic groups as well as indigenous groups. In order to effectively target a specific disease or behavior, behavior change approaches need to be incorporated into a wider, comprehensive policy framework rather than implemented as a single intervention [38, 39].

The behavior change approach promotes health through individual changes in lifestyle that are appropriate to people's settings [13]. Prior to changing their lifestyle, people first need to understand the basics of a particular health issue, adopt a set of attitudes, learn a set of skills, and gain access to appropriate services. It stands to reason that certain behaviors contribute to ill-health, and that convincing people to change their behavior directly would be the most effective and efficient method of reducing illness. Decision makers are fond of this reasoning because it promises quantitative results in a short amount of time, deals with health problems that are usually prevalent, is relatively simple, and offers savings in healthcare services, especially for chronically ill individuals [13].

If the following factors are included, behavior change and health promotion can be made more successful and sustainable: a strong policy framework that generates a supportive environment [34] and the ability for people to empower themselves to make healthy lifestyle decisions. Health promotion programs are frequently reliant on the engagement of persons who are specifically targeted. People also want to participate, and if they are appropriately engaged and share a common interest in the program, they will do so in huge numbers. Successful participation should be congratulated. The most successful empowerment programs, in terms of behavior change, are those where people with mutual interests coexist within the same group [40]. Kalantar-Zadeh et al. state that chronic kidney disease is associated with a troublesome daily life for patients and their care-partners [41]. Therefore, empowering patients and their caregivers, which may include family members or friends involved in their care, may help minimize the burden and consequences of the disease on daily life.

When interacting with the stressful and demanding environment of providing care for the sick or disabled, caregivers should adopt health promotion behaviors to maintain their own health. A study on the factors affecting health promotion behaviors in caregivers caring for dementia patients, revealed the complexity and the diversity of those behaviors. Influencing factors that have been identified as part of the study included age, gender of the caregiver, his/her educational level, the financial situation, and family members with dementia and their relationships. In order to improve health promotion behavior among caregivers caring for elderly relatives suffering from dementia, they concluded that strategic tailored care plans were the most effective approach [42]. Further research is required to assess health promotion behaviors for caregivers of various conditions whether chronic or short-term approaches are the most suitable in order to provide appropriate health promotion solutions.

Persons who provide unpaid assistance or supervision with activities of daily living (ADLs) to someone who is incapable of handling these tasks due to cognitive, physical, or psychological impairments are known as informal caregivers (ICGs) [43]. In this context, the stress (e.g., deriving from the responsibility of assuming the role as well as its complexity) of caring for someone with a chronic disease may also contribute to the lack of health knowledge, health behaviors, and screening adherence among informal caregivers. Consistently, researchers have found that informal caregivers are less likely to practice health-promoting behaviors compared to non-caregivers [13, 44, 45]. Other studies have shown a significant association between caregiving level and inadequate exercise and health promotion practices [46–48]. Because of their demanding role that in many cases requires significant changes in their lives (e.g., changes of roles, balancing the tasks of their own family to those of the care recipient), caregivers do not always have time for preventive care. The majority of caregivers of adults with significant caregiving requirements couldn't leave the care recipient alone and had to schedule their time around the recipients' daily activities significantly limiting their own free time [13, 45, 49]. Even the seemingly limited provision of caregiving can have a significant impact on the person who delivers the care. Therefore, studies [46–48] have demonstrated a link between low levels of caring and insufficient exercise and health-promoting habits.

Self-management and self-efficacy have been shown to increase people's motivation and confidence in their own abilities, knowledge, experience, and satisfaction [50]. Interventions aimed at increasing ICGs' self-efficacy have been proven to be effective and more sustainable over time [51, 52]. Supporting people's self-management also helps them to engage in healthier habits and make overall behavioral changes [53]. Several facilitators have been identified in studies on the topic that have been demonstrated to support higher mammography use in women. Perceived benefits of mammography, self-efficacy, and susceptibility to breast cancer [54, 55] are among the reasons that were highlighted.

Limited health literacy has been linked to a reduction in the use of preventive services across cultures and populations [56–58], and women with poor self-reported health literacy were less likely to have a mammogram in the previous 2 years [59]. Furthermore, low health literacy has been associated to an increased risk of cancer and presenting to cancer care systems at later stages of the disease [53]. The significance of health literacy has been acknowledged early on as a potent game changer in promoting preventive practices among women. Explicitly, findings from a variety of studies suggest that health literacy-focused treatments can change women's attitudes toward breast cancer screening [60–63]. For example, early breast cancer screening using technology-based interventions is possible and cost-effective [64, 65]. However, the potential of health literacy supportive interventions can be effective in other cancer diagnoses and population groups. In a two-arm multicentric randomized controlled cluster trial, a combined health literacy intervention (health literacy and CRC training + brochure and video) was able to reduce disparities in CRC screening, increase screening rates among the most vulnerable populations, and increase knowledge and activation (beneficial in the context of repeated screening) [66]. In the same context of colorectal cancer, a multilevel two-arm intervention trial compared the efficacy of two interventions (C-CARES (education+FIT) or C-CARES Plus (C-CARES+personalized coaching [for those not completing FIT within 90 days]) to promote CRC screening (CRCS) with fecal immunochemical test (FIT). Both interventions included low literacy education materials in either English or Spanish plus provision of a FIT and were successful in promoting FIT uptake among patients. The overall initial screening rate of 69% in this study far exceeds the prevailing UDS rates of the clinics, thus supporting potential utility of these strategies [67].

In the early stages of breast cancer [68], caregiving has been identified as a critical factor that can lead to low usage of healthcare services. As ICGs get older, they may be less likely to meet their own health needs, have higher levels of allostatic load, and have higher rates of death and morbidity [69]. In comparison to non-caregivers, studies have found that ICGs exhibit worse health practices, such as missing their own doctor's appointments and refusing cancer screening tests [38, 70, 71]. Data from a variety of studies suggests that health literacy-focused treatments can change women's attitudes toward breast cancer screening [60–63]. As discussed earlier, interventions either based on technology or low-tech interventions can be viable, feasible to integrate in daily practice and provide benefits. The stress of caregiving raises concerns about women's health, especially BC screening and overall preventative practices, because nearly two-thirds of ICGs over 50 are women [72]. One such example is an EU funded project set up in order to identify the need for specific health literacy interventions. The Prolepsis project explored ICGs' knowledge and perceptions regarding BC early detection practices as well as the healthcare professionals' (HCPs') perceptions regarding ICGs. Understanding the perspectives of informal caregivers and healthcare professionals can highlight the areas of concern that can pose a threat to appropriate BC early detection as well as prevention practices.

Health problems are common among caregivers such as indigestion issues, neuralgia, low mood, sleep disturbances, headaches, anxiety and fatigue and fear of dementia [73]. The World Health Organization has promoted an action plan for the health of caregivers of people with dementia. Dua et al. [74] stress the fact that it is vital to supporting informal caregivers' health promotion by means which involve activities that influence their health and empowerment [54]. However, as studies demonstrate, it is not an easy task for the family caregivers to attend to their own health, as they generally don't have enough time to devote to their own health. This is because they turn much of their attention to their loved one which results in the draining of most of their energy [75].

The caregiver's ability to attend to his or her own health needs is rarely the focus in studies examining caregiver stress and burden. Caregivers are burdened in many ways, including the daily number and complexity of tasks and lack of opportunities for social contact (e.g., limited communication and visits to family members and friends, lack of opportunities to attend social gatherings outside their living space). Informal caregivers such as family members are taking over the responsibility of doing highly technical tasks traditionally done by healthcare professionals. For this reason, caregivers providing home healthcare should have access to on-demand information that can facilitate their caregiving role. They should be able to request assistance through a variety of available means and portals so that they can become more knowledgeable medically both for their own health promotion and become more confident in the care they provide to their loved one [76, 77]. One-to-one consultations with medical and other healthcare professionals have been used effectively as a way to achieve health promotion. However, recent advances in technology and e-health promotion include the use of digital tools, such as the use of mobile apps and specialized online platforms, to help caregivers manage their duties and promote their personal (physical and mental) health [78–80].

Behavioral models are intended to assist researchers in better understanding behavior and attempting to explain why people behave in certain ways choosing to adopt or to reject certain practices. Theories of change, on the other hand, try to explain how people's behavior changes over time. Personal elements are those that are unique to the individual, such as their level of knowledge or their confidence in their capacity to change their habits and behavior [81]. There are several such model examples, based on theories of change, that have been used for a range of conditions including long-term and short-term.

For example, there are a variety of strategies and ways to health promotion that encourage and educate the public about Type 2 diabetes and the primary benefits of the prevention of the disease. This model depicts the desire of an individual to avoid sickness, as well as the idea that illness can be prevented and cured and it relies on people's sentiments of vulnerability to protect themselves from illness vary greatly.

The education approach is another way to health promotion. It is one of the most important components of overall patient care in the community. A health education program should empower people to make informed decisions, rather than simply comply with predetermined health goals [82]. For example, educating diabetes patients has been proven to motivate them and strengthen their ability to manage their illness [83, 84]. A meta-analysis conducted in order to assess the effects of health education for caregivers on the oral health condition of the elderly has proven that this approach may be effective for improving the oral health of the elderly [85]. The provision of education from the professional to the community members and caregivers represents the beginning of a lifelong self-care process [86].

Another approach to health promotion is that of effective communication. There is a wide range of communication channels available to disseminate specific information on health issues and these range from basic face-to-face conversations to telecommunications channels such as phones or e-mails, to digital channels such as phone applications and specialized online platforms (e-health literacy). An example is that of the eLILY e-course, funded by the EU, created and delivered by professionals in order to train caregivers of older people and people with dementia [82]. eLILY was developed in order to identify and understand people with low health literacy. To assist health service users in coping with health problems by empowering them and increasing their self-efficacy. To increase nurses' and other health professionals' eHealth literacy [87].

The most extensively utilized theory in health education and promotion is the Health Belief Model (HBM). This paradigm was created by social psychologists working for the US Public Health Service in the 1950s. Since then, the HBM has been tweaked to fit a variety of situations in order to investigate a number of long- and short-term health behaviors. Individual behavior, according to the HBM, is influenced by a variety of beliefs about risks to one's well-being, as well as the effectiveness and results of specific actions or behaviors [78, 88]. It is important to note that family caregivers' medical information seeking behavior can have an impact on both their health and that of their cancer patients [89].

5   eHealth Literacy

Health technology advances have increased in the past two decades, providing educators and healthcare professionals with the opportunity to make them as accessible as possible to groups with vulnerability. It would be beneficial to provide caregivers with access to web-based services, as caregivers face the consequences of caregiving, such as anxiety, depression, guilt, higher use of antidepressants, and an increased risk of infection more than the general population. Support services by way of the web may include training platforms, disease-specific websites, forums, social networks and other interactive online services, telehealth, telemedicine, and mobile applications. These services are offered and demanded in different ways across European nations, influenced by the people's digital skills and attitudes toward technology. Both health literacy (HL) and e-health literacy (eHL) provide caregivers with the ability to search, assess, and apply health-related information from a variety of sources (e.g., friends, family, neighbors, health professionals, the internet) [90–92].

Over the past few decades, distance self-education for health has become widespread due to the proliferation of patient information websites [90–92]. Providers can use this method to provide patients with an "information prescription" about their condition and how to manage it [93]. In addition, remote educational interventions may require less time of providers (in comparison with traditional methods of face-to-face learning) if they are automated very well [94].

6   The Prolepsis Project: An Example of a HBM Intervention

The promotion of alternative, technology-enhanced tools could facilitate the empowerment of caregivers in changing interventions. The importance of health literacy on health outcomes, within the context discussed in this chapter, has led to a study exploring the knowledge and attitudes of informal caregivers. The study that is presented below was part of the Prolepsis project (Co-Funded by the Erasmus+ Programme of the European Union), which was based on the principles of the HBM (https://prolepsis.eu/). The HBM strategy was used in this project because this model acknowledges and addresses the social context in which health behaviors take place, while focusing on the individual. Health belief models guide or influence interventions aimed at enhancing knowledge of health challenges, enhancing perceptions of personal risk, encouraging actions to reduce or eliminate that risk, and promoting a sense of self-efficacy required for outcome changes. The end-product of this project was the creation of a mobile application developed in a co-designed approach. The philosophy of the creation of this mobile application is to provide caregivers the carefully selected and personalized (i.e., tailored to the person's needs) information for the adoption and maintenance of health behavior in relation to breast health. Prolepsis aimed to develop a mobile phone-based health intervention, through the creation of an Application (App) for tablets and smartphones, to enhance preventive healthcare behavior among informal caregivers. This included tailoring individual messages across broad content areas while bypassing restrictions on where and when messages should be delivered.

Project consortium members believed that providing health information and teaching skills in a text-based format is most effective for helping people with high levels of health literacy. Additionally, participants may benefit from receiving straightforward written information accompanied by graphics and audio narration. As part of the Prolepsis project, participants receive health information aimed at enhancing their ability to adopt preventive measures against breast cancer and be able to timely diagnose it. The Prolepsis project defines precision health information as providing patients with the information they need, when they need it, in a format that they can understand and use.

The study objectives were to investigate the knowledge and perceptions of ICGs, including educational and training opportunities or barriers, regarding BC early detection practices, and the HCPs' perceptions about ICGs to determine the need for specific health literacy interventions.

In order to meet these objectives, a qualitative focus group study was implemented. The focus groups offered the ideal means to retrieve caregivers' perspectives on the needs, attitudes, knowledge, beliefs, and perceptions of breast cancer prevention. A health promotion program's success often depends on the participation of the targeted population. The researchers decided to utilize this method for obtaining the research data as the researchers believe that through this method the data could be obtained in a more appropriate environment because it allows an open discussion with the participants and between the participants themselves (this also allowed the sharing of personal experiences of the barriers and enables of health promotion practices). As described in the previous section, people with mutual interests coexist within the same group of empowerment programs, behavior change is more likely to be successful. The participants in the focus groups were motivated to express their feelings, ideas, agreements, or disagreements. Furthermore, group discussions stimulated memories for the participants, which facilitated the exchange of views and opinions, leading to a more in-depth study of the research topic. The recruited participants consisted of female caregivers, over 55 years old, which have been diagnosed with a chronic disease (for example cancer, dementia, myopathy) and healthcare professional and experts on breast cancer with working experience of two or more years. Both groups were recruited from three European countries (Cyprus, Italy, and Portugal) according to the above-predetermined criteria. Each country recruited a person in order to regulate the focus groups. These persons were healthcare professionals with expertise in health promotion issues and had previous experience in focus group regulation. Local language was used for the discussions to maximize the sharing of the perspectives within the group.

The study results showed that caregivers are fully informed about breast cancer in general and understand routine screening's benefits. Understanding their health literacy needs is important for the implementation of an intervention that is based on the education approach as a way to health promotion. Women are more likely to maintain breast cancer screening habits if they are familiar with the disease and receive specific advice and encouragement from their doctors and nurses. Papadakos et al.'s [53] systematic review of 17 articles referring to health literacy related to cancer, report that there were several significant self-management behaviors and related outcomes that were associated with health literacy, which included cancer screening, chemotherapy, and postoperative complications. The authors concluded that these are associated with significant self-management behaviors and that inadequate health literacy among individuals has significant implications on the healthcare system.

Consequently, women take precautions against breast cancer because they believe they are susceptible to it. The Health Believe Model indicates that women's perceptions of breast cancer based on their knowledge of the disease can predict their engagement with mammography and ultrasound [95–97].

Caregivers understood the value of screening and were fully informed about breast cancer in general. When women had personal or familiar experience with breast cancer and when their doctors provided specific advice and encouraging words, they were more likely to comply with the recommended screening methods. According to Hassan et al. [98], similar findings were found. The reason for this behavior is that women may perceive themselves as susceptible to breast cancer so they take action to prevent it. According to the Health Believe Model, women's perceptions of breast cancer are predictive of their engagement in mammography and ultrasound [95–97].

The Prolepsis study also found that women who are at increased risk for developing breast cancer or who have a prior history of breast cancer do not incorporate breast cancer screening into their daily routines. Perhaps this is due to the fact that caregivers consider this procedure time-consuming, and also feel unprepared for successfully completing this procedure. It is consistent in the relevant literature that most women are unaware of how to perform breast self-examination appropriately, highlighting the lack of promotion and education regarding breast self-examination among women [99–103].

The Prolepsis app[1] aims to educate and enhance caregivers to be able to control disease through changing their lifestyles and living practices. (More information on this and for downloading the app, can be found at https://prolepsis.eu/documents/). Modifying their lifestyle habits, self-monitoring, self-assessment, and enforcing positive behaviors, as well as inviting them to use preventive breast cancer services, are among these. The development of a mobile application for informal caregivers supports self-care and behavior change in illness prevention, based on the characteristics, needs, and preferences of each caregiver. A handbook was also developed that describes how the app can be used in health literacy reinforcement programs targeting not only informal caregivers, but women in general. As an e-book, the handbook presents practical suggestions and guidelines for both target groups.

The educational materials were developed based on the results of the focus group in accordance with the HBM model. The educational material aimed to increase female carers' awareness on breast cancer symptoms, on screening exams (i.e., mammography) and to promote a culture on preventive behavior practices, such as exercise, healthy diet, and stress management techniques.

All training modules are guided by the premise of increasing perceived sensitivity and seriousness about the threat of breast cancer, as well as the carers' understanding of the barriers which prevent them from implementing breast cancer

---

[1] The Prolepsis App can be downloaded here https://play.google.com/store/apps/details?id=eu.singularlogic.prolepsis&hl=en&gl=US

preventative behaviors. These constructs, in turn, may aid women in strengthening their capacity and instilling positive views about preventative behaviors such as breast self-examination, clinical breast examination, and mammography. The educational material was created in multiple stages (conception, peer review, translation) and required 8 months to complete. Initially, the training modules were created by studying reputable and trustworthy sources from which to compile the information. The pedagogical material covers a variety of intervention areas, including:

- *Information on Breast Cancer*: the theory and definition of Breast Cancer, the risk factors, epidemiology, and prevention methods.
- *Preventive lifestyle*: implementation and modifications of lifestyle habits in order to prevent breast cancer (e.g., healthy diet and exercise, psychological well-being, stress management, meditation).
- *Self-monitoring*: self-monitoring methods of the caregiver's own health, benefits of regular mammography.
- *Self-efficacy*: managing feelings of tension prior to mammography screening reduce anxiety-related screening methods. The mobile app will provide information to carers about practical steps that can be taken to maintain breast self-examination habits and incorporates a reminder system (based on the user's personalized preferences) whereby the app sends notifications to women carers about their next scheduled screening test.

The educational material created is reinforced via the app and by healthcare professionals through training seminars. The Prolepsis project creators firmly support the education approach as an important mode of health change promotion and as one of the most important components of overall patient care in the community. The seminars offered the opportunity to caregivers to download the app and try it out. The implementors of this program used these training seminars as a pilot study in order to evaluate the usefulness and the effectiveness of the app. The aim of the Prolepsis training was to build an educational program (and eventually an e-health program) which enables participants to increase their knowledge on breast cancer and understand the importance of prevention. Furthermore, it aimed to promote health change behaviors according to the HBM method by providing them with the skills to self-manage their own health monitoring. The overall effect is to encourage caregivers through a change of behavior to be vigilant about breast cancer prevention and thus lead to an early detection of breast cancer.

Pop-up messages were incorporated in the app as a form of reinforcement of health change. The purpose of the pop-up messages is to encourage self-care such as healthy nutrition, physical exercise, meditation, relaxation exercises, and send reminders to caregivers about their next screening appointment.

Effective communication is another mode of healthcare promotion. The use of the app also creates a supportive environment through communication via a chat feature that enables caregivers and professionals, family and friends, to engage with each other, offering the opportunity of mutual support (though the formation of selective supportive groups). As previously mentioned in this chapter, the most successful empowerment programs which promote behavior change, are those where people with mutual interests coexist within the same group.

The above was incorporated in the Prolepsis app aiming to continue the reinforcement of the inventions, based on the HBM method and the results of the study, through e-learning, based on various modes of health promotion—education, effective communication, and a strong policy framework that creates a supportive environment. Prolepsis aims to continue to promote health change via the app for the early detection of breast cancer.

7   Apps in Health Literacy Programs

Approximately 100 million people worldwide live in extreme poverty and 50% are unable to access essential healthcare services due to out-of-pocket health expenses. Mobile technologies are essential for developing sustainable health systems and promoting health literacy programs. As 80% of the population in developing countries owns a mobile phone, mobile technology can help reach them [104]. A smartphone with notable advanced technology can be useful to support behavior change [105].

In order to increase preventive healthcare in informal caregiver populations, Prolepsis developed a mobile phone-based health intervention. It is likely to provide low-cost and successful methods of reaching out to hard-to-reach people with customized individual communications spanning a wide range of topics, while also overcoming delivery constraints such as location and time [106]. In the sphere of health behavior change, the emerging eHealth and mHealth fields have already proven to be beneficial [107].

"The ability of individuals to find, understand, and use information and services to inform health-related decisions and actions for themselves and others" is defined as "the degree to which individuals have the ability to find, understand, and use information and services to inform health-related decisions and actions for themselves and others" [108]. This is an important component in health outcomes because it affects patients' ability to manage their relationships with healthcare systems [94].

Studies show that low health literacy is linked to poor health outcomes, such as an increased risk of death [109], difficulty finding, understanding, and acting on health-related information [110], cancer screening adherence [111], and influencing cancer patients' behaviors and healthcare service use [111, 112].

The intervention of mHealth interventions is a promising mean of empowering people; experts and locals dealing with preventable health risks related to chronic diseases; allowing people to be actively engaged in the prevention of chronic conditions, providing feedback on the quality of health and care, facilitate early detection of symptoms and thus timely treatment. This will potentially lead to an improvement in health behavior [113].

Having developed this application, the entire philosophy was to provide informal caregivers with carefully selected information for their adoption and maintenance of health behaviors related to breast health. Additionally, it guides users through the right steps for early detection of breast cancer and promotes breast health. An important objective of this mobile application is to provide caregivers with well-selected information so they are not overwhelmed or confused by the abundance of free information available online. Based on this study, the barriers that affected the behavior of ICGs in regard to early screening might have arisen from the misconception women hold about the diagnosis of BC. Thus, providing health literacy programs designed to address BC, including BSE screening, could reduce concerns and motivate individuals to practice BSE on a systematic basis [60–62]. By promoting alternative, technology-enhanced tools, women may be empowered on this basis [65, 114].

8   Conclusion

Caregivers are a vital and resourceful member of the society. Commitment of caring for a close member can pose as a deterrent to adopting preventive health behaviors because they may feel guilty about taking time for themselves and for their own screening, or they don't have time so they go to the doctor only when absolutely necessary. Modifying behavior is complex and challenging but at the same time it has the greatest prospect for adopting healthier behaviours by informal caregivers. The health belief model can be used as a theoretical framework to guide the process of modifying behavior. The Prolepsis example is a completed program which was developed based on this theoretical model to promote and encourage the adoption of preventive healthcare behavior among caregivers and other groups of women, by providing information, education, effective communication ways, empowerment programs, mutual support and encouraging lifestyle change, which can have an impact in preventing the onset of serious healthcare conditions.

References

1. Reimann Z, Miller JR, Dahle KM, Hooper AP, Young AM, Goates MC, et al (2020) Executive functions and health behaviors associated with the leading causes of death in the United States: a systematic review. J Health Psychol [Internet] 25(2):186–196. https://doi.org/10.117 7/1359105318800829?casa_token=wik_ozWs-_YAAAAA%3AdiD0gRHaE99klXJsrJ6-_8c4C az2ahZvaELuUxaoYdVmaFvC9hn3QeJdc7kPgWH2nUb2DbXhbQ
2. Dempsey PC, Friedenreich CM, Leitzmann MF, Buman MP, Lambert E, Willumsen J et al (2021) Global public health guidelines on physical activity and sedentary behavior for people living with chronic conditions: a call to action. J Phys Act Health 18(1):76–85
3. Underwood JM, Brener N, Thornton J, Harris WA, Bryan LN, Shanklin SL, et al (2020) Overview and methods for the youth risk behavior surveillance system - United States, 2019. MMWR Suppl 69(1):1–10. https://pubmed.ncbi.nlm.nih.gov/32817611/
4. Davis R, Campbell R, Hildon Z, Hobbs L, Michie S (2015) Theories of behaviour and behaviour change across the social and behavioural sciences: a scoping review. Health Psychol Rev 9(3):323–344. https://pubmed.ncbi.nlm.nih.gov/25104107/

5. Johnson-Shelton D, Ricci J, Westling E, Peterson M, Rusby JC (2022) Program evaluation of healthy moves™: a community-based trainer in residence professional development program to support generalist teachers with physical education instruction. J Phys Act Health 19(2):125–131. https://pubmed.ncbi.nlm.nih.gov/35061999/

6. Xiong C, Biscardi M, Astell A, Nalder E, Cameron JI, Mihailidis A et al (2020) Sex and gender differences in caregiving burden experienced by family caregivers of persons with dementia: a systematic review. PLoS One 15(4):e0231848. https://doi.org/10.1371/journal.pone.0231848

7. Everett T, Bryant A, Griffin MF, Martin-Hirsch PPL, Forbes CA, Jepson RG (2011) Interventions targeted at women to encourage the uptake of cervical screening. Cochrane database Syst Rev (5). https://pubmed.ncbi.nlm.nih.gov/21563135/

8. Brouwers MC, De Vito C, Bahirathan L, Carol A, Carroll JC, Cotterchio M et al (2011) What implementation interventions increase cancer screening rates? A systematic review. Implement Sci 6

9. Khani Jeihooni A, Bashti S, Erfanian B, Ostovarfar J, Afzali HP (2022) Application of protection motivation theory (PMT) on skin cancer preventive behaviors amongst primary school students in rural areas of Fasa city-Iran. BMC Cancer 22:21

10. Cutrona SL, Choudhry NK, Stedman M, Servi A, Liberman JN, Brennan T, et al (2010) Physician effectiveness in interventions to improve cardiovascular medication adherence: a systematic review. J Gen Intern Med [Internet] 25(10):1090–1096. https://pubmed.ncbi.nlm.nih.gov/20464522/

11. Fuller C, Michie S, Savage J, McAteer J, Besser S, Charlett A, et al (2012) The feedback intervention trial (FIT)--improving hand-hygiene compliance in UK healthcare workers: a stepped wedge cluster randomised controlled trial. PLoS One 7(10). https://pubmed.ncbi.nlm.nih.gov/23110040/

12. Bavel JJV, Baicker K, Boggio PS, Capraro V, Cichocka A, Cikara M, et al (2020) Using social and behavioural science to support COVID-19 pandemic response. Nat Hum Behav 4(5):460–471. https://www.nature.com/articles/s41562-020-0884-z

13. Ross A, Lee LJ, Wehrlen L, Cox R, Yang L, Perez A, et al (2020) Factors that influence health-promoting behaviors in cancer caregivers. Oncol Nurs Forum 47:692–702. https://eds.s.ebscohost.com/eds/pdfviewer/pdfviewer?vid=4&sid=4f9d4fc5-4930-4240-8f7d-404a3b294acf%40redis

14. Beesley VL, Price MA, Webb PM (2011) Loss of lifestyle: health behaviour and weight changes after becoming a caregiver of a family member diagnosed with ovarian cancer. Support Care Cancer 19(12):1949–1956. http://www.deepdyve.com/lp/springer-journals/loss-of-lifestyle-health-behaviour-and-weight-changes-after-becoming-a-GKIenT9lgy

15. Nguyen M, Pachana NA, Beattie E, Fielding E, Ramis MA (2015) Effectiveness of interventions to improve family-staff relationships in the care of people with dementia in residential aged care: a systematic review protocol. JBI Database Syst Rev Implement Rep 13(11):52–63

16. Chiou CJ, Chen IP, Wang HH (2005) The health status of family caregivers in Taiwan: an analysis of gender differences. Int J Geriatr Psychiatry 20(9):821–826. https://pubmed.ncbi.nlm.nih.gov/16116570/

17. Yee JL, Schulz R (2000) Gender differences in psychiatric morbidity among family caregivers: a review and analysis. Gerontologist 40(2):147–164. https://pubmed.ncbi.nlm.nih.gov/10820918/

18. Schölzel-Dorenbos CJM, Draskovic I, Vernooij-Dassen MJ, Olde Rikkert MGM (2009) Quality of life and burden of spouses of Alzheimer disease patients. Alzheimer Dis Assoc Disord 23(2):171–177. https://pubmed.ncbi.nlm.nih.gov/19484919/

19. Thompson RL, Lewis SL, Murphy MR, Hale JM, Blackwell PH, Acton GJ, et al (2004) Are there sex differences in emotional and biological responses in spousal caregivers of patients with Alzheimer's disease? Biol Res Nurs 5(4):319–330. https://pubmed.ncbi.nlm.nih.gov/15068661/

20. Cepoiu-Martin M, Tam-Tham H, Patten S, Maxwell CJ, Hogan DB (2016) Predictors of long-term care placement in persons with dementia: a systematic review and meta-analysis. Int J Geriatr Psychiatry 31(11):1151–1171

21. Hughes TB, Black BS, Albert M, Gitlin LN, Johnson DM, Lyketsos CG, et al (2014) Correlates of objective and subjective measures of caregiver burden among dementia caregivers: influence of unmet patient and caregiver dementia-related care needs. Int Psychogeriatrics 26(11):1875–1883. https://pubmed.ncbi.nlm.nih.gov/25104063/

22. Givens JL, Mezzacappa C, Heeren T, Yaffe K, Fredman L (2014) Depressive symptoms among dementia caregivers: role of mediating factors. Am J Geriatr Psychiatry 22(5):481–488. https://pubmed.ncbi.nlm.nih.gov/23567432/

23. Joling KJ, Van Marwijk HWJ, Veldhuijzen AE, Van Der Horst HE, Scheltens P, Smit F, et al (2015) The two-year incidence of depression and anxiety disorders in spousal caregivers of persons with dementia: who is at the greatest risk? Am J Geriatr Psychiatry 23(3):293–303. https://pubmed.ncbi.nlm.nih.gov/24935785/

24. Etters L, Goodall D, Harrison BE (2008) Caregiver burden among dementia patient caregivers: a review of the literature. J Am Acad Nurse Pract 20(8):423–428

25. Craig P, Dieppe P, Macintyre S, Mitchie S, Nazareth I, Petticrew M (2008) Developing and evaluating complex interventions: the new Medical Research Council guidance. BMJ 337(7676):979–983. https://www.bmj.com/content/337/bmj.a1655

26. Glanz K, Bishop DB (2010) The role of behavioral science theory in development and implementation of public health interventions. Annu Rev Public Health 31(1):399–418. https://doi.org/10.1146/annurev.publhealth.012809.103604

27. Michie S, Johnston M (2012) Theories and techniques of behaviour change: developing a cumulative science of behaviour change. Health Psychol Rev 6(1):1–6

28. Michie S, West R (2013) Behaviour change theory and evidence: a presentation to government. Health Psychol Rev 7(1):1–22

29. Rothman A, Baldwin A, Hertel A, Fuglestad P (2011) Self-regulation and behavior change: disentangling behavioral initiation and behavioral maintenance. https://psycnet.apa.org/record/2010-24692-006

30. Gardner B, Wardle J, Poston L, reviews HC-O (2011) Changing diet and physical activity to reduce gestational weight gain: a meta-analysis. Wiley Online Libr 12(7). https://doi.org/10.1111/j.1467-789X.2011.00884.x

31. Anderson CB, Bulatao R (2004) Behavioral health interventions: what works and why? In: Critical perspectives on racial and ethnic differences in health in late life. https://www.researchgate.net/profile/David-Cutler-4/publication/228378967_Behavioral_Health_Interventions_What_Works_and_Why/links/004635241b582a4295000000/Behavioral-Health-Interventions-What-Works-and-Why.pdf

32. Michie S, Johnston M, Abraham C, Lawton R, Parker D, Walker A (2005) Making psychological theory useful for implementing evidence based practice: a consensus approach. Qual Saf Heal Care 14(1):26–33

33. Kwasnicka D, Dombrowski SU, White M, Sniehotta F (2016) Theoretical explanations for maintenance of behaviour change: a systematic review of behaviour theories. Health Psychol Rev 10(3):277–296

34. Bernier J, Kumar A, Ramaiah V, Spaner D, Atlin G, Bernier J, et al (2007) A large-effect QTL for grain yield under reproductive-stage drought stress in upland rice. Wiley Online Libr 47(2):507–518. https://doi.org/10.2135/cropsci2006.07.0495

35. Challenges GL (2017) The challenge of behaviour change and health promotion. mdpi.com 8:25. https://www.mdpi.com/230490

36. Laverack G (2007) Health promotion practice. https://books.google.com/books?hl=el&lr=&id=nKhEIv-wnNMC&oi=fnd&pg=PP1&dq=Laverack+health+promotion+practice&ots=3CeYJwLQQw&sig=nRISG5bTU58698rSY-iqHPj5ia4

37. Braveman P, Gottlieb L (2014) The social determinants of health: it's time to consider the causes of the causes. Public Health Rep 129(Suppl. 2):19–31. Available from: /pmc/articles/PMC3863696/

38. Dixon D, Johnston M (2021) What competences are required to deliver person-person behaviour change interventions: development of a health behaviour change competency framework. Int J Behav Med 28(3):308–317. https://doi.org/10.1007/s12529-020-09920-6

39. Bull ER, Dale H (2021) Improving community health and social care practitioners' confidence, perceived competence and intention to use behaviour change techniques in health behaviour change conversations. Heal Soc Care Community 29(1):270–283

40. Trisnowati H, Gadjah Mada U, Padmawati RS (2022) Health promotion through youth empowerment to prevent and control smoking behavior: a conceptual paper. https://www.emerald.com/insight/0965-4283.htm

41. Kalantar-Zadeh K, Li PKT, Tantisattamo E, Kumaraswami L, Liakopoulos V, Lui SF et al (2021) Living well with kidney disease by patient and care partner empowerment: kidney health for everyone everywhere. Transpl Int 34(3):391–397. https://doi.org/10.1111/tri.13811

42. Cho A, Cha C (2021) Health promotion behavior among older Korean family caregivers of people with dementia. Int J Environ Res Public Health 18(8). https://eds.s.ebscohost.com/eds/pdfviewer/pdfviewer?vid=2&sid=df8420d0-3393-449c-902c-0250513859ee%40redis

43. Suter N, Ardizzone G, Giarelli G, Cadorin L, Gruarin N, Mis CC et al (2021) The power of informal cancer caregivers' writings: results from a thematic and narrative analysis. Support Care Cancer 29(8):4381–4388

44. Sugiyama T, Tamiya N, Watanabe T, Wakui T, Shibayama T, Moriyama Y et al (2018) Association of care recipients' care-need level with family caregiver participation in health check-ups in Japan. Geriatr Gerontol Int 18(1):26–32

45. Roth DL, Haley WE, David Rhodes J, Sheehan OC, Huang J, Blinka MD et al (2020) Transitions to family caregiving: enrolling incident caregivers and matched non-caregiving controls from a population-based study. Aging Clin Exp Res 32(9):1829–1838

46. Barbosa F, Voss G, Delerue MA (2020) Health impact of providing informal care in Portugal. BMC Geriatr 20:440

47. Rha SY, Park Y, Song SK, Lee CE, Lee J (2015) Caregiving burden and health-promoting behaviors among the family caregivers of cancer patients. Eur J Oncol Nurs 19(2):174–181. http://www.ejoncologynursing.com/article/S1462388914001604/fulltext

48. Adashek JJ, Subbiah IM (2020) Caring for the caregiver: a systematic review characterising the experience of caregivers of older adults with advanced cancers. ESMO Open 5:862

49. Caputo J, Pavalko EK, Hardy MA. The long-term effects of caregiving on women's health and mortality

50. Tan GTH, Yuan Q, Devi F, Wang P, Ng LL, Goveas R et al (2021) Factors associated with caregiving self-efficacy among primary informal caregivers of persons with dementia in Singapore. BMC Geriatr 21:13

51. Yildiz E, Karakaş SA, Güngörmüş Z, Cengiz M (2017) Levels of care burden and self-efficacy for informal caregiver of patients with cancer. Holist Nurs Pract 31(1):7–15. https://journals.lww.com/00004650-201701000-00003

52. Hendrix CC, Bailey DE, Steinhauser KE, Olsen MK, Stechuchak KM, Lowman SG et al (2016) Effects of enhanced caregiver training program on cancer caregiver's self-efficacy, preparedness, and psychological well-being. Support Care Cancer 24(1):327–336

53. Papadakos JK, Hasan SM, Barnsley J, Berta W, Fazelzad R, Papadakos CJ, et al (2018) Health literacy and cancer self-management behaviors: a scoping review. Cancer 124(21):4202–4210. https://doi.org/10.1002/cncr.31733

54. Kim JH, Menon U, Wang E, Szalacha L (2010) Assess the effects of culturally relevant intervention on breast cancer knowledge, beliefs, and mammography use among Korean American women. J Immigr Minor Health 12(4):586–597. Available from: /pmc/articles/PMC2902721/

55. Ghaffari M, Esfahani SN, Rakhshanderou S, Koukamari PH (2019) Evaluation of health belief model-based intervention on breast cancer screening behaviors among health volunteers. J Cancer Educ 34(5):904–912. https://pubmed.ncbi.nlm.nih.gov/29987586/

56. Liu L, Qian X, Chen Z, He T (2020) Health literacy and its effect on chronic disease prevention: Evidence from China's data. BMC Public Health 20(1):690. https://doi.org/10.1186/s12889-020-08804-4
57. Goto E, Ishikawa H, Okuhara T, Kiuchi T (2019) Relationship of health literacy with utilization of health-care services in a general Japanese population. Prev Med Rep 14
58. Vandenbosch J, Van den Broucke S, Vancorenland S, Avalosse H, Verniest R, Callens M (2016) Health literacy and the use of healthcare services in Belgium. J Epidemiol Community Health 70(10):1032–1038. https://jech.bmj.com/content/70/10/1032
59. Fernandez DM, Larson JL, Zikmund-Fisher BJ (2016) Associations between health literacy and preventive health behaviors among older adults: findings from the health and retirement study. BMC Public Health 16(1):596. https://doi.org/10.1186/s12889-016-3267-7
60. Sinicrope PS, Bauer MC, Patten CA, Austin-Garrison M, Garcia L, Hughes CA et al (2020) Development and evaluation of a cancer literacy intervention to promote mammography screening among Navajo women: a pilot study. Am J Health Promot 6:681–685
61. Noman S, Shahar HK, Rahman HA, Ismail S, Al-Jaberi MA, Azzani M (2021) The effectiveness of educational interventions on breast cancer screening uptake, knowledge, and beliefs among women: a systematic review. Int J Environ Res Public Health 18:1–30
62. Luque JS, Logan A, Soulen G, Armeson KE, Garrett DM, Davila CB, et al (2019) Systematic review of mammography screening educational interventions for hispanic women in the United States. J Cancer Educ 34:412–22. Available from: /pmc/articles/PMC6043417/
63. Bashirian S, Mohammadi Y, Barati M, Moaddabshoar L, Dogonchi M (2020) Effectiveness of the theory-based educational interventions on screening of breast cancer in women: a systematic review and meta-analysis. Int Q Community Health Educ 40(3):219–236. https://doi.org/10.1177/0272684X19862148
64. Marino MM, Rienzo M, Serra N, Marino N, Ricciotti R, Mazzariello L et al (2020) Mobile screening units for the early detection of breast cancer and cardiovascular disease: a pilot telemedicine study in southern Italy. Telemed e-Health 26(3):286–293
65. Holt CL, Tagai EK, Santos SLZ, Scheirer MA, Bowie J, Haider M et al (2019) Web-based versus in-person methods for training lay community health advisors to implement health promotion workshops: participant outcomes from a cluster-randomized trial. Transl Behav Med 9(4):573–582
66. Durand MA, Lamouroux A, Redmond NM, Rotily M, Bourmaud A, Schott AM et al (2021) Impact of a health literacy intervention combining general practitioner training and a consumer facing intervention to improve colorectal cancer screening in underserved areas: protocol for a multicentric cluster randomized controlled trial. BMC Public Health 21:1684
67. Christy SM, Sutton SK, Abdulla R, Boxtha C, Gonzalez P, Cousin L et al (2022) A multilevel, low literacy dual language intervention to promote colorectal cancer screening in community clinics in Florida: a randomized controlled trial. Prev Med (Baltim) 158:107021
68. Kinnear H, Connolly S, Rosato M, Hall C, Mairs A, O'Reilly D (2010) Are caregiving responsibilities associated with non-attendance at breast screening? BMC Public Health 10(1):749. https://doi.org/10.1186/1471-2458-10-749, 10
69. Sheets DJ, Black K, Kaye LW (2014) Who cares for caregivers? Evidence-based approaches to family support. J Gerontol Soc Work 57:525–530. https://www.tandfonline.com/action/journalInformation?journalCode=wger20
70. Son J, Erno A, Shea DG, Femia EE, Zarit SH, Parris Stephens MA (2007) The caregiver stress process and health outcomes. J Aging Health 19(6):871–887. https://doi.org/10.1177/0898264307308568
71. Kim SY, Guo Y, Won C, Lee HY (2020) Factors associated with receipt of mammogram among caregivers: a comparison with non-caregivers. BMC Womens Health 20(1). https://pubmed.ncbi.nlm.nih.gov/32993760/
72. Carretero S, Stewart J, Centeno C, Barbabella F, Schmidt A, Lamontagne-Godwin F, et al (2012) Can technology-based services support long-term care challenges in home care? Analysis of evidence from social innovation good practices across the EU: CARICT Project Summary Report. https://publications.jrc.ec.europa.eu/repository/handle/JRC77709

73. Park M, Go Y, Jeong M, Lee S, Kim S, Lee D et al (2017) Influencing factors and risk of caregiver burden of family caregivers for patient with dementia. Korean J Fam Welf 22(3):431–448

74. Dua T, Seeher KM, Sivananthan S, Chowdhary N, Pot AM, Saxena S (2017) [FTS5–03–01]: World Health Organization's global action plan on the public health response to dementia 2017–2025. Alzheimer's Dement 13(7S_Part_30)

75. Kim EK, Park H (2019) Factors associated with burden of family caregivers of home-dwelling elderly people with dementia: a systematic review and meta-analysis. Korean J Adult Nurs 31(4):351–364. https://synapse.koreamed.org/articles/1135954

76. Chen MY (1999) The effectiveness of health promotion counseling to family caregivers. Public Health Nurs 16(2):125–132. https://doi.org/10.1046/j.1525-1446.1999.00125.x

77. Chen MY, Liao JC (2002) Relationship between attendance at breakfast and school achievement among nursing students. J Nurs Res 10(1):15–21. https://europepmc.org/article/med/11923897

78. Edwards EA, Lumsden J, Rivas C, Steed L, Edwards LA, Thiyagarajan A, et al (2016) Gamification for health promotion: systematic review of behaviour change techniques in smartphone apps [Internet]. vol 6, BMJ open, p e012447. https://bmjopen.bmj.com/content/6/10/e012447.short

79. Tiffany B, Blasi P, Catz S, JM-J mHealth, 2018 undefined (2022) Mobile apps for oral health promotion: content review and heuristic usability analysis. https://mhealth.jmir.org/2018/9/e11432/

80. Tiffany B, Blasi P, Catz SL, McClure JB (2018) Mobile apps for oral health promotion: content review and heuristic usability analysis. JMIR Mhealth Uhealth 6(9):e11432. https://mhealth.jmir.org/2018/9/e11432

81. Ngigi S, Busolo D (2018) Behaviour change communication in health promotion: appropriate practices and promising approaches. Int J Innov Res Dev 7. https://www.researchgate.net/publication/328568750

82. Nutbeam D (2018) Health education and health promotion revisited 78(6):705–709. https://doi.org/10.1177/0017896918770215

83. Jarvis J, Skinner TC, Carey ME, Davies MJ (2010) How can structured self-management patient education improve outcomes in people with type 2 diabetes? Diabetes, Obes Metab 12(1):12–19. https://doi.org/10.1111/j.1463-1326.2009.01098.x

84. Marks R, Allegrante JP, Lorig K (2005) A review and synthesis of research evidence for self-efficacy-enhancing interventions for reducing chronic disability: implications for health education practice (part II). Health Promot Pract 6(2):148–56. http://www.ncbi.nlm.nih.gov/pubmed/15855284

85. Wang TF, Huang CM, Chou C, Yu S (2015) Effect of oral health education programs for caregivers on oral hygiene of the elderly: a systemic review and meta-analysis. Int J Nurs Stud 52(6):1090–1096

86. Long MM, Cramer RJ, Jenkins J, Bennington L, Paulson JF (2019) A systematic review of interventions for healthcare professionals to improve screening and referral for perinatal mood and anxiety disorders. Arch Womens Ment Health 22(1):25–36. https://doi.org/10.1007/s00737-018-0876-4

87. Elily [Internet] (2022). https://elily.eu/course/

88. Green EC, Murphy EM, Gryboski K (2020) The health belief model. Wiley Encycl Heal Psychol 2 211–214. https://doi.org/10.1002/9781119057840.ch68

89. Kim H, Paige Powell M, Bhuyan SS, Bhuyan SS (2017) Seeking medical information using mobile apps and the internet: are family caregivers different from the general public? J Med Syst 41(3):1–8. https://doi.org/10.1007/s10916-017-0684-9

90. Miller MP, Arefanian S, Blatnik JA (2020) The impact of internet-based patient self-education of surgical mesh on patient attitudes and healthcare decisions prior to hernia surgery. Surg Endosc 34(11):5132–5141. https://doi.org/10.1007/s00464-019-07300-0

91. Masic I (2008) E-learning as new method of medical education. Acta Inform Medica 16(2):102. Available from: /pmc/articles/PMC3789161/

92. Valizadeh-Haghi S, Rahmatizadeh S, Soleimaninejad A, Mousavi Shirazi SF, Mollaei P (2021) Are health websites credible enough for elderly self-education in the most prevalent elderly diseases? BMC Med Inform Decis Mak 21(1):1–9. https://doi.org/10.1186/s12911-021-01397-x

93. Burke M, Carey P, Haines LL, Lampson AP, Pond F (2010) Implementing the information prescription protocol in a family medicine practice: a case study. J Med Libr Assoc 98(3):228. Available from: /pmc/articles/PMC2901015/

94. Ownby RL, Acevedo A, Waldrop-Valverde D, Woodruff NH (2019) Enhancing the impact of mobile health literacy interventions to reduce health disparities. Q Rev Distance Educ 20(1):15. Available from: /pmc/articles/PMC6752043/

95. Hsieh HM, Chang WC, Shen CT, Liu Y, Chen FM, Kang YT (2021) Mediation effect of health beliefs in the relationship between health knowledge and uptake of mammography in a national breast cancer screening program in Taiwan. J Cancer Educ 36(4):832–843. https://doi.org/10.1007/s13187-020-01711-7

96. AlJunidel R, Alaqel M, AlQahtani SH, AlOgaiel AM, ALJammaz F, Alshammari S (2020) Using the health belief model to predict the uptake of mammographic screening among Saudi women. Cureus 12(10). https://www.cureus.com/articles/44024-using-the-health-belief-model-to-predict-the-uptake-of-mammographic-screening-among-saudi-women

97. Darvishpour A, Vajari SM, Noroozi S (2018) Can health belief model predict breast cancer screening behaviors? Open Access Maced J Med Sci 6(5):949. Available from: /pmc/articles/PMC5985873/

98. Hassan N, Ho WK, Mariapun S, Teo SH (2015) A cross sectional study on the motivators for Asian women to attend opportunistic mammography screening in a private hospital in Malaysia: the MyMammo study health behavior, health promotion and society. BMC Public Health 15(1):1–8. https://doi.org/10.1186/s12889-015-1892-1

99. Akhtari-Zavare M, Juni MH, Ismail IZ, Said SM, Latiff LA (2015) Barriers to breast self examination practice among Malaysian female students: a cross sectional study. Springerplus 4(1):1–6. https://doi.org/10.1186/s40064-015-1491-8

100. Kumarasamy H, Veerakumar A, Subhathra S, Suga Y, Murugaraj R (2017) Determinants of awareness and practice of breast self examination among rural women in Trichy, Tamil Nadu. J Midlife Health 8(2):84. Available from: /pmc/articles/PMC5496285/

101. Gan YX, Lao CK, Chan A (2018) Breast cancer screening behavior, attitude, barriers among middle-aged Chinese women in Macao, China. J Public Health (Bangkok) 40(4):e560–570. https://academic.oup.com/jpubhealth/article/40/4/e560/4993735

102. Taleghani F, Kianpour M, Tabatabaiyan M (2019) Barriers to breast self-examination among Iranian women. Iran J Nurs Midwifery Res 24(2):108. Available from: /pmc/articles/PMC6390439/

103. Baloushah S, Salisu WJ, Elsous A, Muhammad Ibrahim M, Jouda F, Elmodallal H et al (2020) Practice and barriers toward breast self-examination among Palestinian women in Gaza City, Palestine. Sci World J 2020:1

104. Aregbeshola BS, Khan SM (2018) Out-of-pocket payments, catastrophic health expenditure and poverty among households in Nigeria 2010. Int J Heal Policy Manag 7(9):798. Available from: /pmc/articles/PMC6186489/

105. Peixoto MJP, Duarte PAS, Araújo PT, Pinto PIC, Sarmento WWF, Trinta FAM et al (2020) Teaching ubiquitous computing using simulations based on smartphone sensors. Informatics Educ 19(1):129–57. https://eds.p.ebscohost.com/eds/detail/detail?vid=8&sid=12f779a3-5 2b3-46eb-8b34-935af6da4acd%40redis&bdata=JnNpdGU9ZWRzLWxpdmU%3D#AN=E J1248142&db=eric

106. Griffiths F, Lindenmeyer A, Powell J, Lowe P, Thorogood M (2006) Why are health care interventions delivered over the Internet? A systematic review of the published literature. J Med Internet Res 2006;8(2):e10–e498. https://www.jmir.org/2006/2/e10

107. Wei J, Hollin I, Kachnowski S (2011) A review of the use of mobile phone text messaging in clinical and healthy behaviour interventions. J Telemed Telecare 17(1):41–8. https://doi.org/10.1258/jtt.2010.100322

108. Santana S, Brach C, Harris L, Ochiai E, Blakey C, Bevington F et al (2021) Practice full report: updating health literacy for healthy people 2030: defining its importance for a new decade in public health. J Public Heal Manag Pract 27(6):S258. Available from: /pmc/articles/PMC8435055/

109. Fan Z ya, Yang Y, Zhang F (2021) Association between health literacy and mortality: a systematic review and meta-analysis. Arch Public Heal 79(1):1–13. https://doi.org/10.1186/s13690-021-00648-7

110. Bo A, Friis K, Osborne RH, Maindal HT (2014) National indicators of health literacy: ability to understand health information and to engage actively with healthcare providers – a populationbased survey among Danish adults. BMC Public Health 14(1):1–12. https://doi.org/10.1186/1471-2458-14-1095

111. Oldach BR, Katz ML (2014) Health literacy and cancer screening: a systematic review. Patient Educ Couns 94(2):149–157

112. Samoil D, Kim J, Fox C, Papadakos JK (2021) The importance of health literacy on clinical cancer outcomes: a scoping review. Ann Cancer Epidemiol 5:3. https://pdfs.semanticscholar.org/d08c/e156357cee8a9c73f9beb8a26c76a0e78f39.pdf

113. Ghose A, Guo X, Li B, Dang Y (2021) Empowering patients using smart mobile health platforms: evidence from a randomized field experiment [cited 2022 Feb 10]. https://eds.p.ebscohost.com/eds/detail/detail?vid=1&sid=9df25081-e558-4e09-9448-af0ac7a094a5%40redis&bdata=JnNpdGU9ZWRzLWxpdmU%3D#AN=edsarx.2102.05506&db=edsarx

114. Demiris G, Washington K, Ulrich CM, Popescu M, Oliver DP (2019) Innovative tools to support family caregivers of persons with cancer: the role of information technology. Semin Oncol Nurs 35(4):384–388

Future Directions

Andreas Charalambous ⓘ

1   Introduction

Even with modest projections, it is anticipated that healthcare challenges such as the ageing population, higher rates of chronic diseases (e.g. cancer, dementia), widening inequality gaps and resource constraints will intensify in the years to come. These challenges are complemented by the reforms across health systems towards a wider home-based care approach as well as the socialisation and extramuralisation of care. These will in turn increase the significance of informal caregiving in maintaining sustainable as well as resilient health systems. Informal caregiving ranges from assistance with daily activities and provision of direct care to helping the care recipient to navigate within complex healthcare and social services systems. Over the years, informal caregivers have assumed more intensive, complex and longer lasting tasks compared to the past, and caregivers rarely receive adequate preparation for their role. This has increased the likelihood that these informal caregivers will experience at some point the negative effects of caregiving with varying levels of impact on their lives.

Although, specific estimates are sensitive to the usual uncertainties of making projections, it has been predicted that demand for informal care by older people will exceed supply and by 2060 there will be a deficit of approximately 20,000 caregivers in the Netherlands, 400,000 in Germany, and over a million caregivers in Spain [1, 2]. It is expected that the number of available informal caregivers per 85-year-old person will decrease from 30 in 1975 and 15 in 2015, to 6 in 2040 [3, 4]. Therefore

A. Charalambous (✉)
Department of Nursing, School of Health Sciences, Cyprus University of Technology, Limassol, Cyprus

Department of Nursing Science, Faculty of Medicine, University of Turku, Turku, Finland
e-mail: andreas.charalambous@cut.ac.cy

the "care gap" is expected to reach significantly high levels especially in the countries where there is heavy reliance on informal care in the long-term care systems.

The invisibility of the contribution made by informal caregivers, and the burden they carry, may seem surprising given the sheer number of people who play this role. Several reports estimate [5, 6] that a percentage ranging from 60% to 80% of long-term care in Europe is provided by informal caregivers. In other words, patients with chronic support needs receive 4 hours of support from informal caregivers, on average, for every 1 hour provided within the formal service. People with cancer may have especially high needs for support, because it is a particularly stressful diagnosis, it impacts on so many aspects of life, and treatments are often long, toxic and demand multiple hospital visits [7, 8]. It is challenging for informal caregivers to cover short-term care needs for a family member, neighbour or friend. It becomes even more demanding the longer this activity has to be performed, especially when informal caregivers might themselves be of advanced age and care recipients themselves. The absence of a legal framework in place in the member states to provide recourse and support to Europe's more than 100 million informal caregivers complicates the role of the caregivers even more.

2 The "Invisible" or "Hidden" Role of Informal Caregivers

Although evidence show that a great part of the care needs is covered by informal caregivers, they are often called the "invisible workforce" in long-term care systems as they are rarely registered or counted, and their status as informal care provider is often not formally recognised. There appears to be several fundamental ambiguities in relation to the positioning of caregivers within the social care system. Whilst in some senses are considered to be within its remit, part of the subject of its concern and responsibility, and yet are at the same time beyond its remit, part of the taken-for-granted background to provision of care. Furthermore, caregivers are considered to have an "off-centre" character, considering that their outcomes are in a sense only "by-products" of the care system and not its main focus [9]. Due to this consideration as "by-products" of the long-term care system [9], informal caregivers and their needs had long been ignored by policy-makers [5, 10, 11]. These ambiguities resulted in the lack of a single and straightforward model to guide social care agencies' relationship to informal caregivers, often relying on different models, or rather, frames of reference. Each of these different frames of reference conceptualises the subject differently, and each has different implications for policy and for intervention [9].

A clear definition of informal care and of the status of informal carers at national level is an important step in acknowledging the unpaid contribution by informal carers as it forms the basis of formal entitlements relating to financial support, employment regulations and respite care services. Informal care provision and the situation of unpaid carers need to be better understood to provide the support needed in a timely manner. Research, awareness raising and education on informal care among the general public and health and social care professionals can contribute to a greater acknowledgement of informal carers as co-producers of social services.

3   Models of Informal Caregivers' Involvement in Care: Not All Models Were Created Equal

As discussed in previous chapters the contribution of informal caregivers to care and their collaboration with formal caregivers is significant and it includes a broad area of tasks and responsibilities. Preceding studies have provided specific frames of reference that can guide the collaboration of informal care with formal care, including: caregivers as resources, caregivers as co-workers and caregivers as co-clients.

In the "caregivers as resources" model, it is evident that formal and informal care are not of equal normative status. Twigg [9] argues that due to this different normative status, although in theory there can be substitution between the two forms of provision, such substitution is in fact quite narrowly constrained by normative assumptions that give preference to informal caregiving provision. This implies, in terms of informal caregivers, the adoption of an essentially residualist model in which the formal healthcare providers respond to the deficiencies of the care network aiming at care maximisation. This can be achieved through the better understanding of the nature of the informal caregiver, to appreciate its character and to understand its structure, both in its potentialities and its limitations. Twigg [9] asserts that within this resource frame of reference, the main task from a policy and clinical perspective is focused on the maintenance and marginal increase of levels of informal support.

The second model of collaboration is that of carers as co-workers whereby formal healthcare providers work in parallel with the informal caregivers, aiming at a cooperative and enabling role. When it comes to the implications for policy and practice, the aim in this co-worker model is to maintain and enable informal care, but in ways that recognise the importance, particularly the instrumental importance, of carer morale [9].

In the third model, that of "carers as co-clients", the informal caregiver moves over into the realm of formal healthcare providers, with caregivers become fully integrated into the concerns of the formal healthcare providers. This model signifies a distinct difference with the other two models where informal caregivers were regarded them as resources to be exploited or workers to be co-opted [9]. Within this framework, from a policy and practice implication, the aim of intervention is the relief of caregiver burden.

Subsequent studies on the relationship between informal and formal network care services have provided two distinct models to elicit the better understanding of such interaction [12]. According to the dual specialisation model, a coordinated interaction between informal and formal networks is suggested when each assumes varying responsibilities according to their capacity [13]. Informal caregivers are considered suitable to address the unplanned and unscheduled needs, whereas formal network expertise is used to provide scheduled and structured care service. The supplemental model considers a supplementary relationship between informal and formal networks where the availability of a formal network can complement any deficiencies of an informal network to meet the needs of a care recipient [13].

The models discussed above provide an overview of the different ways that informal and formal care can coexist. However, the type of this coexistence (i.e. substitute or complementary) will depend on the exact purpose of using it as well as the context where it will be implemented. In traditional societies for example, informal care mainly comes from within the family. Parents have strong motivations to raise children and to care for them when they are old [14]. Despite there is great variation of formal care systems around the world, a significant percentage of these systems provide formal care which can be significantly insufficient and fragmented. This insufficiency can also generate inequalities in accessing the necessary healthcare services across the disease continuum, including within the context of home-based care. With the formal care being unable to address the needs of people requiring care at the home setting across diseases and conditions, this increases the need and the level of informal care involvement. Another aspect to be considered is that the level of care required by the person can fluctuate over time, with more intensive and specialised care being required at some points especially during disease exacerbation. These are factors that in the course of the disease will also reflect on the input of the informal care required. Therefore, it is not infrequent that in the course of the disease the frames of reference in terms of informal care have to change (for example moving from caregiver as resource to caregiver as co-worker) so that the requirements of the person in need are better met.

4   Supporting Informal Caregivers in Their Role

The complex task of caregiving requires adequate and ongoing preparation of the person who will assume the role. Preceding studies have demonstrated that training informal caregivers does have a clearly measurable positive impact on their ability to perform specific caregiving tasks [15], quality of life, skills and self-reported burden [16, 17], as well as on their ability to cope and resilience to depression. Furthermore, better preparing informal caregivers for their role can make people more confident about their own abilities [18]. However, informal caregivers tend to consider the current support systems insufficient to address their needs: continuous information provision seems to be missing, and services might be difficult to access due to opening hours and lack of flexibility.

A report by EUROCARERS [19] acknowledged the increasing availability of training opportunities for informal caregivers mainly provided by civil society organisations and healthcare institutions. The training needs of informal caregivers are traditionally addressed through formal and informal training and education programmes. However, the content of such training courses should be based on a context-specific Training Need Analysis (TNA), namely the empirical examination of training needs at the care context [20–22]. Such analysis expands into the identification of specific shortcomings in informal care practice and contributes to the better understanding of the needs and expectations of care and support in everyday life among informal caregivers.

In the context of civil society organisations, these training programmes are developed with an emphasis on the needs of caregivers. In the context of healthcare institutions and in most cases in parallel, initiatives are developed within the health and/or social care sector, on the initiative of healthcare institutions which aim both at improving the health status of patients who are discharged after having been hospitalised, and at improving the well-being of caregivers. Despite the availability of such training opportunities, there are significant barriers that limit informal caregivers' accessibility, leading to learning opportunities not being taken up to their full capacity. Such barriers include geographical inequalities with regard to the accessibility of training (e.g. situational barriers have been obstructing caregivers' access to it, when delivered in its traditional face-to-face modality), poor or lack of information on the existence of such training programmes, time-constrained organisational issues and the lack of self-identification as carers [19]. Furthermore, the offer of such training programmes can also be hampered by a lack of funds, trained and available workforce, or infrastructures to scale up services [23].

The acknowledgement of the negative impact of situational barriers on informal caregivers' access to training opportunities has facilitated the increasing development and integration of remote online training and support solutions. This modality of intervention has been recognised as advantageous, much due to its convenient and privacy-preserving delivery, ubiquity, great potential for scalability and presumed (cost)effectiveness [24]. For example, in the context of dementia caregivers, meta-analyses on such online interventions reported beneficial effects on self-efficacy which was reflected in the better performance of the person within the caregiver role [25, 26].

Systematic involvement in medical appointments is another way that healthcare providers can help better prepare informal caregivers for the supportive role they have to play. An example where this approach to supporting informal caregivers is the MyHealth trial of nurse-led follow-up after breast cancer [27]. As part of the trial, the patient's closest support person (i.e. informal caregiver) is invited to attend an appointment that is focused on symptom education together with the patient. This trial is based on the principle that by giving both patients and their informal caregivers the skills to recognise and manage symptoms of a side-effect of treatment, this will benefit both patients and caregivers, for example by improving the ability to cope together (dyadic coping) and reducing anxiety.

Innovative solutions such as the in-group social learning have been developed as a response to the needs of informal caregivers for quality training [28]. This group learning method relies on the narration of personal experience and personal knowledge of each participant, moderated by a group leader. By utilising positive experiences and negative experience that were successfully resolved it elicits learning for the participant. It builds on the human ability to experience empathy and solidarity towards others and in turn, develops these two characteristics further [29]. One of the most significant advantages of in-group social learning is a bidirectional link between theoretical knowledge and actual living situation—skills and knowledge needed by participants are simultaneously transferred from and to everyday practice, helping participants to further understand their needs and possible concrete solutions [28].

5   Policy Strategies to Support Informal Caregivers

Policy measures are needed to address the growing need for care in a way that pre-vents strain on families and caregivers and protects their health and well-being. Furthermore, these measures need to ensure that informal caregivers will not be forced to reduce or give up paid employment, face social exclusion and ultimately be caught in a poverty trap. The Europe 2020 strategy on employment and the European gender empowerment strategy (two-thirds of Europe's caregivers are women) are examples of this, as is the European pillar of social rights and 2016 Parliament report on women domestic workers and caregivers in the EU. Both of these have laid the foundation for increased European action to standardise the rights of caregivers across the EU.

There are a number of ways in which informal caregivers can be supported by national and local governments when assuming their roles. The diversity of the informal caregiver role across countries as well as the varying recognition of the role is reflected in the different policy strategies that have been implemented. Regardless of this diversity, the measures need to be aiming at introducing new stability and well-being to caregivers' lives, given the significant contribution they make to health systems. Of the 126 billion euros cancer costs the EU in 2009, patients and their families carried a staggering 75 billion euros. These numbers show that programmes or compensation on behalf of carers are in fact direct pay-ments in support of sustainable health systems.

Informal caregivers need to have the possibility to work within flexible work-ing arrangements (e.g. such as the possibility to reduce working hours or to work from home) in enabling working caregivers to remain in employment when assuming the role of the caregiver. In the same context, it is essential for the infor-mal caregiver to be able to take compassionate care leave to provide care and support to a family member who has a serious medical condition with a significant risk of death. As such arrangements are largely provided at the discretion of employers, the sensitisation of managers to the needs and challenges of informal caregivers can yield positive results towards more employee oriented and support-ive workplace cultures [30]. Flexible working arrangements that allow workers with care responsibilities to alter their work schedule, working time or work loca-tion are important in helping caregivers flexibly juggle their work and care roles and personal lives [30].

The time devoted by informal caregivers to care is significant and can increase at times of disease exacerbation. For working caregivers, this time is provided often at the expense of their working (and reimbursed) time. As a result, a number of ways need to be adopted to allow the financial support of caregivers. This can be done through an attendance allowance that is paid to the care recipient to purchase social and health care services. This allowance can be seen as an indirect acknowledge-ment of the family caregiver's engagement [30]. In order to ensure social security coverage for informal caregivers measures need to be put in place to ensure that they are able to maintain/obtain access to health, pension and accident insurance. Some countries acknowledge informal caregiver's contributions by covering their contributions to social pension insurance [30].

The complexity and the intensity of the tasks that often informal caregivers are called upon to undertake, highlight the need to quality, flexible and accessible formal care services in the community. The availability of such accessible formal services allows to redistribute some of the care tasks and to have time to pursue other activities (e.g. social). Day care services and home care assistance are examples of community-based services that enable informal caregivers to have time for employment or personal lives. Formal care services can also support informal caregivers with tasks they do not have the capacity to carry out to ensure a high quality of care for care recipients [30]. In the UK for example, under the Care Act local authorities are expected: (1) to ensure that caregivers with a need for information and advice about care and support are able to access it; (2) to take responsibilities for caregivers need by assessing "appearance of need"; and (3) to enable caregivers to undergo eligibility assessments, access to information, respite care and employment and financial assistance [31].

6   Conclusion

As governments have reduced their involvement in providing institutional long-term care, leveraging informal care for this work has become a key strategy in maintaining healthcare system sustainability worldwide. As a result, informal caregivers and their contribution to care are being acknowledged much more than ever before. However, the number of informal caregivers in the near future is somewhat uncertain due to the decline of intergenerational co-residency, higher employment rates of women, and rising old age dependency ratios. Projections to 2060 show that the supply of informal care is unlikely to keep pace with the increasing demand in Europe. With some of these challenges already in place, there is need to better support the role of the informal caregiver across the care continuum. Support services for informal caregivers such as caregiver assessments, respite care and financial assistance all need improvements to accommodate the ever-changing role of caregivers on different stages of caring. Sustainable measures that support informal caregivers will need appropriate policy developments, which to this date remain uneven across countries, with some countries having mechanisms in place to assess the needs and support informal caregivers whilst others are only starting to take an interest in developing support services. The informal caregiver is an invaluable resource for the person on the receiving end of the care, the society and the overall health systems. However, in order to preserve its potential, there is an impeding need to support the role accordingly and systematically.

There are only four types of people in the world: (1) those who have been caregivers, (2) those who currently are caregivers, (3) those who will be caregivers, and (4) those who will need caregivers.
    Rosalyn Carter,
    former First Lady of the United States and wife of Jimmy Carter

References

1. Pickard L, King D, Brimblecombe N, Knapp M (2015) The effectiveness of paid services in supporting unpaid carers' employment in England. J Soc Policy 44(3):567–590
2. Pickard L (2015) A growing care gap? The supply of unpaid care for older people by their adult children in England to 2032. Ageing Soc 35:96–123
3. de Jong A, Kooiker S (2018) Regionale ontwikkelingen in het aantal potentiële helpers van oudere ouderen, 1975-2040. Planbureau voor de Leefomgeving. https://www.pbl.nl/sites/default/files/cms/publicaties/PBL_2018_Regionale-ontwikkelingen-in-het-aantal-potentiele-helpers-van-ouderen-tussen-1975-2040_3238.pdf
4. Janssen TL, Lodder P, de Vries J et al (2020) Caregiver strain on informal caregivers when providing care for older patients undergoing major abdominal surgery: a longitudinal prospective cohort study. BMC Geriatr 20:178. https://doi.org/10.1186/s12877-020-01579-8
5. Hoffmann F, Rodrigues R (2010) Informal carers: who takes care of them? Policy Brief 4/2010. European Centre, Vienna
6. Triantafillou J, Carretero S, Cordero L, Mingot K (2010) Informal care in the long-term care system European overview paper
7. Papastavrou E, Charalambous A, Tsangari H, Karayiannis G (2012) The burdensome and depressive experience of caring: what cancer, schizophrenia, and Alzheimer's disease caregivers have in common. Cancer Nurs 35(3):187–194. https://doi.org/10.1097/NCC.0b013e31822cb4a0
8. Wang T, Molassiotis A, Chung BPM et al (2018) Unmet care needs of advanced cancer patients and their informal caregivers: a systematic review. BMC Palliat Care 17:96. https://doi.org/10.1186/s12904-018-0346-9
9. Twigg J (1989) Models of carers: how do social care agencies conceptualise their relationship with informal carers? J Soc Policy 18(1):53–66
10. Naiditch M (2012) Protecting an endangered resource? Lessons from a European cross-country comparison of support policies for informal carers of elderly dependent persons. Questions d'Economie de la Sante 176:1–8
11. Peters M, Rand S, Fitzpatrick R (2020) Enhancing primary care support for informal carers: a scoping study with professional stakeholders. Health Soc Care Community 28(2):642–650. https://doi.org/10.1111/hsc.12898
12. Lin W (2019) The relationship between formal and informal care among Chinese older adults: based on the 2014 CLHLS dataset. BMC Health Serv Res 19(1):323. https://doi.org/10.1186/s12913-019-4160-8
13. Wacker RR, Roberto KA (2008) Community resources for older adults: programs and services in an era of change. Sage
14. Liu H (2021) Formal and informal care: complementary or substitutes in care for elderly people? Empirical Evidence From China SAGE Open April 2021. https://doi.org/10.1177/21582440211016413
15. Klimova B, Valis M, Kuca K et al (2019) E-learning as valuable caregivers' support for people with dementia – a systematic review. BMC Health Serv Res 19:781. https://doi.org/10.1186/s12913-019-4641-9
16. Haberstroh J et al (2011) TANDEM: communication training for informal caregivers of people with dementia. Aging Mental Health 15(3):405, 9p–413
17. Eggenberger E, Heimerl K, Bennett MI (2013) Communication skills training in dementia care: a systematic review of effectiveness, training content, and didactic methods in different care settings. Int Psychogeriatrics 25
18. Peeters JM, Van Beek A, Meerveld J, Francke AL (2010) Informal caregivers of persons with dementia, their use of and needs for specific professional support: a survey of the National Dementia Programme. BMC Nurs 9:9
19. EUROCARERS (2016) Informal caregiving and learning opportunities: an overview of EU countries. TRACK project funded by the Erasmus+ Programme

20. Pavlidis G, Downs C, Kalinowski TB et al (2020) A survey on the training needs of caregivers in five European countries. J Nurs Manag 28:385–398

21. Lethin C, Hanson E, Margioti E, Chiatti C, Gagliardi C, Vaz de Carvalho C, Malmgren FA (2019) Support needs and expectations of people living with dementia and their informal carers in everyday life: a European study. Soc Sci 8(7):203

22. Markaki A, Malhotra S, Billings R et al (2021) Training needs assessment: tool utilization and global impact. BMC Med Educ 21:310. https://doi.org/10.1186/s12909-021-02748-y

23. World Health Organisation (2015) Supporting informal caregivers of people living with dementia. Retrieved from www.who.int/mental_health/neurology/dementia/dementia_thematicbrief_informal_care.pdf?ua=1

24. Teles S, Paúl C, Sosa Napolskij M, Ferreira A (2020) Dementia caregivers training needs and preferences for online interventions: a mixed-methods study. J Clin Nurs 00:1–19

25. Boots LMM, de Vugt ME, van Knippenberg RJM, Kempen GIJM, Verhey FRJ (2014) A systematic review of internet-based supportive interventions for caregivers of patients with dementia. Int J Geriatr Psychiatry 29(4):331–344

26. Parra-Vidales E, Soto-Pérez F, Perea-Bartolomé MV, Franco-Martín MA, Muñoz-Sánchez JL (2017) Online interventions for caregivers of people with dementia: a systematic review. Actas Espanolas de Psiquiatria 45(3):116–126

27. Saltbæk L, Karlsen RV, Bidstrup PE, Høeg BL, Zoffmann V, Horsbøl TA, Holländer NH, Svendsen MN, Christensen HG, Dalton SO, Johansen C (2019) MyHealth: specialist nurse-led follow-up in breast cancer. A randomized controlled trial - development and feasibility. Acta Oncol 58(5):619–626

28. Ramovš J, Ramovš A, Svetelšek A (2019) Informal carers training: in-group social learning as an effective method for quality care empowerment. Front Sociol (4):63

29. Ramovš J (ed) (2013) Staranje v Sloveniji – Raziskava o potrebah, zmožnostih in Stališčih Nad 50 let Starih Prebivalcev Slovenije (Ageing in Slovenia: survey on the needs, abilities and standpoints of the Slovene population aged 50 years and over. Summary of findings). Inštitut Antona Trstenjaka, Ljubljana. Available online at: http://www.inst-antonatrstenjaka.si/repository/IAT_Staranje_v_Sloveniji_povzetek_angl.pdf

30. UNECE. Policy Brief on Ageing No. 22, September 2019

31. Cottagiri SA, Sykes P (2019) Key health impacts and support systems for informal carers in the UK: a thematic review. J Health Soc Sci 4(2):173–198

Printed in the United States
by Baker & Taylor Publisher Services